MEETING THE NEEDS OF PARENTS PREGNANT AND PARENTING after PERINATAL LOSS

Despite research that highlights parents' increased anxiety and risk of attachment issues with the pregnancy that follows a perinatal loss, there is often little understanding that bereaved families may need different care in their subsequent pregnancies. This book explores the lived experience of pregnancy and parenting after a perinatal loss.

Meeting the Needs of Parents Pregnant and Parenting after Perinatal Loss develops a helpful framework, which integrates continuing bonds and attachment theories, to support prenatal parenting at each stage of pregnancy. Giving insight into how a parent's worldview of a pregnancy may have changed following a loss, readers are provided with tools to assist parents on their journey. The book discusses each stage of a pregnancy, as well as labor and the postpartum period, before examining subjects such as multi-fetal pregnancies, reluctant terminations, use of support groups, and the experiences of fathers and other children in the family. The chapters include up-to-date research findings, vignettes from parents reflecting on their own experiences, and recommendations for practice.

Written for researchers, students, and professionals from a range of health, social welfare, and early years education backgrounds, this text outlines what we know about supporting bereaved families encountering the challenges of a subsequent pregnancy.

Joann O'Leary works as an independent trainer and consultant on issues related to pregnancy, early parenting, and perinatal loss and is field faculty at the University of Minnesota's Center for Early Education and Development. Her research focuses on the infant mental health needs of children born into bereaved families.

Jane Warland is a registered midwife and senior lecturer at the School of Nursing and Midwifery at the University of South Australia. Her research focuses particularly on complications of pregnancy and perinatal mental health.

MEETING THE NEEDS OF PARENTS PREGNANT AND PARENTING after PERINATAL LOSS

Joann O'Leary and Jane Warland

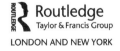
Routledge
Taylor & Francis Group

LONDON AND NEW YORK

First published 2016
by Routledge
2 Park Square, Milton Park, Abingdon, Oxon OX14 4RN

and by Routledge
711 Third Avenue, New York, NY 10017

Routledge is an imprint of the Taylor & Francis Group, an informa business

© 2016 J. O'Leary and J. Warland

British Library Cataloguing in Publication Data
A catalogue record for this book is available from the British Library

Library of Congress Cataloguing in Publication Data
Names: O'Leary, Joann, author. | Warland, Jane, 1957–, author.
Title: Meeting the needs of parents pregnant and parenting after perinatal loss / Joann O'Leary and Jane Warland.
Description: Milton Park, Abingdon, Oxon; New York, NY : Routledge, 2016. | Includes bibliographical references and index.
Identifiers: LCCN 2015050293| ISBN 9781138655065 (hbk) | ISBN 9781138655072 (pbk) | ISBN 9781315622774 (ebk)
Subjects: | MESH: Perinatal Death | Attitude to Death | Bereavement | Parents–psychology | Psychological Trauma–complications | Pregnancy–psychology
Classification: LCC RG648 | NLM WQ 225 | DDC 618.3/92–dc23
LC record available at http://lccn.loc.gov/2015050293

ISBN: 978-1-138-65506-5 (hbk)
ISBN: 978-1-138-65507-2 (pbk)
ISBN: 978-1-315-62277-4 (ebk)

Typeset in Bembo
by Out of House Publishing

Dedicated to Emma and all the babies whose lives were too short; their parents who taught us so much as they braved a pregnancy that followed, and the children in these families who bring many gifts to others because of the loss of a baby sibling.

CONTENTS

ACKNOWLEDGMENTS

There are many people who supported and guided the work of this book; most importantly the parents who shared their story of loss and the journey of the pregnancy that followed.

Special thanks to the early childhood professionals and nurses JOL was privileged to work with and Mary Koloroutis, BSN, MS, Director of Women Care, who never questioned the importance of our work with families experiencing pregnancy after loss; the Bush Foundation, St. Paul, MN, which supported JOL's research with families pregnant after a loss, including families in Australia and collaboration with JW; the School of Nursing and Midwifery UniSA for providing seed funding for JW's research with parents as well as to the UniSA Division of Health Sciences Research for a development grant (2008); Jennifer Huberty, PhD, who reviewed the chapter on CAM; Dr. Emmanuel Gaziano for his review on the twin loss chapter; and Martha Wegner and Sheri Tesch for sharing their stories of loss in their multi-fetal pregnancies.

The content for this book is derived from several sources: a manual written in collaboration with Clare Thorwick, RN, Antenatal Nurse Clinician and Lynnda Parker, BSN, Clinical Nurse Specialist (it was our combined disciplines that developed the prenatal parenting model of relationship intervention); a self-help book written by JW with her husband Mike, which they self-published in 1996, three years after their baby daughter Emma's death; qualitative research which both authors have conducted with bereaved families, both separately and together, over many years; and the extensive clinical and personal experiences of both authors. We therefore acknowledge everyone who contributed their knowledge, expertise, and experiences to enable us to develop the content of this book.

Thanks to our husbands, John Sommerville and Michael Warland, and our children who have supported us in our work with bereaved parents and their children.

1

THE PARENTING EXPERIENCE OF LOSS

The moment pregnancy is confirmed both the woman and her partner begin a complex journey of redefinition, reorganization, and reintegration of self. What parents do not anticipate is perinatal loss, a baby dying during pregnancy or in the newborn period. How does one recover from such a profound loss? How long does such painful grief remain? Most importantly, how does one make sense of self as parent to a baby no longer physically present when parents become pregnant with a new baby? This chapter explores answers to these questions and establishes a theoretical background for attachment-focused representation of prenatal parenting.

Parental perinatal grief

Grief has been defined as the severe and prolonged distress that is a response to the loss of an emotionally important figure, a predictable consequence of the loss of a relationship of attachment (Weiss 2001). Perinatal grief is enduring, exhausting, and has a profound and often lasting effect on both the bereaved and those caring for them:

> *It's really emotionally exhausting to the point of I don't want to do anything except take a nap. I didn't nap every day but I pretty much cried every day and read something related to loss or something on the Internet every day.*

Some parents feel health declines after the loss of a child but most report either level or improved health within four years (Cacciatore et al. 2014). Yet the risk of succumbing to health disorders many years later has been found to be greater in bereaved versus non-bereaved individuals (Mitchell 2012; Song et al. 2010; Stroebe et al. 2007).

Women construct mental representations of the fetus and feelings of affiliation that increase over time during pregnancy (Barone et al. 2014; DiPietro 2010; Fernandez et al. 2011), culminating in the birth of an infant (DiPietro 2010); this has been found true for fathers as well (Condon 2013; Fletcher et al. 2014; Weaver-Hightower 2012). Parents do develop intense and complex emotional feelings about their unborn children, observed in their response to perinatal loss (Badenhorst & Hughes 2007; Brier 2008). How language is used around pregnancy and infant loss is important to parents (Jonas-Simpson & McMahon 2005). The gestational age of the deceased baby is a poor indicator of the strength of the family's reaction to the death as it does not take into account the degree of attachment to and investment in that baby (Moulder 1994; Robinson et al. 2000). Parents rarely say, "I lost a pregnancy" or "I lost a fetus." They usually say, "I was pregnant and my baby died." These feelings speak to an attachment relationship that begins during pregnancy and does not end when an infant dies (O'Leary & Thorwick 2008; Yamazaki 2010).

Grief challenges us to move from loving in presence to loving in separation (Attig 2013), to find an enduring connection with the deceased in the midst of a changed life (Worden 2009). The earlier the loss, the more likely the parents' grief will be disenfranchised, a grief that is not or cannot be openly acknowledged (Doka 2002). It is common to believe parents didn't "really know the baby" so could not have been attached and aren't "really parents," especially if the loss is "managed as a medical procedure, focusing on the 'products of conception' rather than the loss of a hoped for 'baby'" (Fernandez et al. 2011, p. 146). Yet, even mothers who suffer an early loss have been found to develop grief symptoms similar to mothers in a later stage of pregnancy (Kersting & Wagner 2012).

One factor to be considered in response to working with a bereaved parent is whether there has been a failure of their social surround to assist with mourning (Hagman 2001; Lang, Fleiszer et al. 2011; Wood & Quenby 2010). While society relishes the birth of a live healthy baby, too often there is a silent disregard for the grief and despair that pregnancy loss evokes (St. John et al. 2006). Such a loss does not fit the worldview of how things should be, leaving parents with an identity that has "internalized the patterns of parenthood but with the object of their relationship no longer there" (Riches & Dawson 1998, p. 128). When grief occurs, social surroundings need to be re-learned (Attig 2000; Weaver-Hightower 2012), a task rarely done in isolation. Grief should not be expected to follow time limits nor a specific path (McClowery et al. 1987) yet the time limit is often significantly less than what the grieving parent actually requires (Umphrey & Cacciatore 2011). Family and friends want parents to return to their normal self, managing their loss in certain socially approved ways (Corr 2011). Support may quickly dissipate if others feel the parents are grieving too long or talking about the baby too much (Carlson et al. 2012). Avoidance and withdrawal from the bereaved parent are frequently observed due to the anxiety-provoking nature of the loss and intense feelings of personal vulnerability (Lazare 1979). Yet sharing the story of loss is important in healing (Waters 1996) and lack of recognition of the deceased baby can cause parents' grief to be unrecognized as a family tragedy (Fernandez et al. 2011).

The need for a bereaved person to be "normal again" is as old as time, described in a quote from a mother whose son died at three months of age in the early 1800s: "I stifle my grief because it hurts my friends, but alas it preys on the vital part of my afflicted heart, and in spite of all fortitude I can sum up I cannot regain my former feelings" (Lewis 1979, pp.100–101).

Dyregrove and Dyregrove (1999) interviewed parents following the death of their child from SIDS and found two-thirds of both fathers and mothers were still affected by their grief 12 to 15 years after the death. Gold et al. (2012) report a similar finding from an anonymous online survey of over 1,000 bereaved women: parents were still coping with the emotional impacts 5, 10, and even 20 years later, continuing to need a place to acknowledge their deceased child). A bereaved grandfather (whose own four-year-old child had died 30 years earlier), told his daughter-in-law after the loss of her stillborn daughter: *It doesn't get easier. It's going to be like this for a long time. Every time a birthday comes up you're going to be sad. And there's days where you'll just sit there and you'll just start crying, because you know she's not here.* Grief and longing for a deceased child continue throughout the life span, perhaps in a milder manner, but always there (Dyregrove & Dyregrove 1999; O'Leary & Warland 2013).

Finding meaning: the continued emotional bond

> Seeking an answer is the scientific paradigm; finding meaning is quite another.
> (*C. Hammerschlag*, The Theft of the Spirit)

The resolution of parental grief involves a reorganization of the survivor's sense of self to find a new normal (Hagman 2001; Wimmer 2013; Worden 2009) and transformation of the inner representation of the dead child in the parents' social world (O'Leary et al. 2012). Several theorists have suggested that reconstructing a world of meaning is critical for successful adjustment following loss (Gilbert 2002; Grout & Romanoff 1999; Klass 1993; Nadeau 2001; Rochman 2013), and is the central process of grieving (Neimeyer 1998). Klass (2001) defines this process as achieved by an active interaction within one's world where the death is recognized, mourned and the continued bond validated and shared. How the parent attempts to hold onto the tie to the deceased baby is therefore crucial (Hagman 2001). Wheeler (2001) emphasizes that keeping the memory alive is not an attempt to deny the reality of the death but a way of making sense of the trauma in order to reinvest in the world. Parents of deceased children (ranging from prenatal to 48 years) in Wheeler's study described this change as a renewed appreciation of their connections with people and acknowledged positive changes in themselves as a result of the death.

In spite of bereaved parents having no direct life experiences with their deceased baby outside the womb, research suggests that a deep connection develops between the mother and unborn child during pregnancy (Dirix et al. 2009; Sandman et al. 2011; Thomson 2007). Advances in ultrasound imaging, prenatal diagnostics, genetic screening, and fetal surgery have changed the medical and cultural status of the maternal–fetal relationship, suggesting attachment can begin at a much earlier stage in pregnancy (Casper 1998; van Dis 2003; Stormer 2003). Further, because maternal and fetal circulation are connected, fetal cells can enter the maternal circulation during pregnancy (Artlett et al. 1998; Khosrotehrani et al. 2003; Peterson et al. 2012; Simpson & Elias 2006; Williams et al. 2009) and may be considered the biological legacy of pregnancy (Peterson et al. 2013). These microchimeerism cells[1] have been found in the maternal circulation for as long as 27 years after pregnancy completion, after a pregnancy as brief as a few months (Bianchi 2000; Bianchi et al. 1998; Evans 1999) and termination of pregnancy with higher concentrations in pregnancy termination versus miscarriage (Peterson et al. 2012, 2013). This research at the very least suggests that a physical bond between a mother and an unborn child begins prenatally (O'Leary & Thorwick 2008). How grief and the emotional bond are operative in regards to fetal cells remaining may not be known but should not be discounted as playing a role in a mother's continued grief response (personal communication, E. Gaziano, MD). These studies may also provide an explanation for many bereaved mothers expressing, *I still feel the presence of my baby.* It can be argued that mothers are describing an emotional/psychological connection but this information can be useful for partners who may not understand why the mother's grief can be so much more intense than their own. One father, after hearing that the cells of their 14-week miscarried baby might still be circulating in his wife's system commented that it would help him be more respectful of her continued grief.

Integrating attachment theory

It is well known that infant attachment is critical and vital in the formation of a healthy person (Sroufe 2005). The parent or care provider–child attachment is presented as a reciprocal relationship that develops through many day-to-day interactions over time in which both parties are "hard-wired" to engage with each other. This is theorized to be a survival instinct, as the human child is particularly dependent on adults for provision of physical needs (food, shelter, etc.) and safety from harm for an especially protracted period of time. The child draws adults to her through cues such as crying, and adults are primed to respond to the infant's needs. They provide the infant with a "secure base" from which to explore the world and to grow, developing healthy relationships throughout life. Attachment relationships with one's parents help form a mental representation of the experience of being loved and cared for in an intimate context, and are the foundation for much that happens later in life (Ainsworth et al. 1978; Main et al. 1985).

One of the most powerful predictors of an infant's attachment to the parents is the parents' autobiographical narrative coherence (Hesse 1999, cited in Sigel 2001) regarding what they bring into the relationship. This forms our internal working model of who we are and our mental blueprint of how to handle present and future relationships. The care provider's perception of a child as an intentional being lies at the root of sensitive caregiving and is the cornerstone of secure attachment (Fonagy 1998). This relationship can be argued to begin during pregnancy, with research suggesting that the environment in the womb, especially stress in the mother, can alter the development of the fetus and have a permanent effect on the child (Glover 2011, 2012; Hruby & Fedor-Freybergh 2013).

This book is based on a different definition of the term "attachment" to include feelings parents' hold for their unborn children that can impact the attachment process and outcome after birth (Glover 1997). The multidimensional nature of prenatal attachment suggests that there is an interaction between cognitive, emotional, and behavioral components (Doan & Zimerman 2003, 2008), and the cognitive ability to conceptualize the fetus as a person is a prerequisite for prenatal attachment (Doan & Zimerman 2008). The prenatal period and degree of development in-utero enables the human fetus to perceive and process sensory, emotional, and social stimuli, and has been described as a prenatal child (Fedor-Freybergh 2008). This period is a critical phase for brain development and, if going well, continues into the postnatal development of attachment (Hruby & Fedor-Fryebergh 2013). Therefore it is important to understand what prenatal attachment means in regard to the maternal–fetal relationship (Alhusen 2008; van den Bergh 2010; van den Bergh & Simons 2009; Brouchard 2011; Eichhorn 2012; Gaudet 2010; Walsh 2010), especially during a pregnancy following loss.

Some practitioners, theorists, and researchers are exploring the experiences of parents who have suffered a perinatal loss using an attachment lens. John Bowlby's (1969) observations about attachment are often cited as the foundation of this theoretical perspective. He suggested that trauma around loss triggers attachment and can inhibit new coping strategies and activate affectional bonds. A traumatic event happens suddenly and unexpectedly, disrupting one's sense of control, beliefs, and values, and is usually experienced with intensity, terror, and helplessness (Gamble et al. 2002; Landy 2004–2005; Thomson & Downe 2010) or the person fears harm or injury (Black & Wright 2012). The post-trauma experience can threaten the attachment process, inhibit new coping strategies, and activate affectional bonds (Kesternbaum 2011). The trauma of the previous loss, longing for the deceased baby, and fear that an unborn baby that follows a loss might also die can therefore interfere with parents' ability to risk attaching to the new pregnancy.

Moulder (1994) proposed providing a framework for understanding pregnancy loss using integration of the models of attachment and loss. "Attachment and investment are separate but linked processes; attachment is concerned with the development of feelings for the baby, whereas investment is a more active process of involvement in the pregnancy" (p. 66). Bereavement occurs due to the prior formation of attachment bonds and without attachment there would be no bereavement (Bowlby, cited in Balk 2011, p. 48). When attachment definitions include an element of time, there is the potential risk of minimization of a perinatal loss.

In the realm of infant loss any meaningful discussion must inevitably utilize the concept of antenatal emotional attachment and recognize that, psychologically, pregnancy is the gestation of a person who acquires increasing reality, humanness, and emotional relevance (Condon 1987). Archer (1999) integrates aspects of the attachment theory by considering that grief is especially intense following the loss of someone who would eventually have contributed to the bereaved individual's completeness. This may explain why, when parents struggle with their identity after perinatal loss, their grief can be more prolonged, intense, and complicated (Keesee et al. 2008; Lichtenthal et al. 2010).

Examining loss from the perspective of the parent's sense of self from a continued bond and an attachment focused model, attachment relationships are known to endure, with some losses being considered so big and painful that one cannot ever get to a place where grief has ended (Ronen et al. 2009–2010; Rosenblatt 1996a). Parents unable to have a safe place to process their loss and continued parental bond with a deceased baby dismissed by others often cannot address the needs of other children, both living and those to follow, without supportive guidance (O'Leary & Gaziano 2011).

The model put forward in this book aims to help parents, regardless of how their baby died, reframe grief as their parental continued bond, attachment, and spiritual connection to the deceased baby (Klass et al. 1996; O'Leary & Thorwick 2008). The role of parent does not stop when a child dies. Revising grief (as opposed to detaching or getting over the loss) means not needing to have closure but also not denying the loss (Boss 2006). This helps parents develop the emotional energy to develop new relationships (Priegerson et al. 2009; Romanoff & Terenzio 1998), a crucial task as they enter a subsequent pregnancy for the unborn baby who now needs their attention (O'Leary 2004; O'Leary & Thorwick 2006, 2008). In the words of Peter Fedor-Freybergh (1992), "When the It (pregnancy) becomes YOU (my baby) the dialogue begins."

Grief, depression, and anxiety as they relate to pregnancy following loss

Grief, depression, and anxiety often go hand-in-hand in a pregnancy following a loss (Adeyemi et al. 2008; Côté-Arsenault & O'Leary 2015; Couto et al. 2009; Hutti et al. 2015 Côté-Arsenault), yet most parents enter a new pregnancy believing (or at least hoping to believe) that grief for the deceased child will diminish. Instead, however, because what happened at the time of loss is remembered (Chez 1995), it resurrects a layer of grief that cannot be anticipated or prepared for (O'Leary 2004). Parents often feel intense inner conflict as they begin a new pregnancy (Kersting et al. 2011). Rather than putting their grief aside, the new pregnancy becomes a reminder of the loss and the relationship parents continue to have with their deceased baby. This grief can be labeled "unresolved or complicated," but in fact is part of an expected developmental stage parents need to work through as they begin to parent their new unborn baby (Fernandez et al. 2011; O'Leary 2004). Regardless of the gestational age of the previous loss, women are at risk for continuing grief, depression, anxiety, and the symptoms of post-traumatic stress disorder (PTSD) in the subsequent pregnancy (Hutti et al. 2015). Women who have experienced the loss of a prior pregnancy are also prone to higher levels of depression during pregnancy and for up to 33 months post-birth of a healthy child (Robertson-Blackmore et al. 2011). It has also been reported that 10–20 percent of bereaved women are at risk for developing complicated grief, clinically distinct from major depression and PTSD (APA 2013; Hughes et al. 2001; Hutti et al. 2015; Prigerson et al. 2009).

It is important to understand that grief and depression are not the same (Shear 2012a), are culturally determined, and may be virtually indistinguishable from depression (Buckle & Fleming 2011). Grief is the psychobiological response to bereavement; the form love takes when someone loved dies (Shear 2012b). Clinicians should note guidance from the DSM-IV when attempting to differentiate between grief and depression; that is, in grief painful feelings come in waves often intermixed with positive memories of the deceased, whereas in depression mood and ideation are almost constantly negative. In grief, self-esteem is usually preserved whereas in a major depressive illness corrosive feelings of worthlessness and self-loathing are common (APA 2013). In the context of parents who are pregnant after loss, a major depression requires treatment whereas grief requires reassurance and support (Shear 2012b, p. 121).

Similarly it is helpful to differentiate complicated grief (CG) from "normal" grief. Many bereaved parents may have been told that their grief is "complicated" because they are still constantly thinking about and missing their baby. However, grief can only be considered complicated if it involves acute grief symptoms accompanied by an array of complicating thoughts, feelings, and behaviors (APA 2013). Complicated grief can be differentiated from normal grief by the heightened intensity and longer persistence of acute symptoms that interfere with daily functioning and an ability to find meaning in life (ibid). Complicated grief may result from (1) insufficient integration of the loss into one's autobiographical knowledge base, (2) negative global beliefs about and misinterpretations of grief reactions, and (3) anxious and depressive avoidance strategies (Boelen et al. 2006; Neimeyer 2006). All are common issues experienced by bereaved parents during pregnancy with a subsequent baby and support the importance of differentiating grief as "unresolved or complicated" or as a major depression/anxiety that requires treatment or as a normal response given the obstetric history. Barr (2006) found that women in their subsequent pregnancy continued to display active grief but not difficulty coping or despair that are known to be indicators of CG.

Attachment in pregnancy after loss (PAL)

Parental mental representation of and attachment to the unborn child is altered following a previous loss (Doan & Zimerman 2008; Mehran et al. 2013; O'Leary 2004; O'Leary & Thorwick 2008). Loyalty to the deceased baby, anxiety, and fear of loss provide an explanation for why many parents hold back attachment (Armstrong & Hutti 1998; Côté-Arsenault & Donato 2011; Côté-Arsenault et al. 2001; Fernandez et al. 2011; Hughes et al. 2001; Thuet et al. 1992; Zeanah & Harmon 1995).

The mother's ability to make emotional room for the baby during pregnancy first takes place at the imagining level (Slade 2002). These early symbols are created in action between mother and child, with the child forming represention of self from the mother's capacity to make the breadth and depth of the baby's experience real and meaningful (Slade 2000). Leifer (1980) described the progression of parental prenatal attachment as developing in an orderly sequential way during the course of pregnancy (just as does the unborn baby's development). Walsh (2010), citing Bowlby's definition of attachment as the behavior of the child to the parent, suggests that this prenatal relationship is more "about care-seeking as compared to care-giving" (p. 450). We argue that caring for the physical needs of an unborn baby is very different from developing an emotional attachment.

An understanding of how conditions inside and outside a woman's body may affect the development of her prenate (embryo and fetus), as well as knowledge of sensitive and critical periods in the prenatal development of the brain and autonomic nervous system, contribute to an understanding of the psychophysiology of an individual's later interpersonal interactions and the quality of their relationships (Hruby & Fedor-Freybergh 2013; Weinstein 2012). Perry and Szalavitz (2006) write that "even in utero … the brain is processing the nonstop set of incoming signals from their senses" (p. 46). Unresolved histories of early relational trauma often remain actively disregulated in the intra-psychic mind of a parent and may become a powerful source of prenate stress (Thomson 2007). That unborn babies may have a sense of not being welcomed for who they become after birth is difficult to quantify but should not be dismissed.

In the field of pre- and perinatal psychology,[2] prenatal and perinatal events, from conception to birth, are believed to register at deep unconscious levels and lay the foundation for brain development and mental health or illness (van den Bergh & Marcoen 2004; van den Bergh et al. 2008; Costa Segui 1995; Findeisen 1992; Kaplan et al. 2007; Shonkoff et al. 2009; Talge et al. 2007). When the unconscious memory is open to recall during hypnosis, vivid and detailed memories of prenatal life, the birth experience, and early events as a newborn infant readily emerge for many (Phillips 2013; O'Leary & Gaziano 2011). Although the immature brain recalling the memories remains unknown, the vividness and accuracy of specific details and events around memories of intrauterine feelings and pregnancy and birth cannot be denied. Adults who did some type of regression therapy describe a sense of not feeling welcomed (O'Leary 2012; O'Leary et al. 2006b), illustrated by this adult woman born a year after a stillborn sister: *'I went back into the womb and the birth. There was a sense of being all alone and being unaccepted.'*

Can feeling unaccepted continue into postpartum parenting? Allan Shore (1994), a neurobiologist who has been exploring the role of attachment and brain development, explains that the amygdala, involved in emotional learning and memory modulation, is in a critical period of maturation in the first two months after birth; and Phillips (2013, p. 69) suggests that "[s]kin-to-skin contact activates the amygdala via the prefronto-orbital pathway." In other words, babies need to be touched. The following stories are representative of some of the thoughts and feelings these adults (born after a perinatal loss) report, and graphically illustrate what can happen in the early years growing up in a family that did not have the benefit of prenatal relationship-based intervention following the loss of a baby:

> *The story goes I became allergic to my mother's milk, at four months of age. I have touched on this in regressive therapy and it felt as if my mother was rejecting me, that she and her milk, both, were embittered.*

My mom did not want to connect to me. My crying reminded her of him [deceased brother] so she would lay in her bed and have anxiety and I would lay in my crib and cry. And that went on day after day until my dad would come home at night and he would hold me. In my memories I thought it only went on for three months but later when I talked to her, and I was angry at that point, she said, "Well, it was only for a year." I was like WHAT! A year! Half my prime development time! Are you out of your mind? So it's taken, it's been layers and layers and layers of work and time healing from this.

She was never really happy until she had my younger brother five years later. I have a very vivid memory of her giving birth to him; standing in the window of the hospital holding the baby up to show us down below and just this beaming smile on her face, that made me feel … I don't know how it made me feel. I would have to say that, in what memories I have of my early childhood, I'd never seen her that happy.

Patterns of intimate relationships, mental expectations about life, and one's own sense of self have been suggested to develop prenatally (Chamberlain 1997, 2003; Emerson 1998; Lipton 2005; McCarty 2000, 2004), as these quotes from adult subsequent children attest:

I'd always felt like my mother and I weren't really connected. That played out in my own life as feeling like I was a disappointment. And that I was invisible.

My own sense of self is I'm a burden, I'm not pretty enough, the notion that she [deceased sister] was angelic and perfect and I'm just a really lousy substitute.

I always thought that I was trying to please my mother.

Other adults described their need to be okay, not make waves, be "good enough," and, above all, be the child who stayed alive:

I didn't cry. I was not a child that cried. In fact, my childhood model was "Never let them see you cry." My family model is, "Always be okay." I couldn't go to my parents for comfort. I resented not having a place to go to cry.

I resented having to be the good one, the perfect child, the straight A student. I never feel like I've achieved, even when I got my PhD. That's an impossible task.

These adults provide insight to those working with parents in pregnancy after loss to help parents recognize the unborn baby's individuality, to separate one baby from another, and to trust their ability to parent this new baby, beginning in pregnancy. Their stories support Glover's (2011, 2012) belief that stress and support are potentially modifiable targets for intervention in the prenatal period. They help us gain an understanding of why attachment-focused intervention benefits parents in pregnancy after loss. The parents of these babies (now adults) were not provided with prenatal therapeutic intervention, and often were told to move on as if the birth, death, and baby never existed (O'Leary & Warland 2013). One cannot retrospectively examine the attachment history of these adults' own mothers or fathers or whether their parents experienced unresolved grief, acute fear, and high anxiety behaviors during their pregnancies, all of which would impact the adults' intrauterine experience. Nor can we know how these adults would have scored on Mary Ainsworth's Strange Situation paradigm/experiment at one year of age (Ainsworth et al. 1978). We can only know how these adults describe their lived experience as a child who followed the loss of a sibling. Because maternal psychological distress adversely affects early parenting, and prenatal maternal distress predicts postnatal maternal distress, pregnancy provides a key opportunity for maternal mental health interventions, particularly given the number of provider contacts that occur in routine prenatal care (DiPietro 2012).

Foundation of the intervention

Winnicott et al. (1987) describe the "holding" environment (the uterus during pregnancy) provided by the nurturer as the infant's first experience with extra uterine life (p. 96). Thayer and Hupp (2010, p. 11) suggest that "the process of the holding environment may be influenced early by the mother's psychological adaptations to pregnancy and the emotional development that she experiences as she comes to accept or not, the infant developing within her." Parents are changed in profound ways as they enter a new pregnancy, and so is the "holding environment" (the parents' mental representation) for the unborn baby.

Working with parents who are pregnant following a previous loss involves uniquely different tasks from those observed by Rubin (1975) in normal pregnancy. The tasks we now address in a pregnancy after loss (PAL) support group are based on listening to parents' stories and observing behaviors that reflect their continued grief for the deceased baby alongside fear and anxiety regarding attachment to a new unborn baby. These tasks are:

- Working with the fear of another abnormal pregnancy
- Working through the avoidance of attachment for fear of future loss
- Moving past the unwillingness to give up grieving out of loyalty to the deceased baby
- Attaching to the unborn child separately from the deceased baby
- Grieving the loss of self, the part that is a parent.

(O'Leary & Thorwick 1997)

Learning what parents require to break through these barriers and trust the woman's body to safely carry a baby to term became the guiding force in merging the continued bond and attachment theory for the prenatal parenting relationship-based intervention with the medical model of care. Parents needed help to understand their role as a parent for two babies and affect change in maternal/paternal behaviors (O'Leary & Thorwick 1997, 2008).

The intervention

A relationship-based prenatal attachment framework using a cognitive structured educational focus on fetal competencies was developed to support mental representations of the parenting role in relation to both the deceased baby and the unborn baby. The intervention drew on the pioneering infant mental health work with parents experiencing attachment difficulty postpartum, unable to hear "the cry of the baby," described in Selma Fraiberg's "Ghosts in the Nursery" (Fraiberg et al. 1980b, 1980c). In a pregnancy after loss, the "ghost" of the deceased baby can interfere with the parents' ability to embrace their new child. Unless parents are able to find meaning and understand their continued bond with and attachment to the deceased baby, this "ghost" pregnancy and baby in the past may interfere with their ability to pay attention to the physical and emotional needs of the unborn baby that follows. The intervention uses the unborn baby "as center" or "leading the way" as an essential component facilitating changes in the parents (Fonagy 1998; Fraiberg & Fraiberg 1987; Fraiberg et al. 1980b, 1980c; O'Leary & Thorwick 1997; Pawl 1995; Weatherston 1998). As Fraiberg et al. (1980a, p. 53) state: "When a baby is at the center of treatment something happens that has no parallel in any other form of psychotherapy."

In pregnancy after loss the physiology of a healthy unborn baby's development doesn't change but parents' behavior and response to the pregnancy and unborn baby change significantly. Contrary to the past belief (Bourne & Lewis 1984) that parents cannot grieve and attach at the same time, the intervention demonstrates the necessity of working with grief and attachment simultaneously. Therapeutic developmental guidance (Pawl 1995) is provided using an interactive-focused prenatal intervention that focuses on the behavior of parents as it relates to their feelings toward the unborn baby (Barnett 2005; Condon 1987; Condon et al. 2013; O'Leary 2004; Raphael-Leff 2004).

Research on the unborn baby's connection with the mother's emotions and on prenatal attachment forms the foundation of this intervention. As such, the intervention integrates continued bond/attachment theory into an infant mental health model of care during pregnancy. It combines this with an early childhood model that helps parents to understand the development of their children. One way to facilitate intuitive prenatal parenting is to think about how children's postnatal development influences parenting behaviors. For example, in a healthy parent–child interaction, parents respond to their child based on his developmental level. Obviously, the needs of a child are different at three months and three years of age, and parents respond accordingly; this is also true prenatally. Parents' behaviors, normally viewed as "psycho-social changes of pregnancy," are reframed as parenting behaviors driven by the developmental stage of the unborn baby "because *in utero* the foetus has already anticipated to a great degree the reactions of early neonatal life … the very arrangement and relationships of his neurons have pointed to the future" (Gesell 1940, p. 12).

The cycles/phases of development begin during pregnancy and continue throughout one's lifetime. Gesell demonstrated how humans cycle through phases of disequilibrium (break-up, inwardizing, "neurotic" fitting together), whereby bodies grow and change and then stabilize; equilibrium (smooth, sorting out, expansion). At the same time growth is never stagnant; a three year old shows the solid development of a two and a half year old (disequilibrium), lots of three-year-old behaviour (equilibrium) and pieces of being three and a half (disequilibrium). Under stress, a child reverts back to a younger phase until stable again. Gesell's neurological phases of development showing these orderly sequential shifts in children's growth (see Table 1.1) were adapted for the prenatal period and integrated into the medical model of pregnancy (see Table 1.2) (see the flow diagrams at the beginning of Chapters 2, 3, 4, 5, 6 and 8). Initially adapted for parents in a "normal pregnancy" (O'Leary & Thorwick 1993), this framework illustrates how, from the moment pregnancy is suspected, the neurological and behavioral growth and development of the unborn baby elicits physical, emotional, and behavioral changes in the mother and her partner (O'Leary et al. 2012a). Regardless of the outcome, the baby leads the way as parents learn to advocate for themselves and their baby (O'Leary & Thorwick 1993; Verny 2002). The guide to facilitate parents developing an emotional attachment to the new unborn baby uses cognitive-based education on fetal development (Doan & Zimerman 2008; O'Leary & Thorwick 1997). The intervention conceptualizes the presence of a growing and developing baby (fetus) influencing parental behaviors, not just a pregnancy or imagined baby to meet at birth. It is a practical application to help parents understand that they can influence their unborn child's development (O'Leary et al. 1993, 2012; Thompson 2007) and why perinatal loss does not take away their role as a parent.

Cognitive-behavioral education on the developmental milestones at each stage of fetal development explores behaviors of the unborn baby (whose development doesn't change) with parents whose own behaviors are altered as a result of previous loss (see Table 1.3). The unborn baby's competencies become the focus of 'leading the way' as parents learn to trust the process of pregnancy and advocate for themselves and their baby. This framework helps parents understand that the unborn baby is already present while simultaneously reinforcing their prenatal parenting relationship with the deceased baby. This follows the model for resolution of complicated grief; that is, to conceptually process and integrate one's loss with existing autobiographical knowledge (Boelen et al. 2006) in order to help organize one's responses to the experience (Thomas 1996).

The information on the unborn baby's fetal development at each gestational stage guides parents as they undertake the emotional and psychological work necessary to embrace the subsequent baby following a perinatal loss who now needs their attention (O'Leary et al. 2012). Parents learn that the unborn baby knows their voices, has an awareness of their emotions, and needs to hear the words expressing the parents' fears and anxieties. The prenatal interventionist becomes the voice of the unborn child, gently providing information on the baby's development within the uterus.

TABLE 1.1   Phases & cycle of developement

Smooth	Break-up	Sorting out	Inwardizing	Expansion	"Neurotic" Fitting together
1	2	3	4	5	6

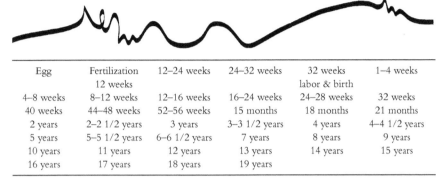

Egg	Fertilization 12 weeks	12–24 weeks	24–32 weeks	32 weeks labor & birth	1–4 weeks
4–8 weeks	8–12 weeks	12–16 weeks	16–24 weeks	24–28 weeks	32 weeks
40 weeks	44–48 weeks	52–56 weeks	15 months	18 months	21 months
2 years	2–2 1/2 years	3 years	3–3 1/2 years	4 years	4–4 1/2 years
5 years	5–5 1/2 years	6–6 1/2 years	7 years	8 years	9 years
10 years	11 years	12 years	13 years	14 years	15 years
16 years	17 years	18 years	19 years		

Joann O'Leary, PhD. Prenatal adaptaion of Gesell's stages, (c) 1986

Parents' responses can be quite varied based on their cultural background, personality type, life situation and experiences, financial status, and partner relationship, status and these details must be taken into account. All affect the ability to adapt to the life-altering experience of parenthood and the style in which a person does so. For teenagers, adaptation to the parenting behaviors in the cycle can be noticeably different depending on their own stage of development. For example, a pregnant 15 year old will be in disequilibrium, a physiological time when her body is growing and she has less control of her emotions so will not be as open to helpful suggestions. She will react differently from a pregnant 16 year old in equilibrium, whose physiological growth has stabilized and is thus more open to information on pregnancy and her baby.

Honoring and integrating the parenting role with the deceased baby

Some parents feel that grief is their only connection to the deceased baby when others want them to move on as they enter a pregnancy after loss. Letting go of grief can imply they are being disloyal because they do not understand that the parenting relationship with the deceased baby remains in the new pregnancy.

To facilitate parents' awareness of their developing relationship with the new baby, they are asked to revisit the deceased baby's competencies by evoking memories of

TABLE 1.2 Developmental cycles of parenting during "normal" pregnancy

Phases of Cycle	Smooth Conception	Break-Up Blastocyte – 12 Weeks	Sorting Out 12–24 Weeks	Inwardizing 24–32 Weeks	Expansion 32 Weeks Labor/Birth	"Neurotic" Fitting Together PP–4 Weeks
Caplan's Psychological Tasks	Acceptance of Pregnancy: Emotional affiliation with baby			Perception of baby as separate individual		
Fetal Physiology	Conception	• All organ systems forming & differentiate • Most vulnerable to adversity	• Rapid growth • Placental functions in relationship with mother	• Baby assumes fetal position • Growth spurt • Fetal heart rate (FHR) reacts to activity	• Lungs mature • Settles into mother's pelvis	• Transition from fetal circulation extra uterine life re: resp. HR. temp
Fetal Behavior Baby	Potential	• **Energy:** Baby forming into who she is; reflex actions more differentiated • **Mouth:** Opens; jaws snap rapidly • **Fingers:** Close incompletely • **Body:** Generalized movement • **Extremity:** Isolated arm or leg movement • **Eyes:** Move	• Grasp with hands • Sucks & swallows • Coordinated hand to mouth movements • Reacts to sounds • Limb movments both reciprocal & symmetric • Breathes	• Movements pattern stronger	• Consciousness more closely defined after 38 weeks • Sleep/awake cycles; awake longer • Stretch & extend limbs with contractions • Hearing more acute • Much more aware of intrauterine life • Competence increases	• Copes with gravity; still flexed & mobile • Shuts down if unfamliar sounds • Needs soft light • Slow pace to see & hear together • Movement more purpose & less reflective

Maternal Physiology	Ovulation & conception	• Impantation • HCG rises • Progesterone, estrogen rise • Breast size increases • Fatigue	• Quickening • Placenta functions • Becomes used to pregnancy • Looks pregnant • Fewer disruptive symptoms	• Abdominal size & weight increase • Notices fetal movements, uterine contractions	• Uterine contractions blood volume increase • Cervical ripening • Labor & birth	• Involution • Lochia • Lactation • Maternal hormones decrease
Behavior & Psychosocial Partner & Family	Calm, satisfied & in harmony with body & environment Uncertain, variable	• Oppositional • At odds with self & environment • Emotional roller coaster • Ambivalence • Own framily background resurfaces	• Temporary • What fits • Seeking out others • People & support • Discover & explore • Problem solving • Time of questioning • Mother sorts uterine contractions from baby movements • Prepare finacially • Dream • Prenatal Testing	• Restriction of view • Work with parts to create new whole • Introspective • Concentrates energy on child within • Can feel left out • May distance self • Seek help to affiliate with baby • Fewer people around, now future oriented	• New energy burst • "Nesting" • Prepares for birth, ready for birth class, ready to release baby to outside • Seeks safe place & people to birth with	• Emotional • Sleep deprived • Identity change "Mom" & "Dad" not couple • Let baby lead into roles

TABLE 1.3 Developmental cycles of parenting during subsequent pregnancy

Phases of Cycles	Smooth Conception	Break-up Blastocyte – 12 Weeks	Sorting Out 12–24 Weeks	Inwardizing 24–32 Weeks	Expansion 32 Weeks Labor/Birth	"Neurotic" Fitting Together PP–4 Weeks
Subsequent pregnancy	• "Should we get pregnant? What if something happens?" "I feel empty. I need a baby!" • "We have to get pregnant right away." "I'm a failure…. I won't ever have a baby." "My body kills babies."	• Excitement can turn to panic and fear. "I'm going to lose this baby too" • Aware of every ache & pain while tying not to think about being pregnant • Continually checking for bleeding • Fear of moving her body • Need to hear heartbeat or see baby on scan	• Maybe I really am pregnant • Fear of losing this baby too. Is this baby OK? • Mother's movements can be frozen, uanble to deep breath or touch abdomen. • Fetal movement both reassuring yet not—is it too much or not enough? • Sorting out this is not the deceased baby causing loyalty to the deceased baby to surface • Conflict in attaching	• Want to rush through this time. • If well supported it can be a time of reduced anxiety—if the baby is born now parents know he/she can survive in NICU • Baby's movements begin to be more predictable so a good time to help separate the personalities of the babies • Narrow life, turn more inward • Increased anxiety can cause contractions, especially around time of previous loss	• May be the first time they reach out for help as reality of the pregnancy is "full front." "I really am going to have a baby!" • Anxiety can rise; "Get the baby out while he/she is still alive!" • Have to face labor • Often increased grief over the deceased baby	• New layer of grief can surface; see what they missed in the death of their other baby and the deceased baby is still not here • Grief is still there and can be more intense, surprising to many • Normal postpartum issues can be alarming • Breast feeding can be more difficult; they have to keep this baby alive • Fear this baby will die too can cause parents to be afraid to sleep • Trust in the world again takes a long time
Partners	• Can feel the same or be asynchronous because of past loss	• Fear to touch partner • May not want to talk about the baby • Fearful every time the phone rings	• Continued fear of loss • Ambivalent about attachment • May seen unsupportive, not wanting to think about pregnancy	• May withdraw feel even more left out • Struggle to know what to do with feelings in order to protect their partner	• Often first encounter if/when they come to birth class • May be first time they get in touch with their grief as reality of previous loss becomes real	• Can be very optimist during the pregnancy and fall apart after the baby is born alive • Same fears that this baby might die too • Can take a long time to trust again

their psychological proximity to her; as Field (2006) notes, doing so is fully compatible with the knowledge and acceptance that the other baby is dead. Exploring the deceased baby's competencies during the previous pregnancy provides a cognitive model of understanding why their grief and feelings of attachment and loyalty continue. Parents gain new information to re-conceptualize the nature of the relationship, reframing their grief as parenting feelings providing a "durable biography" (Walters 1996) or narrative story (Neimeyer 1996, 2002) that organizes the prenatal story of the deceased baby's life into a healthy connection (Armstrong & Shakespeare-Finch 2011). This cognitive model can help lessen negative feelings (Michael & Snyder 2005) such as fear of attachment to a new baby from a sense of loyalty to the deceased baby. It internalizes the parents' continued bond, legitimizes their grief, and recognizes that the deceased baby was a sentient being in utero and, at some level we cannot qualify, knew them as his parents.

Such intervention provides a new way for parents to think about their deceased baby beyond grief. They can then understand that their grief is not "unresolved" or "complicated" but represents their continued bond and attachment to this much missed baby. Parents can then gain emotional comfort, fond memories, and a symbolic connection with their attachment relationship to a baby who left an indelible mark in their lives (Rochman 2013). Without this focus, parents' grief can be vague or shadowy, which may in turn interfere with the current unborn baby's needs and impact his future emotional development. Sharing the experience of the deceased baby's prenatal life helps parents process, understand, and eventually accept the loss (Lepore et al. 1996). Parents learn that they do not need to give up their attachment to and relationship with the deceased baby in order to embrace the unborn baby who follows. Grief is then less likely to become "pathological" or "complicated" when parents are given focused intervention on fetal competencies for both the deceased baby and unborn baby. The interventionist moves "back and forth between the present and past through interpretations which will lead to insight" (Fraiberg et al.1980a, p. 61) that give meaning to their mutually incompatible and intertwined feelings of grief and attachment in the new pregnancy, always returning to the unborn baby in the present.

Attachment theory supports parental love for both babies. The parents' continuing bond and prenatal attachment relationship with the deceased baby are made part of the socially shared reality, transforming in the parents' psychic life the inner representation of the deceased baby. They realize they are parents to two babies, the one who has died and the one in the present pregnancy, an important message to help the new unborn child not become a replacement baby:

> Learning to love those who have died in separation gives them a new and welcome presence in our lives. We give their legacies places in our memories, practical lives, souls, and spirits. As we do, we realize how much of value in their lives has not been lost.
>
> *(Attig 2000, p. 13)*

Summary

This chapter has introduced the reader to how the loss of a baby during pregnancy alters self as parent forever but does not dismiss one's role of being a parent. We have made a case that parental attachment to an unborn baby begins during pregnancy regardless of the length and outcome and on-going grief for a deceased baby is legitimate when framed as parents' attachment and continued bond. Integrating the continued bond/meaning-making theories with attachment theory is an important concept for bereaved parents who need to understand that the unborn baby carried in the new pregnancy needs more than being cared for physically. Babies needs parents engaged in helping them grow to term and know they are important individuals in their own right.

This chapter has also addressed the themes found in research with parents pregnant after loss and the stories of adults who were the child in their family born after loss. Their stories provide insight for the benefit of attachment-focused intervention for parents during their pregnancy following loss.

Finally, this chapter introduced the rationale for the attachment-based intervention described in the first section of this book. The chapters that follow will address how to gently guide parents to work with their fears and anxieties using the relationship-focused attachment intervention at each gestational stage of pregnancy.

Notes

1 The presence of a small amount of genetically foreign material within the circulation or tissues of a person.
2 An interdisciplinary field commonly defined as the study and clinical practice relating to our earliest development to include pre-conception, conception, gestation, birth, postnatal experience, and the infant's first postnatal year (Glenn & Cappon 2013).

2

SMOOTH PHASE

Preconception

Phases of cycle

Smooth	Break-up	Sorting out	Inwardizing	Expansion	"Neurotic" fitting together
1	2	3	4	5	6
Egg	Fertilization–12 weeks	12–24 weeks	24–32 weeks	32 weeks–labor and birth	1–4 weeks

This chapter provides suggestions to help parents make a decision about when to try again. All of the phases experienced in pregnancy are shown above, and the smooth phase of prenatal parenting is normally a time of equilibrium. For parents who have had a previous loss, however, the driving force is loss of naivety. Pre-pregnancy counselling and questions to discuss as well as emotional and physical issues to consider are suggested. Insights from other parents on decisions to try again are provided.

Decisions, decisions

One of the biggest decisions parents face after a baby has died is whether to have another. They have lost their innocence; babies do die, and they fear it can happen again. Can they go through all that pain again? Usually a cycle of equilibrium prevails when a couple is ready to start a family, but not for parents who have suffered loss. They are grieving for the loss of their previous baby and often believe getting pregnant again will take away some of the grief. The focus of the intervention is to confirm that they are still parents to their deceased baby while they begin to prepare for a new pregnancy and baby. Parents struggle with the turmoil resulting from the following thoughts:

- Should we get pregnant?
- What if it happens again?
- We need to get pregnant!
- I feel empty … I need a baby!
- I'm a failure … I won't ever have a baby.
- My body kills babies.

As a result of this turmoil, questions in their mind might be:

- Can I get pregnant again or was that the only time?
- Can I carry a pregnancy to term?
- Can I have a healthy baby this time, or at least one that lives?

These fears are very common, as expressed by one mother:

> *We haven't experienced success yet. We've watched everybody else experience it. We've had one pregnancy and it was a bad outcome.*

Inter-conception counseling: planning the next pregnancy

Interconception refers to the time period between pregnancies (McCain et al. 2013); a time for parents to have a detailed discussion with their proposed obstetrician and a possible referral to a genetic counselor. This provides an opportunity for parents to gather as much information as possible on the cause of death and what preventive measures could be taken for the next pregnancy (Bhattacharya et al. 2010; Lee et al. 2013; Moore et al. 2010). It is important to temper information with hope (Roscignol et al. 2012). A consensus statement now being developed by international experts confirms that parents want to hear about the full range of treatment options available and honest accounts of possible outcomes together with any negative statistical information (Heazell et al. 2015).

In order to gauge their readiness, professionals should assess the parents' openness to expressions of grief and support systems in place (Moore et al. 2010). Some parents may have been given a cause of death (COD) that differs from what they actually believe caused their baby's death (Warland et al. 2015). This may reveal implausible reasons for the baby's death that may be useful to air as well as feelings of guilt and regret that could be discussed. This conversation may also provide clues to potential trauma triggers to be aware of in the next pregnancy.

While it is true that the later the loss occurred during pregnancy the more women express a significant state of distress (Gaudent 2010), it is also important to ascertain the parents' view on the meaning of their prior pregnancy loss as that may be more relevant for planning and counselling than gestational age at the time of the loss (Swanson 2000). For example, some parents view an early miscarriage as a flux, knowing it is common, while others have named the baby and memorialize the date on which the baby should have been born. Alderman et al. (1998) found in a study of 19 bereaved parents that 95 percent of the mothers and 79 percent of the fathers feel the need to mourn their miscarriage.

Trust in the smooth phase: risk of repeat loss?

Painful memories of the past alter parents' ability to trust the process of pregnancy and the belief they will bring a live baby home (Côté-Arsenault & Donato 2011; Mills et al. 2014; O'Leary & Thorwick 1997). They may be scared to give up any sense of control and need help to build a trusting relationship that enables them to move through the subsequent pregnancy (Soliday & Tremblay 2013).

Their ability to trust reflects a relinquishing of some personal control and intensification of associated vulnerability for the mother, her partner and the unborn baby (ibid). Along with discussing risks, it is also important to discuss the emotions that will surface in a pregnancy after loss (Lee et al. 2013) and the support system available to them (Moore et al. 2010).

Assessing how parents were treated at the time of their pregnancy loss can be important in terms of their perception of care in the pregnancy that follows, particularly around emotional support (Simmons et al. 2006). The disparity in health care providers' ability to provide compassionate care in terms of education related to this type of loss continues to be a problem (Earle et al. 2008). Stray-Pedersen and Stray-Pedersen (1984, 1988) divided 195 women with a history of miscarriage into two groups: one receiving routine obstetric care during the next pregnancy and the other given psychological support with weekly medical and ultrasonographic examinations. Among the couples with no abnormal findings, women receiving specific antenatal counselling and psychological support had a pregnancy success rate of 86 percent, as compared to a success rate of 33 percent in women who were given no specific antenatal care, a highly statistically significant finding ($p < 0.001$). Two other randomized studies also found significant improvement of subsequent pregnancy outcomes as a result of close monitoring and support (Clifford et al. 1997; Brigham et al. 1999).

Fear of another loss is real and needs to be processed with parents' health care provider, supportive family and friends. Recurrent miscarriage is more uncommon and their chance of having a live healthy baby next time is quite good. For example, research shows that recurrent miscarriage affects just under 1 percent of couples and is thought to be the result of genetic abnormalities, and sometimes age of the mother (ASRM 2012). According to Rubio et al. (2003), the cause of recurrent miscarriage can be found 60 percent of the time; however, other research suggests that up to 50 percent do not have a known etiology (ASRM 2012). With no treatment after recurrent loss, couples still have a 60–70 percent chance of delivering a live infant (Lund et al. 2012).

Women who have experienced one stillbirth are nearly five times more likely than women without that history to lose another baby in that way (Lamont et al. 2015), suggesting that their subsequent pregnancies should always be managed as high risk (Heazell et al. 2015). Parents should be encouraged to receive counselling with a maternity care provider who has an understanding of the exact circumstances of their previous stillbirth and can counsel them regarding their individual level of risk (Reddy 2010):

> *We had to take into consideration that I may again have an abruption. I had been told I had a 12.5 percent chance of it happening again.*

However, consistency between care provider advice is also key for parents' peace of mind:

> *Why did it happen? Give us some answers. Can we have another baby? One doctor might tell you, "Well, it's a complete fluke, this happened to you once, so the odds of this happening again to you are probably slim to none." And another doctor might say, "Well, since it happened to you once, it could happen to you again."*

Other risks

These parents also have an increased incidence of preterm birth, assisted and operative birth, induction of labour, and caesarean section (Black et al. 2008; Crowther 1995), in our experience more likely if they do not receive caring support throughout pregnancy. Prior loss is also associated with an increased risk of subsequent babies being small for gestation age (SGA); for Caucasian mothers nearly a three-fold and African-American mothers a four-fold heightened risk (Salihu et al. 2013). Inter-conception care and ongoing PAL support may assist in reduction of these poor pregnancy outcomes (Bassam et al. 2011; Mahande et al. 2013; Ouyang et al. 2013).

> *We didn't know why Emma died and realized that the likelihood of another baby dying inexplicably at term was probably remote. However, this head knowledge didn't ever filter through to my heart and my next pregnancy was a very anxious time for me.*

Health risks associated with a pregnancy after loss

Perinatal loss also puts parents at risk of mental health issues such as depression, post-traumatic stress disorder, complicated grief, and anxiety (Bennett et al. 2005; Cacciatore et al. 2013). Studies of health issues in parents who have suffered a perinatal loss have found overall increased mortality from both natural and unnatural causes in mothers, and an early increased mortality from unnatural causes in fathers who have suffered the loss of an older child (Li et al. 2003, 2005). This research reinforces the importance of care and intervention in a subsequent pregnancy after loss to minimise poor health outcomes.

Readiness: continued bond with and attachment to the deceased baby

"Letting go" or learning to accommodate their loss in the past has been described as part of parents' grief work and may be made more difficult by a subsequent pregnancy (Lewis 1979). The continued bond theory suggests that, rather than "letting go," parents need to understand that their bond with and attachment to the deceased baby remains as they plan their readiness for another baby.

It takes time and cannot be rushed. Integrating their loss into their life is not something that is easily achieved and will continue into and beyond the next pregnancy. It cannot be hurried. The prenatal parenting framework helps parents integrate memories of the deceased child's life as still an important member of their family, accept what has happened and move forward. It is *not* forgetting; it is saying goodbye to what could have been.

Parents cannot force themselves to move forward any more than they can force themselves to stop grieving. When they are usually able to accept that outside life goes on; when their day is no longer always dominated by thoughts of their dead child; when they feel they can get involved in life again and learn to be happy once more—then they are well into the hard and ongoing process of moving forward:

> *I realized I was somewhat better when I found myself in the middle of the baby section in the local department store. Previously I had consciously avoided it.*

Parents can be helped through this time by understanding that the commonly-held notion and belief that the passage of time "heals" grief should be questioned (Rando 1986). Instead, parents should be helped to create meaning of their experience. Rosenblatt (1996a) suggests that making meaning is a long-term project but necessary in order to connect to the deceased in such a way that the past is validated. With this validation, parents can be more receptive to opening their hearts to a subsequent child.

Listening to parents with the intention of understanding their stories and exploring the relationship they still want to have with the deceased baby has been described by bereaved parents as a "life-saving" experience (Jonas-Simpson et al. 2005). Asking them to share the name and story of their deceased child to develop an understanding of the specialness of that baby's life, though brief, is an important part of the process of making meaning (Keyser 2002) and preparing for a new baby. The desire to have another baby can be utterly overwhelming. Many women find it completely irresistible:

> *I am not sure I was really ready to have another baby but the feelings were so strong I had no control. I had been told to wait a year but I couldn't wait that long. I had intentions to, but as time went on I couldn't.*

The desire to have another baby can be viewed by both mothers and fathers as an act of disloyalty to their dead baby (Côté-Arsenault & Donato 2011;

O'Leary & Thorwick 2006, 2008). This intense inner conflict between mourning the loss of an unborn baby and going on with the next pregnancy has also been reported in women who experienced an early miscarriage (Kersting et al. 2011). It is helpful to normalize feelings of loyalty by reminding them that most parents who are not bereaved also wonder if they can feel the same sense of attachment to their second baby as to their first when they are planning and preparing for its birth. The professionals' job is to help parents begin to understand that they do not have to give up loving their deceased baby in order to embrace a new baby:

> I began counselling before I was pregnant again and this continued throughout the pregnancy. At our sessions some time was devoted to "grief work" and some for preparation for the new baby. I was therefore facing issues related to both, meaning that grieving wasn't "shelved" because of the closeness of the pregnancies.

So, how can parents tell if they are ready? When they can say they are on the road to wholeness and have begun the process of "moving" forward: *'I felt ready to take the risk again although I was still anxious and sad.'*

How long to wait and why?

It is estimated that 86 percent of women become pregnant again within 18 months after perinatal loss (Cuisinier et al. 1996). Advice given to parents varies from waiting one to twelve months following the loss (Radestad et al. 2010). The reasons behind the suggestion to wait are usually twofold. First, their body needs time to physically recover. Second, and probably more importantly, the parents need time to process the shock and trauma of what happened when their baby died as they embark on planning a new pregnancy:

> Should we try to have another one? Is it worth the risk? We finally decided let's just go for it. In the back of my mind no matter how much we wanted the pregnancy to be normal it just wasn't going to be.

Once the decision is made to go ahead the next issue is when. Some women are ready well before others. For some parents there is no question that they will try again:

> If I could have had another baby the next day, I would have. While feeling scared about the outcome I just wanted another baby as soon as possible.

> We knew we wanted to have another baby. That was never a question after Micah was born and died. We gave ourselves time to go through the grieving process both emotionally and physically. I felt confident we could have a healthy baby. I trusted what our care providers told us—that Micah's condition was an anomaly, not genetic.

Others, however, may be fearful from the beginning:

> *My sister had said to me, "What are you scared of?" I said, "What do you mean?" She said, "You're scared. You need to acknowledge that and accept that and figure out what you need to do with that for this next pregnancy." So that was really hard for me, because she was right. The bottom line was, I didn't want to get pregnant again, because I was too scared. And when I started to work on that, then I got pregnant.*

In reality, parents will make their own decision, one study finding that parents tend to disregard advice to wait longer than six months, believing that the decision about when to get pregnant again is a deeply personal one which is only theirs to make (Davis Stewart & Harmon 1989; Gaudet 2010; Lee et al. 2013; Radested et al. 2010). A recent survey conducted with more than 800 US obstetricians examining advice given to parents regarding inter-pregnancy interval confirms the most common response was "when the parents feel ready" (Gold et al. 2010). It is also recommended that women avoid getting pregnant three months after the loss in order to avoid having a similar due date with a subsequent pregnancy because it can be psychologically confusing (Côté-Arsenault (2003):

> *Our obstetrician said wait three months. I had my first period after 11 weeks. We decided that was close enough!*
>
> *I didn't have the mindset of "Well we have to get pregnant right away." We just realized that the plan isn't ours so we're just going to live our lives and whatever happens, happens. We thought if we don't have any control we might as well do what we want to do.*

Couple preparedness

One issue that many parents face is that one partner may be ready ahead of the other. A helpful technique used more generally in couples counselling (Connolly et al. 2003) may be to set a timeframe within which to discuss a future pregnancy:

> *Initially after Emma died I wanted a hysterectomy I felt so strongly that I never wanted another pregnancy. Mike on the other hand was quite keen to have another baby virtually immediately. Because our feelings were completely different it was helpful for us to decide not to talk about it for a month. This avoided the potential for nagging and conflict whilst still maintaining the commitment to talk at some time in the future. When we did come to talk about it, the major issue that helped us decide to go ahead and risk another pregnancy was the realization that we had made a carefully thought-out decision to have a fourth baby. In lots of ways we probably thought more carefully about having Emma than we did our other children. None of these reasons died with her. Hence we were able to come to the decision to try again.*

When to time a subsequent pregnancy after perinatal death is complicated by the varied grief and emotional responses of bereaved parents to the loss and psychologic challenges of the next pregnancy (Gold et al. 2010). It is fair to say that stress levels can impact on fertility (Wilson & Kopitzke 2002). If either of the parents are over age 35 they may be conscious of their biological clock ticking: *'I felt pressured by my age [38] and the fact I might be taking other risks if I left it too long. I probably would have left it longer if I was younger.'* They may also consider the impact of raising active teenagers when they are themselves older than 50. They may not feel they have the luxury of being able to wait, because they risk other age-related problems such as lowered fertility and age-linked chromosomal disorders such as trisomy 21:

> We certainly didn't expect we would conceive again so quickly, given the amount of stress I was feeling and the fact it had taken me almost a year to fall pregnant with Thomas.

If they are having difficulty falling pregnant, particularly if they have not had trouble before, it may be appropriate to advise parents to seek professional counselling or consultation with a fertility specialist.

Anticipatory mourning

When pregnancy ends in loss, death comes before birth. Parents know pregnancy has no guarantees of ending in a healthy baby (Fernandez et al. 2011). Parents' auto-graphic memory and maternal/paternal representation of an unborn child in pregnancy often becomes one of "babies die" (Côté-Arsenault 2007; Côté-Arsenault et al. 2006; O'Leary 2004; O'Leary & Thorwick 2008). Parents need to think seriously about how they might feel if they lost another baby. Do they think they have recovered enough to cope with the resulting compound grief? Is their relationship able to withstand a further blow? Have they started to piece their life back together? Parents have received a blow to their assumptive world. Rando (2000b, p. 8) describes the assumptive world as "the mental schema containing everything a person assumes to be true about the world and self on the basis of previous experience," including psychological reorganization that begins in part with the awareness of the impending loss. Many parents undergo anticipatory mourning defined as

> the phenomenon encompassing seven generic operations (grief and mourning, coping, interaction, psychosocial reorganization, planning, balancing, conflicting demands, and facilitating an appropriate death) that, within the context of adaptational demands caused by experiences of loss and trauma, is stimulated in response to the awareness of life-threatening or terminal illness in oneself or a significant other and the recognition of associated losses in the past, present, and future.

> *(Rando 2000a, p. 4)*

For one mother, this entailed letting go of hopes, dreams, and expectations of a long-term future with a person and accepting death as an outcome:

If I didn't have an understanding that [death] is an outcome as well as an outcome of having a live baby, then I couldn't have made that conscious decision to try for another baby. We did have a miscarriage [before our daughter's death] so it does happen again that you lose a pregnancy. For me to be sane during the pregnancy, I needed to accept that the outcome could be death or else I couldn't have done it.

This thought, that anxiety, anticipatory grief (expecting another loss), and issues with maternal attachment during the next pregnancy may all be designed to prepare for the danger of losing the pregnancy, thereby reducing the traumatic impact should the worst fear actually materialize (Gold et al. 2010). This paradox has also been found in patients with a terminal illness, which helped the physician and family have a deeper conversation on giving equal time to hope and preparation (Black et al. 2003). While these intense reactions are often labeled as abnormal behaviors, they may be better understood as adaptive (Côté-Arsenault & O'Leary, 2015; O'Leary & Thorwick 1997).

BOX 2.1

What can parents do to prepare?

- Decide what care provider will meet their needs. Some parents continue with the same doctor because it can be a healing experience for both. Others want a fresh start with a new doctor.
- Review with their provider details of the prior loss, including cause, if known, and any preventive measures that might apply to their new pregnancy.
- Discuss a plan for their needs in each stage of pregnancy for the best possible outcome both physically and psychologically.

BOX 2.2

When deciding which doctor or midwife will support them, parents may need to consider whether their physician/midwife:

- Have knowledge regarding high-risk medical factors and specialists if needed?
- Initiate discussions about the medical issues pertaining to the previous loss?
- Seem attentive and sensitive to their emotional needs around perinatal loss and pregnancy after loss?
- Encourage them to phone or come in for reassurance when needed?

BOX 2.3

The professional must be the voice of the deceased baby and tell the parents what the baby might want for them. For example, the baby would:

- Encourage her parents to seek support from family, friends, support groups, and professionals when needed.
- Want her parents to know she still loves them.
- Want her parents to find their way back home with those who survive, embrace life in the human condition, keep love for her alive in their hearts, and cherish her legacy.

CASE STUDY

This family's previous loss was a son who had undiagnosed hydrops fetalis, was delivered by emergency Cesarean, and died seven hours after birth in another hospital. This case study describes the process the parents went through when deciding to try for another baby.

Kathy joined the infant loss group while her husband stayed home with the other children. She processed both the trauma around his death and the fact that she had not trusted her intuition that something wasn't right, which was dismissed by her health care provider as "just your fourth pregnancy." Kathy wanted another child but her husband had been adamant he did not. In preparation she explored other health care providers, asking group members for recommendations. She and her husband attended a "Meet the Midwives" evening to decide if another hospital would desensitize them to memories of their son's death. They spent a weekend at Faith's Lodge,[1] a retreat center for bereaved parents, where her husband was able to share the story and began to heal. They kept in touch with another couple, and, when her husband found out that they were pregnant, he agreed to try again, saying, "If they are brave enough to try with no other children, we can try again too as we know we can have healthy children." She joined the PAL group as soon as she achieved pregnancy.

Summary

This chapter has provided an overview of what helps parents as they make their decision about when to try to become pregnant again. As bereaved parents prepare for a new baby in the smooth phase of prenatal parenting, loss of naivety, fear, anxiety, hope, and ongoing attachment are all important elements in their journey as they plan and begin a new pregnancy. Pre-pregnancy counselling and questions and discussion points were suggested. Insight from other parents on how they made their decision to try again and prepare for their next pregnancy was provided.

Note

1 http://www.faithslodge.org/contact-us/

3

BREAK-UP PHASE

Disequilibrium

Smooth	**Break-up**	Sorting out	Inwardizing	Expansion	"Neurotic" fitting together
1	**2**	3	4	5	6
Egg	**Fertilization–12 weeks**	12–24 weeks	24–32 weeks	32 weeks–labor and birth	1–4 weeks

This chapter introduces the unborn baby's stages of growth and development that influence parenting behaviors in the "break-up" phase (disequilibrium) and explores the range of common emotions parents might experience in the first weeks of prenatal parenting as "the baby leads the way." Other content covered includes coping strategies to share as parents begin the journey of a pregnancy after loss.

The first trimester: the presence of a third person[1]

The developmental cycle of "break-up" is initiated when the egg and sperm unite, beginning the process of fetal motor and sensory development, stage by stage. There is tremendous disequilibrium as the fetus/unborn baby and the placenta begin to form.[2] Movement begins around 7–7.5 weeks (deVries et al. 1982). The heart has a definite form by week 8 and by week 10 the peripheral vascular system is complete. By week 9, the third and lateral ventricles are formed, and the fingers are distinct. By week 10, the anal membrane perforates. The kidneys ascend from the pelvis in week 8 and are in their adult location by week 11. At 10 weeks after fertilization the human fetus is able to change its position in utero and by 15 weeks displays a wide range of behavior (16 different kinds of movement), including independent movements of extremities, rotation, head movements, yawning, swallowing, breathing, and so on (Fedor-Freybergh & Maas 2011, p. 124). By week 12 the mid-gut herniates into the base of the umbilical cord and the baby is structurally formed, in that it looks like a very tiny baby.

From the moment pregnancy is suspected, the neurological and behavioral growth and development of the unborn baby during the break-up cycle elicits a reciprocal interaction between heredity and environment, thus fetal and maternal programming occur in parallel (Sandman et al. 2011) and they are bidirectional (DiPietro 2010; Thomson 2007). The physical, emotional, and behavioral changes in the mother and her partner parallel the development of the unborn baby as dramatic hormonal changes in the mother initiate break-up. The mother may experience symptoms of nausea, tender breasts, and an increase in blood flow and uterine bulk causing her to urinate more frequently as her body begins adjusting to the presence of the unborn baby and takes on the pregnancy. If all goes well, the unborn baby at 12 weeks, now at a very immature level of development, will be the same baby at birth, not just an imagined baby they are "expecting."

Discovery of the pregnancy

The dynamics of the break-up phase are exacerbated when conception follows loss. While there is much hope and expectation, fear of another loss can be paralyzing to both parents. "Keeping the baby in mind" (Slade 2002) becomes a complex developmental process, encompassing diverse and shifting feelings. As one mother noted: *'What did I get myself into? Nothing is gone* [the grief] *and I have nausea on top of it.'*

Initial feelings

Parents can exhibit many emotions; feelings of happiness mixed with fear can cause parents to feel "tentative" (Katz Rothman 1996) or "cautiously optimistic" about the new pregnancy. "Watch and worry" has been described as a hallmark of these pregnancies (Côté-Arsenault et al. 2006). Often parents wonder, "Is this going to be the day that something goes wrong?" Most women are likely to be feeling a range of emotions:

> I didn't really believe that I was pregnant. We had even seen and heard the heartbeat and still it was really hard to accept that we were pregnant again.

> I was really happy to be pregnant again but I also knew I was in for a long worrying nine months.

> There was some denial. It was weird. After the first day I found out I was pregnant, he was excited, and we hugged, and then didn't talk about it again for a couple of months. It became just this thing that was going on that we did not want to bring up in case something happened.

Other parents will think about "looking after the pregnancy" but not "having a baby":

> I think I was too scared to really have a lot of emotions when I was pregnant. My approach was more mechanical: Am I eating the right things, am I sleeping enough [or] too much?

> I took care of myself but I didn't want to believe there was a baby inside.

Fathers can have just as many mixed feelings upon hearing of the pregnancy:

> *I don't know how you can be happy and scared as hell in one moment. What's going to happen is the next thing. So you put those two emotions together. It's not that you don't want this new baby; you want both babies. Your initial excitement may turn to fear that this baby could die too.*

Another father debated with himself about how he would cope during this new pregnancy:

> *It's a matter of, okay, do I fully accept it and embrace it and then something happens or do I just kind of not get too attached if something happens and it's not as bad. So if you won't accept it or embrace it, it's tough to visualize what's going to happen. Even though you don't know what's going to happen. You're kind of caught between a rock and a hard place.*

Common feelings and behaviors early in a new pregnancy can be described as emotional cushioning (Côté-Arsenault & Donato 2011):

> *It's still hard to make that full commitment to the happy pregnancy, I guess. It's weird. It's like there's this bubble that I've created around myself that sometimes is stifling because it feels like I'm being really negative about the pregnancy. But then at the same time it's kind of comforting that it's there, kind of like a protection.*

Other common thoughts and feelings are fear and anxiety, the mother's mistrust in her body as a safe place for a baby to grow, and wanting the pregnancy to be over:

> *My womb killed my last baby so it's not a comfort for me to know my baby is there. This is where my last one died. And it's really, really hard.*

For others, protective parenting behaviors, a phenomenon found in many parents of deceased children (Rosenblatt 2000b), begins during pregnancy. Both parents can display behaviors indicating their need to control and protect the baby (Armstrong 2001; Armstrong & Hutti 1998; Côté-Arsenault & Mahlangu 1998; O'Leary & Thorwick 2006).

> *I [can] be very assertive when I need to know something and I'm concerned. I feel like this is my body, my life, and my baby's life on the line* [mother].
>
> *I'm just not there sitting in the corner, basically for support. I want to know what's going on, how come, why. Ask more questions* [father].

One of the most difficult things with a pregnancy after a loss is other people perceiving that the parents are "finally happy again," and over their grief. This thought process becomes complicated when others do not understand that the crisis of the past intrudes. Family and friends may believe that the bereaved parents are replacing the deceased baby as a means of recovery (Powell 1995):

> *I had mixed feelings and people have a hard time understanding that. I told my relatives, Ann's pregnant. Oh congratulations. And I'm like, well thank you, but…. I mean I'm happy, I'm looking forward to being a father. At the same time, there was so much pain involved with the last experience. And it happened so quickly; from elation to "We're having twins" to a week later Ann's in labor, preterm labor, and then both babies are dead.*

> *'Oh, you're back to normal, you've moved on'; so now we can put aside our grief and memories of our loss. For me, it's still vivid every day. If I forget Derek, who will ever remember him? [They] think, 'Look they have another child so everything's hunky-dory.' And it's not.*

Some parents share the pregnancy right away, knowing they will want support if they experience another loss:

> *We told everyone straight away as most people had shared our sorrow and now we wanted them to share our joy.*

Others electively tell people on a need-to-know basis:

> *I had to tell my boss at work because he'd wonder why I was taking so much time off.*

> *She had to tell her boss because they were expecting her to take on some extra duties, which was the opposite of what our doctors were saying, only work eight to five and go home and rest. But family and friends, we didn't tell anybody until we were 22 [weeks], not even our parents.*

One mother sensed that her husband's family did not understand the depth of her feelings because no one had "seen" her miscarried babies and thus did not want to share the news. This insensitive behavior from others has been decribed as empathic failure, a failure to understand another's suffering and hurt, the gravity of what happened or the anguish and loss of meaning in the mourner's life (Neimeyer & Jordan 2002). Others have said that their parents and in-laws did not want to talk about their deceased baby, making it difficult for them to announce the pregnancy and share feelings about the current unborn baby (O'Leary et al. 2011). This can isolate parents from social support, in turn increasing reliance on external and professional interventions (Mills et al. 2014).

Attachment in break-up

Knowing that adequate support has an important influence on grieving (Cacciatore et al. 2008; Carlson et al. 2012; Umphrey & Cacciatore 2011) and buffering of complicated grief during the weeks of "break-up," professionals can begin the work of a relationship-based intervention by introducing the notion of the continued bond and attachment theories. This honors the parenting role to the deceased baby and helps parents begin to process the unborn baby as separate. The message is that they are parents of two babies. The new unborn baby needs their attention now in order to mature optimally until birth. Suzanne Higgins (personal communication, 2012) eloquently describes the work "as 'holding' the bereaved mother (it is usually the mother) while she journeys in the exquisite pain of transitioning from mothering one (deceased) baby and welcoming another." The professionals provide the "holding environment" as sensitive listeners, able to hear the parents' story of loss and their fear of attaching to a new baby who could also die:

> *I look at the first trimester a lot like the first seven or eight months of grief (from my previous loss). It was feeling like I need to keep a grip on basic mental health. I need to not break with reality. My psychological stress felt that stressful, and really wondering about myself, like how far can I push myself, are there limits where you don't get to come back and become a different person or lose part of your sanity and you can't find it again? It just felt like a daily struggle to stay in touch with what has to happen that day; like we were ticking off time. That's how we ended every day; we never have to do this day again. It was really hard.*

> *I think the hardest part for me was the first trimester because you hear of so many people having miscarriages. I knew that this was kind of our last ditch effort. I knew that if we were to miscarry then all of our hopes for a biological child would be gone. We haven't experienced success yet. We've watched everybody else experience it. We've had one pregnancy and it was a bad outcome.*

Building trust

The first visit to confirm the pregnancy and discuss care options is likely to be an anxious and emotional time. A sensitive care provider should be able to give reassurance, as this mother found:

> *I went to see the doctor yesterday [who] was completely understanding. I voiced my concern over not really feeling pregnant. He immediately went and got the portable ultrasound machine. When I saw our new [unborn] baby I cried with relief and also anxiety.*

Living with pregnancy-specific anxiety and worry about the outcome should be viewed as a hallmark of pregnancy after perinatal loss (Côté-Arsenault 2007; Côté-Aresenault & O'Leary 2015; Côté-Arsenault et al. 2006; O'Leary 2004). This seems to be the case regardless of cultural background (Sutan & Miskam 2012) or if parents are the same gender (Cacciatore & Raffo 2011). Côté-Arsenault and colleagues (2006, 2007) suggest that giving false reassurance that "everything will be okay this time" is not helpful and it is inappropriate to provide care without addressing the previous loss(es). They further caution that an absence of questions or statements of feigned calm may be indicators of parents trying to cope rather than evidence of actual feelings. Professionals need to be willing to form a therapeutic relationship and take time to assist parents in processing the past pregnancy. Forming a therapeutic relationship means to promote, guide, and support the healing of another person through knowledgeable and authentic connection (Koloroutis & Trout 2012, p. 53), not owned by any one profession. Therefore encouraging parents to choose a care provider who will provide this type of care and understand their anxiety and fears is foremost in developing trust (Soliday & Tremblay 2013). However, because previous anxiety disorders have been found to be exacerbated in pregnancy after loss (Austin & Priest 2005), this situation should be closely monitored.

Fear of miscarriage

Statistics suggest that one in five confirmed pregnancies ends in miscarriage (Tsartsara & Johnson 2006). Miscarriage is a risk factor for higher anxiety and depression in a pregnancy after loss, especially if the mother responded to the miscarriage with more depressive coping and anxiety (Bergner et al. 2008). Anxiety has been found to decrease by the third trimester when there was a known cause for the miscarriage but not in parents when there was no known cause (Nikcevic et al. 2007).

Irrespective of knowing the cause of their loss, parents can expect a surge of anxiety around the time their loss occurred. Parents who had a miscarriage before 12 weeks may find their level of anxiety may settle to a more manageable level but often will not dissipate until a live baby is in their arms. Those whose loss was later will still fear miscarriage and carry it farther into their new pregnancy. There is often little that can be said during the first 12 weeks to reassure them. It is a matter of weathering the storm and hoping they are indeed in the successful group this time, as these women attest:

> *The first three months were very stressful. I had very little support around me. I was sure that I would lose this baby too.*

Unfortunately, a small percentage of women do lose another pregnancy (Bhattacharay et al. 2008; Frias et al. 2004; Nijkamp et al. 2013). Here are stories from women who experienced this grim reality:

> *Since having a [repeat] miscarriage I feel I have been pushed back somewhere to that place where I can't believe that anything will go right. I had believed that I was ready to take the risk of a new pregnancy and accept the outcome, good or bad. In reality the bad outcome has knocked me about. This "regression" has led me to conclude that when you make a decision to "risk" you actually do so on the basis of believing that "it" won't happen to you.*

A mother of three miscarried babies now pregnant again adds:

> *The first miscarriage I had no conception that this could happen to me. I had heard the word but I didn't really know what it meant. I was shocked that it could happen to me. Now it feels so possible, almost probable. I don't want to feel that way but it does.*

It is helpful for the care provider to ask about and take note of the deceased baby's birth/death date that will fall in the current pregnancy. Parents will need increased support at those times and care providers should reassure the bereaved couple that they are aware that it is approaching. Of all the "anniversaries" the baby's death is usually the one that has the most impact on the bereaved parents, especially during the pregnancy after loss when they are already struggling with loyalty issues. Often the lead-up to any anniversary is worse than the actual day so suggesting that parents take control of it by planning something so as not to be caught off guard by the resurfacing of grief is a good idea. On the actual day there is usually something concrete they can do such as visiting the cemetery, buying some flowers, or burning a candle to help them through the day. One mother scheduled an extra appointment just to hear the new baby's heartbeat on the anniversary of her son's loss.

Anticipatory mourning

Just as in the smooth phase, it is common to hear parents express anticipatory grief in many ways, as these quotes attest:

> *I was anxious and feared this baby would also die. I also thought about other causes for a baby to die like congenital abnormalities and prematurity. Nothing anybody said could allow me to believe I could have a positive outcome.*
>
> *When we got pregnant with this one it was like, I'll wait until the end of 40 weeks before I get too excited.*

Bereaved fathers can feel the same:

> *Initially I was excited, thrilled. After about one month, it sunk in. This is real. Hey, this can happen again. No matter what, you are paranoid in any pregnancy. When you have lost one you have a lot more [paranoia]. You don't want to set yourself up for disappointment so pregnancy is bittersweet.*

Anticipatory mourning in order to cope can also be viewed as healthy and constructive (Corr 2011). Rando (1986b) points out that this type of reaction can bring some parents closer to a child who is dying, knowing they may only have a few weeks or months. For example, one family had not known the gender of their previous baby, believing she would become a member of the family at birth. So now knowing pregnancy may be the only time they might have, they included their unborn son as part of their family from the beginning:

> *As soon as we knew, he became us. We named him. That has helped us accept that if something could go wrong we wouldn't say that he wasn't part of our family. He's our son.*

Rebuilding trust during "break-up": how professionals can help

Rebuilding trust for parents during break-up can be a challenge. Corr (2011) provides guidelines to providers caring for people who are experiencing anticipatory grief and mourning, three of which are important for parents pregnant after a loss: (1) be available, be present, listen; (2) meet people where they are at; and (3) expect to encounter different perspectives (pp. 26–27). Professionals working with these parents should be aware that people in this phase are often resistant to active intervention. They are at odds with their self, their environment, and even other people. The "break-up" phase is about listening, not fixing, as there is usually too much disequilibrium in the parents' state of mind. Parents do better with people who will ride out this period of disequilibrium with them, providing steady, accepting support.

Regardless of how the previous loss occurred, most mothers have a heightened awareness of every ache and pain and will check for bleeding persistently. Partners talk of getting reassurance if the mother has morning sickness as this is perceived as a sign of high level pregnancy hormones. Partners may also avoid touching the mother's body, fearing harm to the baby as a result of sexual activity. Many experience panic when the phone rings: *Every time the phone rings I think she's calling about another loss. Every time she gets up to go to the bathroom at night I think this is the end.*

Health care providers should discuss with both parents what will be helpful in this pregnancy (DeBackere et al. 2008). One family had been going to their small town doctor when their previous baby died. When they became pregnant again, the doctor immediately sent them to a high risk center:

> He said basically "I'm the bread and butter cases. I'm sending you right to a high risk center." So that was reassuring in that they weren't even going to try. I mean, I respected him for that; that he wasn't going to get something out of his league. He just didn't want to take the risk.

At the first visit it is helpful to ask the parents if they are comfortable sharing the story of their previous loss/es. They can be invited with a gentle, "Tell me about your loss/es" cognizant to cultural differences. The care provider must be open to the possibility that parents may have felt unheard in the previous pregnancy, which may have been mismanaged and contributed to the pregnancy outcome. Parents may be carrying anger, described by this mother during her subsequent pregnancy:

> There were a couple of weeks before when he had slowed down and I got really scared. And I called the doctor and they would be saying, "Oh just drink some orange juice and lay on your side. The baby will move within 30 minutes and everything will be fine." I just wish that they had said, "Why don't' you just come in and we will hook you up to the fetal heart rate monitor. Why don't we just do a non-stress test, you know, and see if anything's going on." I really feel that the health care system just really failed us.

There is no need to defend previous medical management; the care provider can just listen. Conversation should follow the parents' lead to avoid probing so much that they feel exposed and vulnerable. The issues they raise must be accepted, however painful, and specific clues listened for that will help care for the family. The care provider should not be afraid to be with them in their pain and be willing to tolerate enduring discussions of negative affective states resulting from the previous loss (Cacciatore et al. 2014). Showing empathy allows the family to feel safe in venting their feelings and begins to build trust.

One of the most caring interventions is to ask if they named the deceased baby and then to use the baby's name in conversation. This is a simple thing and usually means a tremendous amount to the parents. It means that the care provider is listening and recognizes that they are still parents to this baby. Using the deceased baby's name also begins to separate the babies as individuals.

Distrust of the medical community is common (O'Leary & Thorwick 2006a, 2006b), so accepting this can be the first step in reestablishment of their trust in this pregnancy (Côte-Arseneault & Morrison 2001). As one perinatal nurse articulated; "You can expect someone who's had a loss to be very anxious. You must expect them to be very suspicious, and you must expect to do more for them and that is still within normal for their situation" (Thorwick, personal communication). The care provider must offer reassurance while also watching the parents closely, knowing that they cannot help compare pregnancies and feel anxious. As one father stated:

> I don't know how many times I've heard people at the perinatal clinic say already, do not compare this pregnancy to the other one because they'll be different. But at the same time, you compare it to the previous pregnancy because that's how we learn from our mistakes.

The care provider must explore what will help the parents feel comfortable, such as coming in more often for heartbeat checks in the early weeks. These parents need hope and, regardless of the care provider's professional discipline, that person is in a position to help them with this. As found in a study of cancer patients coping with loss and associated negative emotions, families who have suffered trauma need people who will provide medical information, show that they care about them as individuals, balance hope and realism while expressing empathy, and help them discover and identify realistic expectations (Evans et al. 2006). One mother's doctor understood her fears and acknowledged this by saying, "You'll be all right, but you won't believe anyone until you have the baby in your arms." This was his first step in respecting that she would be anxious in the new pregnancy and he would support what she and her partner might need.

Studies have found that women who have experienced stillbirth are likely to consider they played a role in their baby's death (Duncan & Cacciatore 2015; Warland et al. 2015). Regaining sense of self as mother to protect this new baby and for the father to protect the mother and baby can be daunting. Finding a care provider who will join in a therapeutic relationship with the parents is crucial in helping share the burden of responsibility. "A therapeutic interchange is fundamental to gaining the knowledge essential to care and greater understanding" (Koloroutis & Trout 2012, p. 104). One perinatologist offers the following suggestions to providers caring for these parents:

> Encourage the parents to ask questions. It's very important for them to tell us how they are feeling about it and to communicate what happened with the previous loss, what it means to them. If we can build bridges that way, understanding what their fear is and understanding what their trust is then we can go much further in taking care of the current pregnancy.

This type of care is described below:

> *Frequent ultrasounds and monitoring helped tremendously. I often went in just to hear the heartbeat and be comforted by knowing that, for at least that moment, my baby was alive … I felt fortunate that my care providers were very understanding and supportive.*

People under stress are often unable to take in complicated information. During the trauma of their previous loss parents may not have understood all that happened. Therefore it is common for parents to ask their care provider the same questions during visits in order to understand everything that may have gone wrong in the previous pregnancy for the sake of the new baby and their stress levels. Parents need concrete, specific information from their health care provider on what will be done differently and how they can know their unborn baby is safe. Helpful boundaries must be set to separate the past from the current experience by reassuring parents that this is a different pregnancy and a different baby:

> The most important message I could give parents is to be upfront with their care providers at the beginning of the pregnancy. They may have to say to the provider, "We had this loss and this is going to be a different pregnancy for us and we don't feel a sense of trust." They then need to tell their health provider that it's nothing personal. That's the way they're going to feel about it.
>
> *(Personal communication, Dr. Manny Gaziano)*

One study (Hutti et al. 2011) found an increase in utilization of health care in parents pregnant after loss and recommended referral to support groups as one way to help decrease their need for constant medical reassurance:

> *I've actually had three scans already. I had one at six weeks. I wanted to be sure in fact that I did have a baby with a heartbeat, so that early on, you know it was as okay as it could be. And also that it was developing normally maybe. My husband found that really helpful because he figured if it was going well at 12 weeks it would be alright.*

I just thought, I've got to get to 12 weeks. Even at 12 weeks I started to think, even though we'd seen the heartbeat, we'd seen this baby three times now, 7 weeks, 9 weeks, and 12 weeks and I know she's okay, I'm not going to feel better until I get to 20 weeks.

Parents may feel alone and therefore may appreciate having a safe place for processing their emotions with other parents pregnant after loss. They can be referred to a support group so that they can focus on *this* baby and *this* pregnancy. It also helps to provide consistent care providers to help parents build trust and avoid having to retell their story to successive people.

CASE STUDY

The following case illustrates a mother's lack of support during her loss because they were "early miscarriages" that continued in her subsequent pregnancies after loss.

Alice had a miscarriage between the births of two children and then two more miscarriages during a nine-month period, when she joined the infant loss support group. She expressed a lot of anger over her loss of control in spacing children two years apart and anger at her parents and a woman, who she had considered a friend, for dismissing these losses. During the conversation in which Alice told her about the miscarriage, rather than recognizing Alice's grief, her "friend" announced that she herself was pregnant.

Once pregnant, in addition to not trusting the pregnancy would last, the anger towards unsupportive people and those who had become pregnant before her dominating her feelings in the PAL group. At this stage she needed a safe space to share and vent while receiving much needed support. The facilitators held these emotions, acknowledging how painful it must be to have no outside support.

Summary

This chapter has reviewed common feelings of parents during the first trimester 'break-up" phase as the unborn baby is developing from an embryo to a fetus. It is a time when most parents realize they are pregnant, which brings a resurgence of grief accompanied by anxiety and distrust. During these weeks parents need support and understanding as they start to process fear, anxiety, and grief. They appreciate others understanding they will be anxious and need strategies for managing the new pregnancy. They need a care provider who will listen to their fears and provide information on how the pregnancy will be managed to keep the unborn baby safe. Professionals working with these parents should be aware that the new pregnancy does not take away the pain of their previous loss; therefore they will be working with parents who are still grieving.

Notes

1 Throughout this book we will refer to the fetus as unborn baby because, when parents suffer a loss (including a miscarriage), they talk of losing a "baby" not a "fetus."
2 Information on fetal development is drawn from www.obimages.net and used with the permission of Dr. Emanuel Gaziano.

4

SORTING-OUT PHASE

12–24 weeks gestation

Smooth	Break-up	**Sorting out**	Inwardizing	Expansion	"Neurotic" fitting together
1	2	**3**	4	5	6
Egg	Fertilization–12 weeks	**12–24 weeks**	24–32 weeks	32 weeks–labor and birth	1–4 weeks

This chapter explores parental feelings as they move into the second trimester and begin to "sort out" (equilibrium) the reality of the pregnancy; that perhaps a baby is truly present. The many issues parents face in regard to the risk, benefits, and meaning of prenatal diagnostic testing offered, which tests might provide more information or reassurance, and how to clarify questions put to their care provider will be covered. Fetal movement becomes more consistent during these weeks so this is a time in which to help parents learn ways to trust in the process of pregnancy and "sort out" the difference between fetal movement and contractions. A common dilemma that merges with fetal movement is parents questioning loyalty to their deceased baby.

The baby's "sorting out"

After the disequilibrium of break-up, the sorting-out phase is a time of tremendous growth for the unborn baby.[1] Babies are "sorting out" the inter-uterine environment, using energy to explore the world (the uterus) through their senses of touch and hearing (parents and siblings on the outside). By week 13 babies display creeping, climbing motions, and can move their elbows and knees, open and close their hands, open their mouth, stick out their tongue, and place fingers in their mouth. They are sucking and swallowing amniotic fluid, moving the diaphragm during breathing movements, the beginning, practice, behavior for breathing after birth.

The baby has mastered basic patterns of movement, as the fetus is able to extend her body, and she uses the remainder of the pregnancy to refine and master these motor abilities. Somewhere during these weeks the mother begins to feel "flutters" of movement.

Tests and screens

During these weeks parents are generally more task-oriented, open to cognitive problem solving, exploring options, and eager to establish relationships with providers to achieve specific goals. Testing can provide reassurance and bonding or deliver life-changing news (McCoyd 2010). While the majority of parents believe prenatal screening is related to bonding rather than health assessment of the baby (McCoyd 2013), most parents pregnant after loss choose testing for information that will help reduce anxiety. Parents have to "sort out" whether they want to undergo testing and what type, seek information on diagnostic and screening tests that may be offered, and revisit questions regarding what happened last time. Parents should receive additional information on risks, reliability of testing, including false positive and false negative rates and outcomes, before deciding to have screening tests (McCoyd 2010). Parents' understanding of the implications of each test and what choices they will face pending the outcome of each test must be assessed. Parents must also be encouraged to ask for more information such as, "What does each test mean and what is it for? What information will I gain?"

Understanding the cultural issues around testing is also important. For instance, Sutan and Miskam (2012) reported that decision making in regards to testing for Muslim women was dependent on the partner and family. It can be helpful for parents to discuss "what ifs" before testing. Parents pregnant after loss may also forego testing if their previous baby died because of ruptured membranes following an amniocentesis for genetic screening, only to find out the baby had been healthy.

One father going into testing at 18 weeks who had experienced a loss at 22 weeks gestation and already had a son born at 26 weeks who was blind and had cerebral palsy, stated:

> *My fear of having another child like our son is stronger than my fear of loss. If we can just get through to 26 weeks gestation I will feel safer.*

Amniocentesis

Amniocentesis is currently able to detect around 5,000 different disorders. This test cultures cells from the amniotic fluid and can accurately pick up any chromosomal abnormality, and certain other genetic diseases as well as determine the gender of the baby.[2] Parents need to sort out whether or not they wish to know this information. The procedure involves passing a needle through the mother's abdomen to draw a small amount of fluid from around the baby. Depending on the skill and experience of the operator, there may be a slightly increased risk of miscarriage associated with this test. One study with Latina women (Seth et al. 2010) found that the risk of procedure-related complications played a more concrete role in the decision to undergo this test than spiritual beliefs. Irrespective of their obstetric history, waiting for results is a very anxious time.

Ultrasound

Another screening test is diagnostic Level II ultrasound, offered as a matter of routine in most high income countries at around weeks 18–20. In a metasynthesis of 14 PAL studies (Mills et al. 2014), parents expressed discontent with aspects of care, one being that they were ill-prepared for the anxiety generated around appointments. Most parents learned about the death of their baby or that their baby had a severe disability through ultrasound imaging. The ultrasound examination can carry embodied memories for these parents as it engages all of the perceptual senses: lived body, lived time, lived space, and lived relations; flashbacks are thus common for parents pregnant after loss and will risk activation of sad memories (O'Leary 2005). It is critical that parents have an awareness of this before the examination and also that health care providers understand that symptoms of PTSD are normal under these circumstances. Sensitive intervention such as acknowledging they will be anxious until they see the heartbeat and may experience reliving events in the form of flashbacks can be helpful in alleviating symptoms (Yehuda 2002).

> *The way we lost her was so sudden and out of the blue, lying on the ultrasound table. The ultrasound tech never said a word. The doctor came in and said the baby was dead.*
>
> *I get the gut ache because you're always waiting for the bad news. "Okay, what's going to be wrong? So you sit there for an hour and they measure the toes and the bones and they look at the kidneys, she'd start zooming in on the heart and you'd see the chambers going. I couldn't wait for the doctor to come in and officially go through things and tell us it looks like we have a very healthy little girl in there, which she did. It was very exciting even with all the stress.*

Parents who have ended pregnancy due to their baby's abnormality often need more support (Rillstone & Hutchinson, 2001). Pregnant after termination of a baby who had hydrocephaly and spina bifida, the ultrasound in their subsequent pregnancy created ambivalent feelings for this father:

> *I needed to know that every vertebrae looks fine, the brain and the head, everything looks fine there. So even when we got the phone call saying the numbers were elevated for Down's Syndrome and we need to check further for that, it was like bringing up the memories of the past. While they validated everything we were saying, they still said your risks are really low. I just kept thinking over and over, we were that one person. Somebody's got to be that one person.*

It can be helpful for parents to bring a supportive person with them to ultrasound appointments. Such support can sometimes help parents "stay focused in the present" while being mindful of their past, which lessens the risk of flashbacks occurring. Parents must be reminded to tell care providers that they have experienced a previous loss and to ask to see the heartbeat first (O'Leary 2005). Some sonographers now have the ability to make a short DVD of the scan. If this can be arranged, it will be a useful memento to refer to throughout the parents' new pregnancy:

> It was a relief to see a strong heartbeat and see a healthy baby on the screen.

As the health care provider, it is important to review the testing to provide reassurance and reconfirm the positive results and how the woman's body is growing and nurturing the baby. This can help parents begin to learn ways to let "the unborn baby lead" by visualizing a baby growing and staying healthy. If all is well, parents often feel relieved but this may also cause mixed feelings. Sometimes the father may not be able to be supportive for fear of another loss, as this mother found:

> Mike brought me back to earth with a thud after my ultrasound. I expressed how relieved I felt that everything seemed okay and he said, "Yes, but everything seemed okay with Emma's ultrasound too." Wonderful man!

It is common for parents to experience anxiety during ultrasounds throughout the entire pregnancy:

> I was hysterical. Every time I went I thought it would look the same and the baby would be dead.

> All of those same feelings that you have in that ultrasound room, turn off the lights, all of those same emotions, fears and anxieties, just by the sake of association, they're all you know about being in a room. They all come back, same as going into a hospital and seeing the machine. You can't help but have those emotions come back.

Sharing the news

Parents are often well into the sorting-out phase before they want to share the news of the pregnancy:

> We decided to delay telling anyone until 20 weeks [because] we felt that we would be misunderstood. We imagined statements like "Haven't they had enough – they already have three children, why take the risk again?" We felt anxious enough without adding other people's opinions and anxieties to our own. From 16 to 20 weeks there were some glances at my waistline, but no one actually asked directly.

Although not carried out with parents pregnant after loss, one study found that higher maternal pregnancy-specific anxiety between 13 and 17 weeks' gestation was associated with increased negative temperament in children (Blair et al. 2011; Christian 2012). This is a period during which parents pregnant after loss can experience a high level of anxiety concerning the risk of miscarriage:

> *I'm concerned about the health and welfare of the baby I'm carrying. Yet you try not to be negative and have a lot of anxiety. At least for myself, I worry if I have too much anxiety, what it's doing to my baby. Some books say any anxiety is normal, but, if you have too much, you're wondering if it's going to affect the health of your baby. I feel like sometimes I worry too much. Is my blood pressure going to start rising? Is that going to affect the health of my baby?*

Use of Complementary Alternative Medicine (CAM), discussed in Chapter 16, also helps parents who may be demonstrating detachment or emotional cushioning (Campbell-Jackson et al. 2014; Côté-Arsenault & Donato 2011), holding back attachment out of loyalty to the deceased baby (O'Leary & Thorwick 2008). Professionals hearing this fear can gently guide parents using attachment-focused interventions such as "Of course you want that baby back but this is a new baby, a younger sibling who will always miss his/her older sibling too." As information on the unborn baby's competence is explored (that is, hearing the outside uterine environment, sensing the emotions of grief), the care provider also reinforces that the parents' continued bond and attachment remains and the deceased baby knew them as parents too. They need to talk about the deceased baby as they reconstruct their new identity (Walter 1996):

> *I chose not to tell anyone until I was 20 weeks for a number of reasons. First I was trying to ignore it and telling them would make it real and put the spotlight on me. I felt people would expect me to be happy and excited (which I wasn't). I didn't want to risk a new baby. I wanted our other one back. When we finally did tell other people we lied about the due date, telling them a month later than I actually was, to protect our privacy.*

Many parents whose loss was defined as a "miscarriage," often managed as a medical procedure (Fernandez et al. 2011), would be particularly anxious during these weeks. The miscarriage can be engraved in their minds in much the same way as parents who suffer a full-term loss (Gerber-Epstein et al. 2009). Alderman et al. (1998) found that, although men and women who had experienced miscarriage did not significantly differ from each other on the Avoidance Scale, women were more in touch with their feelings and willing to admit to them than their partners, possibly because males are socialized to control their emotions. Others have also found that fathers experience depression after miscarriage (deMontigny et al. 2013). When parents pass the gestational age of the previous loss they need more support and education on the normal physiology of pregnancy as the woman's uterus expands to accommodate a growing baby.

An unexpected hospital visit is not unusual if symptoms similar to the woman's former pregnancy occur (that is, increased or decreased fetal movement, suspicion of ruptured membranes). One bereaved father describes his feelings as his partner approached 22 weeks, the time when ruptured membranes resulted in the death of his son:

> *I just can't wait for week 22, because I feel if we get to that point, we're pretty much home free. You get through each milestone. Call me at 30 weeks and I'll probably be having a party because I'll just believe, at that point even if she did have to come out that's nothing compared to what we've been through and she would have so many chances to be okay.*

Anticipating the anniversary of the previous loss and offering extra office visits can prevent the expense of a hospital visit: *I've had several unscheduled appointments. They don't need to do an ultrasound but they need to hold my hand and get me through today.*

Hearing the fetal heartbeat

Parents often need frequent heartbeat checks in the early weeks of "sorting out" until they feel regular fetal movements. Regular doctor's visits often are not enough so parents should request more for reassurance.

> *I was actually going to my obstetrician twice a week between 16 and 18 weeks because in between I actually had trouble sort of planning things. I kept thinking. "Oh, I might be going and finding out that it had died again" and then everything was going to start all over.*
>
> *Up to 20 weeks I was going to the obstetrician each time I wasn't sure whether the baby was alive or not. He's been very understanding. It was his idea that I come in…. He'd have a feel and say, "Yes, I definitely feel like [the baby is] growing."*

Sorting out the baby's gender

Having a strong preference for one gender over the other is not confined to those enduring a pregnancy after loss; some societies still practice infanticide if the baby is not the desired sex. If the gender of their baby is important, encourage parents to find out before the birth so they can begin to come to terms with having a baby of the "wrong gender."

> *We had hoped for a girl previously and I felt guilty and devastated when we had a son who died. This time we wanted a live baby and the gender was unimportant.*

Finding out they were having a third girl after the loss of a son, one father explained his feelings thus:

> *Really disappointed; I just had hoped for a brother for Sawyer that was here. But four is definitely a number that I'm not going any higher. We make our peace with it. I also think it could be better than having another baby boy after Lincoln. What you want and what you can handle are sometimes two different things.*

His wife was disappointed too, so they decided to give the baby a name and shared it with their children to help separate the babies and understand that Lincoln would not be coming back.

Differentiating the new baby from the deceased baby takes conscious effort. *You can't really replace him. You can fill in the spot where maybe he left off but you can never replace him.* While some parents want the same gender baby, others want everything to be different. Even if a parent chooses not to learn, knowing the gender can be particularly helpful for parents pregnant after loss:

> *Knowing the sex helped me relate to this little baby who was growing inside me as a very particular person and helped me bond with her. I could call her by name and imagine what she might be like.*

Sorting out fetal movements and contractions

> *I felt stressed until I felt the first movements and greatly relieved every time the baby kicked — he kicked a lot!*

Fetal movements are simultaneously reassuring and yet anxiety provoking if the baby does not move very much. It is never too early to help a mother understand the changes happening in her body and the difference between fetal movements and contractions. This can begin towards the last weeks of the sorting-out phase (16–22 weeks). Partners can be shown how to place their hands on the woman's abdomen and recognize that a tight abdomen means a contraction and a soft abdomen with movement indicates movement by the baby. This information can save babies' lives (O'Leary et al. 2012):

> *A big turning point for us was when the baby started moving. They say usually about the 18th week the mothers can start to feel little flutters but it happened a little earlier for us. There wasn't a whole lot of movement but there was a definite shift in our attitude towards the baby, like as long as you can feel the baby moving you're thinking everything's okay.*

Teaching the difference between fetal movements and contractions can help mothers spot the very cues that might reassure them all is well, or, alternatively, identify signs to be concerned about and to present to their care provider. Some parents may have experienced preterm labor that ended in their baby's death, not knowing they would need a cerclage[3] to prevent premature labor. For example, at 22 weeks in their previous pregnancy one father noticed his partner had some back pain that progressively got worse, together with some bleeding:

> *We didn't know it was contractions at the time. So we went to our local hospital and it took four hours for the doctor to show up after we got there. By that time she was dilated four centimeters and the baby was coming out.*

This story is illustrative of other parents who did not get seen in time. A cerclage was put in place in the subsequent pregnancy:

> *We've followed this one much, much closer. Even the doctors and my wife physically pay attention a lot closer to what her body is feeling to see if anything's different, just to make sure that something doesn't happen again. With the cerclage we're a little bit more okay with it but we still watch it pretty closely.*

Rebuilding trust in sorting out

Attig (2000) notes that people experiencing grief often feel anxiety about their own fitness. Pregnancy loss can undermine one's belief in being a woman/mother who can protect her child (Campbell-Jackson et al. 2014; Gerber-Epstein et al. 2009). A woman's ability to trust her body as a safe place for a baby to grow needs to be nurtured in a pregnancy after loss. Mothers question what they might have done wrong in the previous pregnancy: *There had to be something that made it happen. They tell me it's not me but it just happens to be my body that this happened in.* How could they not have known their previous baby had died? Regardless of the gestation of the previous loss, the parents' sense of self (Cumming et al. 2007; O'Leary & Thorwick 2006a) is damaged; not having been stronger advocates for and protected their previous baby can weigh heavily on some parents' minds (O'Leary et al. 2011).

Helping both parents regain trust in the pregnancy, that the mother's body is protecting the baby, and their intuitive knowing of their unborn baby, becomes a part of the interventionist role in reviewing the past to focus on prenatal parenting; advocating for themselves and their baby. This has been described as the professional taking the point of view of the user (parent) seriously to empower them to gain mastery of their lives from a previously suppressed position (Higgins, personal communication 2012) in the previous pregnancy where their intuition of something wrong with the baby was dismissed by others:

> *I'm always paying attention to try and make sure I don't miss something this time. I didn't miss it last time but no one would listen to me. So I told my doctor that she's not moving very much. And he just laughed and said, you're almost dilated to a two and you're going to have this baby in a day, so just don't worry. You're just being silly. And she died.*

Intuition has been described as "an innate capability, specific to each individual, serving as a guide, counselor, and informant—a segment of the universal mind from which all knowing and physical manifestation are derived" (Leviton 2002, p. 29). Professionals need to be respectful of a mother's intuitive knowing. A recent study showed that many bereaved mothers reported having a "gut feeling that something was wrong" during their previous pregnancy (Warland et al. 2015). Others have described mothers who had a premonition their baby was in trouble (Chapman & Chapman 1990); for example, this mother's experience during her 18-week ultrasound:

We had our ultrasound with him. I just remember lying there having this weird feeling like this was the last time that I would ever see my child alive. I never acknowledged it until after everything happened because how can you acknowledge a feeling like that?

Two months later:

The doctor couldn't find the heartbeat so he sent me down to ultrasound. You know. Here's an ultrasound picture of my dead baby. It was like, you know, I remember two months back when I had my first one with him; those feelings just came rushing back again. You sensed this two months ago and here you are.

In the current pregnancy she trusts her intuition, saying *I don't have that when I see this baby on ultrasound*. This illustrates the importance of providers understanding issues from the previous loss and respecting and responding to a mother's intuition regarding her baby in this new pregnancy (O'Leary et al. 2011).

The need to control is foremost in both parents' minds. Fathers no longer view themselves as just the "support person," even as they realize they had no control over the last experience or in this new pregnancy:

For guys, it's all about control. Your job is to manage the upkeep of the house; all the responsibilities of a young father are really impressed upon you. And then to have what happened to our first and you have no control over it.

Nine months is a long time and you realize how much you are not in control of anything. So I'm just excited but I'll really be happy once the baby is born.

Rebuilding trust: the role of self-blame

Regardless of their cultural background, two studies have reported that it is common for women to believe that their body failed to protect their baby as a reason for the previous loss (Duncan & Cacciatore 2015). If the mother is reporting that she feels she played a role in her last baby's death (Warland et al. 2015), it may be particularly difficult for her to trust herself and her new baby. In the bereavement literature self-blame is described as making self-attributions about the cause of death (Davis et al. 1996; Weinberg 1994) that are different than regret, a negative emotion, believing one could have done something different to prevent the outcome (Stroebe et al. 2014).

Self-blame has been correlated with depression and anxiety (Cacciatore et al. 2013; Graham et al. 1987; Sutan & Miskam 2012) but just as there is a fundamental difference between depression (pathology) and grief (normality), it is important to distinguish the difference between the definitions of self-blame and regret. "Regret in bereavement focuses more on a possible better outcome, without impaired sense of self" (Stroebe et al. 2014, p. 2).

Fathers can also feel regret if they dismissed the mother's concerns (O'Leary et al. 2011a). *He kept telling me nothing's wrong. Then we found out the baby's dead and he cried.* Grieving the loss of self as mother (and partner) (Campbell-Jackson et al. 2014; O'Leary & Thorwick 1997) and helping to rebuild trust is an ongoing task throughout pregnancy. Cacciatore and colleagues (2013) stress that it is critical for providers to be aware of the role of self-blame, shame, and guilt in negative psychological outcomes. In applying the prenatal parenting model of intervention with parents who indicate that they are blaming themselves for their baby's death, it may be helpful to suggest that the story of self as parent can be reframed as that of a mother who was very in touch with her deceased baby and did all she could to get help. Her deceased baby felt her emotions, heard her heartbeat, and felt her love as he died and knew, at some level, she was trying to protect him. This is a creative intervention that dispels (ibid) rather than reinforces anger at previous health care management. At the same time, parents understand physicians cannot give guarantees:

> *I didn't think it was fair to ask the doctor to tell me this is going to be alright. He wouldn't be able to answer the question other than saying, "Yes, it is normal for now."*

Most parents pregnant after loss need objective data, such as listening to the fetal heart, undergoing a non-stress test or biophysical profile, explained in layman's terms because they are *so* subjectively involved, and can find it difficult to trust their intuition, especially if it was dismissed previously. Mills and colleagues (2014) caution against parents being over-reliant on technology and instead emphasize the importance of regular contact with their care provider and sustained psychological support.

Attachment and loyalty: learning to love both babies

> *I've had a hard time bonding with this child just because of the fear of loss.*

Helping parents reframe their grief as a continued bond with and attachment to their deceased baby is crucial, especially in light of research with adults who were the child in their family born after loss (O'Leary 2012; O'Leary et al. 2006). Parents pregnant after loss need professionals who are open to letting anxiety and fears surface (Soliday & Tremblay 2013) in order to hear what they are saying about their continued loyalty to the deceased baby. Klass (2001) suggests that care providers who block the attempt of parents to talk about and grieve for their previous child may heighten their need to "hang on" to their grief and complicate the healing process.

Once fetal movement is felt during the sorting-out phase, ambivalent feelings of loyalty are common. Recalling the break-up phase in which people who find out they are pregnant again wish for the return of the deceased baby, parents need help to differentiate this baby as a separate individual. Like any pregnant parents, they may feel that the unknown baby is a stranger, compounded by the fact that they are still more emotionally connected to the deceased baby. It is perfectly natural to wonder if they are capable of loving another baby and it is important for parents to hear: "It's not that you don't want this new unborn baby. You want *both* babies." Parents need help sorting out their feelings, and must be told that there is space in their hearts for more than one child. This mother illustrates why the prenatal parenting intervention focuses on helping parents understand that they are parents to both babies:

> *I felt there was an air of unreality about the pregnancy from the beginning. I really wondered how I would have felt if Samantha [the subsequent child she is carrying] had died. I suspect that I would not have felt too surprised; it was almost as if I had programmed myself for failure. I felt I didn't know Samantha. I knew Edward and was still feeling sad about him so I did not allow myself to emotionally attach to the new baby before her birth.*

If the previous baby died during these weeks, the care provider needs to ask open-ended questions periodically, such as "You're getting close to the time you had trouble in your last pregnancy. How are you feeling?" If the parents initially refuse help, this should not preclude offering access to support systems as the pregnancy progresses.

While honoring the parents' need to continue to talk about their deceased baby, the intervention needs to keep the focus on *this* unborn baby by providing reassurance and leading the way to a healthy outcome. This is when sharing the cognitive structured educational information on the developing fetal competencies can begin. The baby is moving about, flexing, extending his body, and by week 16 can hear things outside the uterus. Most parents know this and some, like this father, actively start interacting with the baby: *We read somewhere that at 20 weeks babies hear so that was our start date to play music and read.* Again, the care provider can help parents to build the autographic memory of the deceased baby by reviewing how he knew them as parents too.

Research indicates that unborn babies at this developmental stage respond to parental stress, which impacts their development during the first year of life and beyond (Glover 2011; Mendelson et al. 2011; Sandman et al. 2012; Tollenaar et al. 2011). This information can be very distressing to parents, who may verbalize that they don't want the baby to know what they are feeling. The care provider must understand that mixed feelings are difficult yet normal after what the parents have been through; they are grieving for their deceased baby and struggling to attach to the new baby (O'Leary et al. 2008). Parents need to be gently reminded: "Do they think it will hurt less if you don't attach and this baby dies too? Your baby needs you now."

> *I'd been reading books on the symptoms of pregnancy— trying to do all that cerebral stuff, but the bottom line is I was terrified, scared to attach and fearful about replacing my son.*
>
> *Neither one of us wanted to attach. Last time I talked a lot more to Nicolas [deceased son]. This baby deserves a chance to get everything we had planned on giving Nicolas. After the 19-week ultrasound we started playing Baby Beethoven and read to the baby every night.*

In doing the work of guiding the attachment relationship with the unborn baby the professional becomes the voice for babies who are at risk for attachment issues postpartum, as recommended in the work of Selma Fraiberg and colleagues (1980a).

Releasing fears verbally gives voice to them and, at some level, gives meaning to what the unborn baby may be feeling regarding the mother's emotions. We cannot quantify that an unborn baby or a pre-verbal baby postpartum understand the words, as an adult would. However, adult subsequent children who underwent regression therapy back into the womb shared stories of feeling the emotions of their mothers, which illustrates the cellular memory they carried (O'Leary 2012; O'Leary et al. 2006). Sharing the story of their continued bond with and attachment to the deceased sibling helps parents learn that the subsequent baby will always miss the deceased sibling too, confirmed by research with adults who were the child in their family born after loss (O'Leary & Gaziano 2011). This mode of healing for pre-verbal babies has been used as an intervention in a newborn intensive care unit with parents, modeling the importance of "giving the baby the words" for the perceived sensations she is experiencing (Szejer 2005). One example Szejer shares is that of having a conversation with a surviving twin, in the presence of the parents: "Of course you can keep her memory alive inside you, but she [deceased twin] will never again be (*physically*) near you" (p. 40):

> *Babies can start to determine sounds and have the ability to hear at approximately 17 weeks. That just coincided with knowing her and it made me want to start talking to her and sharing things with her, letting her know how much we cared about her. I read about a mom who said, "However many days this child has, whether in the uterus or out in the world, I want it to be of a high quality." To me, that made a lot of sense. So whether you lost them shortly after birth again or whether you lost them whenever, you wanted to make sure that child knew who you were and that you loved them, cared about them, and wanted to take the best care of them.*

Other parents report a deeper understanding and appreciation of themselves as a parent to a baby already present, displaying attachment feelings. Now 22 weeks pregnant, this mother shifted her sense of self as a mother to her baby:

> *It was not hard for me to be emotionally attached in the first pregnancy. Then I was so surprised and devastated when I lost it. The second loss, I steeled myself off from it. Early in this third pregnancy, I was hesitant to form too close an emotional bond but this feels so real. I feel a personal and emotional connection, a tie to this baby that I'm going to bring into the world.*

A feeling of being a parent happens for fathers too:

> *I've gotten to know this baby a lot more before birth than I did my other two. One of my ultrasound pictures is just his hand; I treasure everything about him when I see him.*
>
> *What helped me get in touch with the baby was to lie in bed and feel the baby move inside my wife, which scared the crap out of me. Each time the baby would move, I'd jump. Wow! It gave me more appreciation of what my wife was doing, carrying the baby.*

There are some parents who will not want to talk about the deceased baby or attachment issues they may be having with the new baby, often because it is too painful for them. This can be hard to accept in the light of current research suggesting that, if parents are not helped to reframe their grief for a deceased child as their continuing bond and attachment, it can have long-term negative implications for the family system (O'Leary et al. 2006b). It is crucial to respect the parents' boundaries, gently focusing on the unborn baby's competencies to help break down their barriers while providing autobiographical information on the deceased baby's competencies. The process of engaging parents with the new unborn baby should begin in the sorting-out phase and continue throughout the pregnancy. This process takes time and cannot be forced; the parents must lead the way regarding how much they can absorb. Almost always, it is useful to encourage the parents to allow the baby to lead them into understanding that she is a separate sibling who needs their parenting attention now. As they develop trust in the person who is listening to their fears and anxieties, that person can begin to gently nurture and guide them through the pregnancy, keeping the focus on the unborn baby leading the way. Separating the new baby from the deceased baby can be hard work for some parents, who may not be ready until the postpartum period or even months or years later.

Journaling

Journaling offers a way to help parents incorporate and process their very deep feelings, and differentiate the deceased baby and the new unborn baby as they organize their new sense of identity (Neimeyer et al. 2008), supporting Selma Fraiberg's (Fraiberg & Fraiberg, 1987) belief regarding releasing the power of feelings. Writing has been documented since the 1700s as a coping skill to deal with bereavement, illustrated in Rosenblatt's (1983) compilation of nineteenth-century diaries, and is especially appropriate when the death is sudden and unintentional as a means to decrease feelings of emotional loneliness (van der Houwen et al. 2010), as in perinatal loss. It provides a greater sense of control to grieving people, a way to process feelings and reduce the physical and mental stress associated with loss (Smart 1993–94), especially among people with high anxiety (Smyth & Pennebaker 2008).

The direct, non-mediated communication in journaling offers a valuable form of healing for bereaved people (Lander & Graham Pole 2008–2009) and may result in fewer visits to health care providers (Pennebaker 1997; Pennebaker et al. 1997). Pennebaker and Beall (1986) asked individuals to write about their thoughts and feelings around a traumatic event and they showed improved health over subsequent months compared to a control group who wrote about superficial topics. In a cognitive behavioral internet-based therapy specific to perinatal bereaved parents that included 10 writing assignments, overall mental health and depression significantly improved in the experimental group (Kersting et al. 2011) and the follow-up found significantly reduced symptoms of post-traumatic stress, prolonged grief, depression and anxiety compared to the control group (Kersting et al. 2013). Expressive writing as an intervention with mothers of premature babies (Horsch et al. 2014) and an intervention group of mothers pregnant after loss as a way to relieve stress and anxiety was also found helpful (Côté-Arsenault & Moore 2014).

> *During my pregnancy I had a lot of angry feelings toward other pregnant women and families with young children. I would always assume that those women were all so blissful and happy and had never experienced the tragedy that we had. It helped to write down all those angry feelings about how life can be so unfair. I was pleased to find that others in the support group had these same kinds of feelings. I also learned that other people have experienced terrible losses, you just don't know what has happened in other people's lives.*

Writing translates experience into narrative language and helps people to label and acknowledge an emotional event; putting something into words provides a more complex cognitive representation of the event and surrounding emotions (Smyth & Pennebaker 2008). Liefer (1977, 1980) concluded that writing undertaken by mothers during pregnancy that expresses worries about the mental health of the fetus may reflect an emotional investment in the unborn baby.

The process of helping parents journal or use guided imagery to cope with their feelings takes time and involves persistent, gentle nurturing on the part of the professional. While some parents may journal throughout their pregnancy, it is important to explore what the journaling is about, as without guidance a parent may not necessarily be focused on what is most helpful (Lichtenthal & Cruess 2010; Stroebe et al. 2006). Often parents are resistant to writing. They may say, "I don't want this baby to know what I'm thinking." The care provider needs to point out that in any normal pregnancy parents tend to be more attached to the previous child than an unborn baby still developing. A question might be: "Does the baby not hear and feel your thoughts anyway? It's a good thing to tell the new baby you are sad because of their sibling who will not be here to greet them." It is a good idea to suggest to the parents that they first begin to write to the deceased baby, the one they know best, about the sibling who is coming. This can help them appreciate that they are parents to *both* babies. As the new unborn baby's presence gets stronger, most parents are able to shift their writing to the unborn baby about the older sibling who came before: *I began to think of my baby who died as a kind of guardian angel and confidante.* This statement is in line with continued bond/attachment theories, whereby if the deceased can be internalized as a psychologically comforting presence the survivor's emotional (for example, attachment) system is more likely to accept and tolerate the physical unavailability of the deceased (Rochman 2013).

For parents who do not feel comfortable in a group setting writing can be especially helpful. Because most men report that their partner is their main support, writing can be an outlet for fathers to express feelings:

> *As I tossed in my sleep last night, I thought I might enjoy keeping a little diary of how our lives progress during these next few months. Maybe I'll share these with [my wife] sometime, maybe with other expectant fathers.*

BOX 4.1

Parental features during sorting out: 12–24 weeks

- Parents can continue to be surprised that the pregnancy does not help them to feel better. The care provider must be prepared for them to not trust the medical system or technology because it has previously "failed them."
- Parents do not demonstrate the calmness typical of this equilibrium phase in a normal pregnancy, especially if test results raise anxieties.
- Parents may perceive normal procedures as having a threatening impact.
- Parents' loyalty to the deceased baby can interfere with attachment to the new baby.
- Partners may avoid clinic or home visits, or interactions with the mother in denial of their own fears.

BOX 4.2

Helpful interventions for professionals

Professionals can:

- Acknowledge the parents' continued parenting role to the deceased baby.
- Ask parents about their attentiveness to the new baby.
- Affirm that ambivalent feelings are normal.
- Emphasize that this baby is a sibling.
- Assure parents that happiness for the new baby does not negate their love for the deceased baby.
- Recognize that parents may be afraid to trust the medical system even when tests confirm the baby's health.
- Remain aware of impending anniversaries that can open the door for interventions.
- Encourage parents to ask for more unscheduled clinic visits for heart rate checks.
- Teach the difference between contractions and baby's movements.
- Inform parents to report any changes at once to their care provider. Parents are the only constant care provider for the baby.
- Encourage parents to find peer support from in community and/or from groups.

BOX 4.3

The baby leads

The care provider can:

- Gently challenge parents by stating: "The baby, at some level, already knows your fears and anxieties" or "It's okay to give the baby the words for how you are feeling."
- Encourage journaling, first to the deceased baby about the unborn baby/sibling and then, once movements are consistent, to the new baby about the missing sibling.
- Give the baby words about the efforts being made to keep him safe.
- Encourage parents to visualize the baby growing and staying healthy.

The following case study demonstrates how the loss may not affect the first pregnancy that follows a loss but can sometimes impact the second subsequent child.

CASE STUDY

Mrs. Latten was in her third pregnancy, having experienced the loss of a baby girl at 22 weeks gestation in her first pregnancy and the subsequent birth of a healthy son. She had declined any help in her previous pregnancy but was pleased to see the parent–infant specialist now as she shared information about her living child. When asked how she was doing, she began to cry and talk about her fear of getting through the anniversary of the loss of her first baby. She and her husband talked about their deceased daughter every day, wondering what she would be like and what the family would have been like if she had lived. She realized that she didn't fully comprehend the impact of her previous loss until after the birth of a healthy baby. She knew what she had missed and understood why she was now so much more fearful, worrying about every ache and pain, coming in between visits to gain reassurance when she felt "funny." She rearranged her work schedule and began attending the PAL group.

Summary

This chapter has addressed issues parents may face as they come to terms with the reality of the pregnancy and the array of tests that can be offered during the sorting-out phase of prenatal parenting. It is a time when parents may be more open to information on ways to cope with fears and anxieties in relation to trusting the woman's body to keep this baby safe. Parents may voice conflicting feelings of loyalty to the deceased baby, thus ways to incorporate the continued bond and attachment theories into care providers' work with families have been suggested. During this phase parents are learning how to advocate for themselves and the unborn baby, an on-going process until the birth of a healthy baby.

Notes

1 See Hruby and Fedor-Frybergh (2013).
2 See *The Tentative Pregnancy* by Katz Rotham (1993) for information in lay terms.
3 A stitch to hold the cervix tightly closed.

5

INWARDIZING PHASE

24–32 weeks gestation

Smooth	Break-up		Sorting out	**Inwardizing**	Expansion	"Neurotic" fitting together
1	2		3	**4**	5	6
Egg	Fertilization–12 weeks		12–24 weeks	**24–32 weeks**	32 weeks–labor and birth	1–4 weeks

I overanalyze everything. If the baby hasn't moved for a half hour or 15 minutes, I freak out. I wish I could enjoy it more than I do. I feel kind of bad about that. But I just don't see any way around it other than to quit worrying, and that's absolutely impossible.

This chapter discusses the weeks during which the baby's increased movements make his presence more real, drawing the parents to focus inward. Although a time of disequilibrium, especially in relation to the issue of loyalty to the deceased baby, it is also during this period that professionals can more easily incorporate the continued bond relationship with the deceased baby while facilitating the attachment relationship to the unborn baby alongside the medical model of care, specifically during antenatal testing.

Inwardizing: the unborn baby

The average weight of the developing baby at week 26 is two pounds (1000 grams) and the organ system is structurally complete but functionally immature. Breathing movements can be seen on the ultrasound, especially after maternal meals or glucose administration. By week 26 the baby is clearly responding to sounds and, if awake, when a flashlight is directed on the woman's abdomen (Gomes-Pedro et al. 2013). A baby born at week 24 and beyond has a chance of survival but will spend time in a special care nursery for further lung development.

Inwardizing: parents

It can be difficult for parents to focus on the future beyond surviving the pregnancy. It is normal to need more reassurance and to utilize more health care (Hutti et al. 2011).

> *Everything's great for that one day [in clinic] and then you come home and you feel like you're on your own again. You don't want to cry wolf but it's just … every day of this pregnancy we've needed reassurance that everything is going to be okay.*

During these weeks paying attention to the underlying emotions parents may be keeping at bay can provide clues to attachment issues. Many parents are invested in looking good for their health care provider when underneath they may have distanced themselves from the pregnancy and baby. Sowden et al. (2007, p. 91) describe this situation well:

> Women we perceive as "coping well" are likely to be the ones we feel reassured about when they attend clinic. They generate little anxiety for us as clinicians and we feel no need to make special arrangements. We perceive them as initiating contact with health services in a timely way, following reasonable health care advice, seeking information, making rational decisions; they cooperate with us in planning their care.

Underneath this compliant behavior can be a woman and partner avoiding attachment. A woman can be physically caring for herself and the unborn baby but not connecting to "a baby inside." For example, after two unexplained losses at 32 weeks gestation, this mother attended her appointments faithfully, and underwent non-stress tests and biophysical profiles weekly from 28 weeks to the birth of her healthy daughter. Yet underneath her "normal" appearance, she apparently felt *totally detached from that pregnancy. I bought a sports car. I was in denial. I was like "You're [God] going to take this one too, I just know it. I was so angry.* A professional may sense that one or both parents are not engaging to protect themselves from another loss. One technique that has been suggested is to wonder with them. "Wondering is supported by 1) becoming empty 2) using wide eyes, 3) listening and watching with curiosity, 4) noticing and suspending judgment, 4) purposefully eliminating all barriers to the above" (Koloroutis & Trout 2012, p. 51). The care provider can ask how they might be feeling about the pregnancy and unborn baby, guided by the parents leading the responses. Parents who know they are being listened to tend to be more open to trusting guidance. Saying something along the lines of, "Of course you're scared but getting to know your baby's movement patterns can be helpful in providing the reassurance you need."

A minor victory came at 24 weeks gestation for this mother when, with the help of her husband, she accepted some of her fears:

> *One of the revelations I had over Christmas came through Mike on Boxing Day. I was talking to my cousin about how awful Christmas was, how much I missed Emma, and*

> *how fearful I was for this pregnancy. Naturally enough this made me cry so Mike and I went for a walk around a nearby lake. I asked him, "What can I do about my fears?" He asked, "What are you afraid of?" I answered, "I'm afraid of emotionally attaching to this baby lest it die. I'm afraid of the effect of my emotional detachment on the baby's emotional development. I'm afraid that the baby will be a boy and I will have difficulty loving it because it is the 'wrong' sex."*
>
> *Mike said that these were all completely understandable fears. He said I shouldn't feel weak or guilty for having them. I shouldn't continue to punish myself for being unable to let my fear go. With this acceptance of my fears came peace. Yes, it is okay for me to be afraid. Since that day near the lake I have not felt nearly so afraid. It is almost as if by admitting the fear, allowing it to be, not fighting it or feeling guilty about it has caused it to lose its power over me.*

Voicing fear out loud can take away some of its power. "To be in touch with the deepest reservoirs of feeling in oneself can lead to a binding together of the elements of personality, a form of self-healing" (Fraiberg et al. 1980b, p. 54). A victory over fear precipitated a period of peace that lasted several weeks for this mother at 27 weeks gestation, as she described in her journal:

> *Now there is a "lull" period in this pregnancy where I feel like I have dealt with a lot of the issues I faced earlier and now it is a matter of waiting for growth! Although I do not expect this feeling to last for long I am grateful for the reprieve it has afforded me.*

Some parents want time to move quickly in this period, especially when reaching 28 weeks gestation. One father explains:

> *We worked our way up to 24 and every week after that you're just holding on because then you know the baby is growing. Oh, 28 is good, this person has a chance of coming home with you without complications. But 30 is really good so now we're looking from one week to yesterday when we'll be 30.*

Another father knew that past 24 weeks was an important goal:

> *Let's get past 24 weeks because at 24 weeks it's viability. Then if it does have problems they'll just deliver early and get it out of the environment.*

This father let go of some of his fears by beginning to trust the doctors:

> *I think in the second trimester I made a decision with myself, let's not self-diagnose everything. Let's put our faith in the doctors. They treated our first pregnancy, they know what our fears are, they know our history. Let's just put our faith in them and if they say, "We're concerned," there's something to be concerned about. If they say, "Don't*

worry about it," we're not going to worry about it. Can doctors be wrong? Absolutely but every two weeks I listen to what the doctors have to say at the perinatal clinic and go from there.

Regardless of professional role, with each interaction with the family, besides asking about physical needs, the care provider must assess the mother's mood, especially anxiety, as preterm contractions that can lead to labor have been found to be associated with anxiety (Cheek 1996).

Rebuilding trust: learning to know the unborn baby

High quality medical care is achieved through a full connection and partnership with the parents (Koloroutis & Trout 2012). In making decisions about the care and health of their baby, parents will meet and interact with a maze of information, services, places, and faces. Remind parents they are the only consistent figures for the unborn baby; the key source of information and safeguarding when professionals allow them to assume that role (Davis et al. 2013). Tasks during this time include helping parents know what is normal for *their* baby and assessing what the baby is doing (fetal movements) and what is going on within the mother's body (contractions). *It's just the last few weeks where I'm more able to understand when the baby's moving and then I can start feeling where its head is and where the different body parts are.* This mother began to know her unborn twins by paying attention to the difference between their movements and contractions:

> *I think contractions feel like I'm wearing a corset, all the way around, hard to breathe, hard to inhale. Movements almost always feel like bubbling water or being kicked. I'm trying to get a sense of separation from the babies in the sense of where their movements are, where's my body, where's their body, just trying to locate where everybody is. I also think about a sense of connection. I talk about them like we're all on the same team, trying to do something together.*

A mother also needs to pay attention to the difference between Braxton Hicks[1] contractions and early labor. Mothers have been admitted to a high risk unit because they thought they were having "Braxton Hicks" contractions but actually were in true labor and had started to dilate. If contractions become regular (which may be felt more in the back) or don't subside after the mother rests or increases her fluid intake, then she needs to call her care provider.

Most parents struggle with trust issues—in sense of self as mother to protect her unborn baby, in the health care provider to be listened to, and, for the partner, anger and hyper-vigilance to make sure all is being done for the mother and baby. For example, one baby had a blood disorder and the father remembers he and his partner putting all their trust in their local doctors. The baby died at 24 weeks. Referred to a high-risk clinic in their following pregnancy, he wanted all the information he could get:

> *We didn't think anything was going to happen because the doctors reassured us, we're doing everything possible. Then we get up here and we find out there could have been a lot more done.*

On bed rest pregnant with twins, this mother advocated for her babies not to go home just because her contractions had stopped. She was allowed to stay until they were born at 36 weeks:

> *When I was in the hospital they were going to send me home because the babies were "viable." They're viable because they would live and they were going to take me off the magnesium sulphate. I said I'm not leaving because viable is not good enough.*

Attachment and fetal movement: learning ways to let the baby lead

> *Before you just felt that everything should go okay. You have faith, so much blind faith. With this one, I don't feel innocent. I don't feel free. I don't feel I have much faith. Things like when you feel the baby move. You think, "My God. It's still alive! Where before you think, "Isn't that amazing?"*

Parental fear, uncertainty, and the need for reassurance of fetal well-being after a loss are not restricted to Western societies but may be universal because they have also been described by other cultures (Sun et al. 2011). These parents take nothing for granted. Fetal movement can bring a sense of regret that they had taken their previous pregnancies for granted, causing some parents to openly embrace the next pregnancy as a chance to begin a relational engagement with the unborn baby (Côté-Arsenault et al. 2006; O'Leary & Thorwick 2008; Simmons & Goldberg 2011):

> *It was very apparent and clear right away, I felt closer. Being pregnant the first time, I didn't really associate the baby with me or the baby as a person. I just wasn't having my period anymore. This seems like more of a miracle ... not just something biological that was happening to me. I was going to have a baby.*
>
> *Before, with the other two, if I was at work and I felt movement I would just keep on working. "Oh, it's just the baby." But now I actually catch myself stopping just so I can savor every last second of the baby moving inside me. I always think, maybe in the back of my mind, that [this] may be the last time. I think it comes from the fact that I didn't realize Jacob hadn't moved in a day or two. So I stop and take the time to [appreciate it] this time.*

Other parents may cope by trying not to pay attention to fetal movement. *I don't check for fetal movement because I'm afraid the baby won't be alive.* Once the baby is moving, parents should be encouraged to find time each day to try relaxing and paying attention to their baby's behavior. *I just think you're so tuned in to everything; a kick, a hiccup. You know the baby. You could almost lay here and close your eyes and just visualize what they're doing in there.* Ways to facilitate this through guided imagery and relaxation are addressed in Chapter 16. Parental worries can be put to work for them and assist in maternal–infant attachment:

> *I'll go lie down because that's when I feel the baby the most. So for me it's a matter of telling myself to calm down. If I thought every time the baby didn't move it had died I think I'd be a wreck. It's finding a ground between, the baby's sleeping or it's time to go and get checked.*

After the loss of triplets at 22 weeks and now at 24 weeks with twins, this mother began to trust they were going to survive and began to communicate with them:

> *I sing to them. I think about what melodies I want them to know, what type of music we want to influence them to play. I talk to them in a similar way that I talk to the cats. Like somebody doesn't really understand the words you're saying but you say them anyway.*

A helpful strategy to get in touch with the baby is having parents visualize the behavior of a newborn baby, awake and asleep, and relate that to what they feel inside. This allows the unborn baby to lead, giving reassurance throughout each day. *I pay attention more. I know his schedule of when he's going to [be awake and asleep].* When parents become familiar with their baby's normal pattern, they should immediately call their care provider and be seen that day if the pattern changes.

Worth (1997) describes the loss of an infant for fathers as an unfulfilled relationship, especially if they missed out on feeling movement in the previous pregnancy (O'Leary & Thorwick 2006). *I never got to feel the baby the last time because it was just too early.* Fathers are also more motivatated to form a relationship with their unborn baby following a previous loss (Fletcher et al. 2014). Condon and colleagues (2013) suggest that antenatal paternal attachment might reflect a capacity to take the risk of enduring the pain of grief if the object of the attachment is lost. Many fathers take on an active role in the next pregnancy:

> *I want to know what's going on too, how come, why, ask more questions. I'm just not there sitting in the corner for support.*

One father felt that his time to be with the baby was after his wife was asleep, putting his hand over the uterus. The baby's consistent movement each night helped him fall asleep. Other fathers can feel powerless, so reassurance of movement comes only from the mother:

> *It's probably one of the questions I ask her the most, every time I talk to her during the day at work, "Is the baby moving?" Because that was one of my biggest fears. "Yes."*

Several times at night I'll ask her and several times she'll say, "Tom, here, the baby's moving. Feel my tummy." Whenever the baby stops moving she starts to stress and then I start to stress.

When the mother reports that the baby is more active and asks her partner to feel movement, the baby may sense a different hand and stop moving. However, if the father waits and talks to the baby, she usually then responds:

Every day it moves is one good thing. I'm kind of a pain in the butt that way, but I keep asking her every day, "Well, how did it move today?" I'd tell you if something was wrong, she tells me but … I want to know. I'm more aware of it. Before she's said there'd be two, three days where she'd block it out, didn't really pay attention. Now I think we're more aware of it.

Some fathers check the mother's behavior as a way to gauge if all is well. *I look at my wife's face. If she's okay then I know things are okay.*

Fetal testing

Fetal testing provides an ideal opportunity to discuss the baby's competencies and how the reciprocal relationship is developing to enhance the parents' innate know-ledge about the health of the baby. If parents are well supported, this can be a time of reduced anxiety. *I was eager for testing because I knew it would give me some peace of mind and hopefully, prevent future tragedy.*

Fetal testing begins at around 28 weeks (Silver 2007) and is common when there are risk factors such as maternal high blood pressure, gestational diabetes, growth concerns, or previous loss, whether the cause is known or not known. Fetal testing is a way for the baby to demonstrate wellness before birth and can provide reassurance for anxious parents. It includes non-stress tests, electronic fetal monitoring, amniotic fluid assessment, biophysical profiles, and Doppler studies.

The biophysical profile is used as one means to assess fetal wellbeing in most modern obstetric centers across the globe. It provides results based on known healthy parameters for the baby (Stepp-Gilbert 2007). Points for movement, tone, breathing, and fluid indicate wellness and imply fetal wellbeing. Regular (weekly or bi-weekly) biophysical profiles to gain reassurance regarding the baby's health is a normal need for all parents pregnant after loss (Robson 2009) and can reduce the risk of stillbirth in women over the age of 35 (Fox et al. 2013).

They did a lot of things that helped me feel more comfortable. The office visits were of a much longer length than before. We also did a lot of ultrasounds [and] non-stress tests. From 28 weeks on I had an hour and a half ultrasound every week (biophysical profile and non-stress test). That helped me feel more comfortable and was reassuring.

Fetal testing is not always reassuring for some parents, who may present with great fear. Testing can stir up old memories if parents had testing in their previous pregnancy and the baby died:

> *CTGs were bad, as I had one on for three days before I had James and the noise is ingrained in my mind. I still hate the sound of them but in my case it is essential to have them.*

Memories of the previous baby can be an opportunity to carry out a continued bond/attachment focused intervention. Parents can be asked who this new unborn baby is to them, and reminded that this is a sibling who needs their attention now. They may worry about loyalty issues, as one dad shared: *I worry that every time I watch this son playing baseball I will always be thinking about the little boy who didn't make it.* The competencies of this new baby can be reviewed and related to those of the previous baby. That baby knew them as parents, felt their love, and wished to see them at birth too:

> *When I finally got into that thirtieth week I kind of permitted myself to be a little happy and kind of confident that we might take home a live baby this time.*

Testing can increase anxiety for some parents. If the fetal heart rate is above normal it may be because the mother is also tachycardic. If the mother is encouraged to do deep breathing to relax and watch the monitor, she can then see that the baby's heart rate also calms down. This helps her realize she can assist her baby to settle by being calmer herself. A study examining fetal response to induced maternal relaxation found that it assisted the unborn baby to settle, and showed normal increased fetal heart rate variability and fetal heart rate coupling (DiPietro et al. 2008).

Testing can be used in a positive way to enhance parents' innate knowledge of their baby and foster the development of a reciprocal relationship. Before applying the fetal monitor for a non-stress test, the care provider can say to the mother, "Tell me about your baby." Parents can think this is a strange request initially but they are being asked what *they* know about their baby. The mother may answer with what she has been told; for example, *The doctor says the baby is about 4 lbs now.* If the mother provides only factual information, the care provider can follow up by asking whether the baby is a morning or an evening person, a social person who always responds to voices or the father's or siblings' touch, a strong kicker or a gentle flutterer, and if there has been any recent change. By asking what the mother knows about her baby, the professional is also saying, "You know your baby best." After starting a few testing sessions in this manner, the focus changes from using technology to report on what the baby is doing to technology confirming what a mother knows about her baby (O'Leary et al. 2011).

> *I learned a lot about my body in the process of the monitoring. I learned a lot about listening to the heartbeat and the contractions and understanding what to do with the*

contractions, where they stimulated and what happened with that. It built some safety and trust for me in a totally different way.

Through fetal testing mothers learn to appreciate the difference between contractions and the movement patterns of the baby and how they can affect each other. Then, if threatened premature labor occurs, she is more likely to recognize its onset.

There can be many reasons why some mothers are not paying attention to fetal movement so care providers must always enquire. For example, when one mother was asked about fetal movements, she replied that she was too busy with her toddler daughter to notice. She was gently asked if she was afraid to pay attention to the baby in case she could not feel movement. She then cried and replied this was true. Another situation is a mother who had emigrated to the United States with her husband, leaving two older children behind with her mother. She was being tested regularly for high blood pressure. When asked how her baby was doing, she was vague, simply guessing that the baby was moving. The nurse asked about the rest of her family and then heard the story of the children left behind. Her grief for her existing children and focus on being reunited with them was interfering with her ability to pay attention to the current unborn baby. The nurse calmly reminded her, "This baby needs you too." At the next visit she reported with certainty that she knew her baby was fine, which testing confirmed.

Parents are often thinking. *Is the baby still alive and how do you know it won't die when we leave this room?* When the parents leave an appointment having confirmed what they know about their baby, they learn when to come in for more help:

> *Even if it's nothing, I don't feel bad about going in. They say come in and we'll check you out. I don't think they've ever said, "Oh it's nothing, just ignore it." They've never made me feel bad about a false alarm at all. So some of the times I might feel like I'm crying wolf or something but compared to last time I never regret it or feel like I shouldn't do it at all.*

Intuitive knowledge can be a protective behavior that enables mothers to keep babies safe during pregnancy (O'Leary et al. 2011; Warland et al. 2015). A medical practitioner who parents trust will be accommodating of the parents' concerns and fears, and provide a level of support that is both practical and comfortable for them (Soliday & Tremblay 2013).

> *I made sure I got the care I felt most comfortable with. I wanted to see only one doctor who [I felt] was very compassionate. She understood my need for more frequent exams and ultrasounds and was willing to allow extra appointment time to talk with me about my emotional ups and downs during the pregnancy.*

Keeping the baby safe is everyone's goal. Non-medical professionals making prenatal home visits (infant mental health or early head start professionals) should ask if parents are comfortable with them attending their prenatal appointments. This can be an important non-traditional "home visit." These professionals can learn how the mother's body is working to protect the baby and discover with parents the normal movement/activity/behavior for *this* baby at this stage of development just as they help parents understand normal development in the postpartum period. Parents are the constant, as one father states: *She is the only one who really knows what's going on in there. Everybody else, it's just words. They don't feel it.* Collaboration between the health care team and home visitors helps educate each discipline on ways to reinforce the work both are doing for the family.

BOX 5.1

How professionals can help during the inwardizing phase

Professionals can:

- Encourage the mother to rest by explaining that rest increases blood flow to the placenta and she is thus "feeding the baby prenatally."
- Help parents shift their focus on to the new baby, if journaling has not already done so.
- Teach both parents about how the woman's body is working to support the growth of the baby.
- Provide specific reasons and explanations regarding why they know that their baby is safe, for example that the baby is growing as he should be.
- Stress that, although the medical facts in this pregnancy may not support the parents' level of concern, the fact that their previous baby died does. For this reason, the professional should make every *reasonable* attempt to accommodate the parents' need for a higher level of care.
- Encourage parents to make contact if they have any questions or concerns.
- Refer parents to a PAL support group.
- Teach parents how to use guided imagery to relieve stress.
- Avoid talking about birth preparation unless the mother is at risk for preterm labor.
- Appreciate parents' powerful emotions and self-advocacy as protective parenting.
- Help parents realize that they can attach when the time is right while also reinforcing that their parenting role continues with the deceased baby.
- Encourage parents' awareness of the baby's movements as both a welcoming reassurance and a source of empowerment; that is, if they notice a change in their baby's behavior they can seek assistance.
- Encourage parents to maintain routines that give normalcy to their day, and to control what they can control and let go of things that are out of their control.

Parents who visit the clinic once or twice a week should be validated for demonstrating good parenting. Testing can be a time to help a fearful partner learn with the mother how to recognize that their baby is safe. Using words and phrases such as "mom," "dad," and "When this baby decides to be born" helps them emotionally attach to their baby whilst discovering the meaning of fetal testing. Approaching testing as an opportunity for the baby to "tell us" what is going on reassures the parents that the baby is participating (O'Leary & Thorwick 1993). *The baby is center and takes the lead.*

CASE STUDY

This case provides an example of what can lie beneath someone's fears and anxieties. This woman's story supports Selma Fraiberg's (Fraiberg & Fraiberg,1987) belief that giving words to a situation aids healing because one is able to let go of secrets and emotions.

Ms. Peterson was in her seventh pregnancy, with no living children. She was not married to the father of this baby, and had experienced six losses during a previous marriage. She was referred to the support group by her provider but refused. During a clinic visit at 30 weeks, the group facilitator invited her to attend the special birth class for parents pregnant after loss. Ms. Peterson appeared anxious and nervous, but denied any concerns. When invited to bring her partner to show him where she would give birth, she began to sob. She shared that thinking about the birth resulted in nightmares in which six dead babies followed this baby out of the womb. She had had D&Cs[1] following her previous losses so had never seen her babies. Each time she discovered they had died, she would say, "Just leave the baby in" because, in her mind, the baby would then still be with her. The facilitator suggested that attending the birth class might help her partner understand her fears related to the past losses. They began attending the group the following week and entered the birth class. She acknowledged that, after verbalizing her feelings out loud, her nightmares stopped. In follow-up eight years later, Ms. Peterson was still happily raising her daughter with the father but had never married because "being married means dead babies."

Summary

This chapter has addressed issues parents face as they enter the phase of pregnancy during which the baby becomes more active and could survive if born after 24 weeks gestation. This is a time for professionals to help parents learn about their baby's movements and the difference between Braxton Hicks contractions[2] and preterm labor. Information on ways to incorporate prenatal parenting using the continued bond and attachment-based intervention alongside the medical care of fetal testing has been addressed. As parents move from inwardizing into expansion they are getting closer to understanding and accepting that this baby is a sibling to their deceased baby. Unless the baby is at risk for preterm labor, a helpful guideline is to not offer a birth preparation class until at least 32 weeks gestation. Parents are not ready to hear about releasing the baby when they are trying to keep the baby inside to maximize its level of maturity.

Notes

1 Dilation and curettage (D&C) is a procedure to remove tissue from inside the uterus (www.mayoclinic.org).
2 Braxton Hicks contractions are intermittent irregular tightenings of the uterus occurring throughout pregnancy, which are often more noticeable after week 30 (www.abdopain.com/braxton-hicks.html).

6

EXPANSION PHASE

32 weeks–birth

Smooth	Break-up		Sorting out	Inwardizing	**Expansion**	"Neurotic" fitting together
1	2		3	4	**5**	6
Egg	Fertilization–12 weeks		12–24 weeks	24–32 weeks	**32 weeks–labor and birth**	1–4 weeks

This chapter explores parents' last weeks of pregnancy, a time of expansion and rapid growth as the baby prepares for birth. Increased anxiety, common for any pregnant mother and her partner, is exacerbated for parents pregnant after loss. Helping parents trust that the baby is safe until ready to birth is a major task, with the use of technology for reassurance.

The unborn baby

During these weeks the baby usually settles into a birthing position. The baby gains about half a pound (500 grams) a week, which parallels the "expansion" of the mother's uterus. It has been practicing breathing, sucking, and swallowing amniotic fluid from the earliest weeks of pregnancy, demonstrating the motor activities of thrusting and extending her body to prepare for birth (Comparetti 1981). Behavioral states (cycles of sleeping and wakefulness) seen in the newborn period appear at around week 36 (DiPietro et al. 1996), often including the times for feedings at night after birth.

Although it is not completely known when fetal memory emerges, the fetus does respond to auditory experiences during weeks 28–34 (Krueger et al. 2004). Dirix and colleagues (2009) assessed fetal learning and memory, based on habituation to repeated vibroacoustic stimulation, and found that 34-week-old fetuses are able to store information and retrieve it four weeks later. Similar to breathing practice prenatally preparing the baby for breathing postpartum, the near-term fetus shows an orienting response to the maternal spoken voice, suggesting this shapes auditory learning and has implications for attachment and acquisition of language and preference for the maternal voice postpartum (Hepper 2005; 1996; Voegtline et al. 2013). This information—that the deceased baby was aware of his mother's emotional state and responded to the voice of his parents and siblings— also reinforces the parents' attachment, continued bond, and parenting relationship with that deceased baby.

It is crucial to reinforce to parents that it is not normal for fetal movements to decrease in the last weeks of pregnancy (Peat et al. 2012; Stacey et al. 2011) and that they must inform their care provider if they feel that something isn't right (Malm et al. 2010). Bereaved parents will commonly say they noticed that their deceased baby's movements had changed but were not concerned because they believed it was normal for babies to "slow down as they run out of room" (Warland et al. 2015). Studies of parents of stillborn babies have reported that many mothers intuitively feel that something is wrong, well ahead of the stillbirth; sadly, however, some mothers have difficulty communicating their worry to their provider (Malm et al. 2010; Trulsson & Radestad 2004; Warland et al. 2015). The mother below describes regret that she did not advocate more strongly for her deceased baby:

> When I called they wouldn't let me come in because I wasn't in labor. They said there's nothing wrong, she's just not moving a lot. Babies do that. It just frustrates me. So I should have just insisted; just gone in there. Everybody was telling me not to go in. I should have just showed up there because they would have had to do something. But I didn't.

Building trust during expansion: reassurance from the unborn baby

Most parents continue fetal testing at least once a week, many more often, depending on the reason for the previous loss and how the unborn baby is doing. Parents continue to need concrete explanations of the baby's behavior and how the biophysical profile helps assess the baby's readiness for labor and birth. Movement and tone means the baby's muscles are working correctly. Fetal breathing is evidence that the baby is already practicing what is needed at birth. The amniotic fluid volume indicates that the kidneys are functioning, there is swallowing and emptying of the bladder, there is enough blood flow to nurture the baby, and the fluid level is enough to keep the baby protected. A change in score may help clinicians decide to deliver the baby. "The test gives us another way to hear from the baby when is the safest time to be born," is a statement which the parents readily connect to once they understand how testing works.

The mother's trust in herself as able to protect her baby may be fragile, and she may fear missing something, especially if she feels she played a role in the previous loss (Malm et al. 2010; Warland et al. 2015). *While the baby is inside me I don't feel like it is safe.* Telling parents not to be anxious is like telling them not to breathe. Follow, hold, and listen (Koloroutis & Trout 2012) are helpful strategies that enable the parents to share their legitimate fears and anxieties. The care giver must follow the lead of the parents, hold their emotions, and listen to what they are expressing. A statement that sometimes opens the door is, "My expectation is that the baby will be born at the right time and the baby will tell us when that is." The care provider must reconfirm with the parents that they will be the first to notice if the baby's behavior changes and will be empowered to seek care promptly.

As wellbeing of the baby is confirmed through fetal testing, parents begin to differentiate the deceased and current babies more clearly. *I set aside my grief for the moment because I realized this baby needs me now.* Through testing, the mother learns to recognize and trust her perception of the baby's activity, which provides her with daily reassurance. This mother used testing to verify what she knew about her baby when she was at home:

> *I practiced talking to her in utero. I practiced kick counts. I would drink juice and practice what that felt like and interpret that. Then in the office when I would see my midwife, I would watch the monitor during the ultrasounds and watch what the baby was doing. It was an affirmation, a confirmation, that Ah, yes. What she's doing is what I thought she was doing. So I started developing a trust.*

Testing helps share the burden of responsibility that mothers may carry. This mother sought help for her anxiety:

> *I couldn't feel her moving and I thought for sure she had died. I called and said, "I'm scared. I think she's died." And the nurse said, you need to come in and get objective data because you're so subjectively involved. The nurse just fit me right in with all these other women, monitored me right away, and I could see the heartbeat. I was reassured and my husband and I could go home. It's okay, she really is okay.*

Trusting the mother's body and remaining pregnant can become very difficult. Will it all happen again? *I just want it over with because all I do is worry.* Mothers often want to be induced early, saying, *Just get the baby out whilst it is still alive.* Most parents appreciate that, if born at 34 weeks, the baby will battle issues associated with prematurity, yet one mother voices: *I'd much prefer to have a premature baby and know that it's moving than to not have anything kick.*

Expectant fathers can also struggle with waiting:

> *I think this pregnancy will have seemed longer than the other because of the uncertainty of everything. Then from 38 weeks on the fact that the placenta often starts to degenerate, we think that 38 weeks is term. Let's have it now.*

The baby is center and leads

By the expansion phase a mother should have a clear awareness of her baby's sleeping/wakefulness patterns and know intuitively if something is wrong. *I'm very in tune with the rhythm of the baby, very aware of his waking and sleeping patterns, and how he moves and how he kicks me. When I go to bed he is totally active.* It is important to address maternal concerns about a change in the baby's normal behavior rather than to set specific "alarm limits," such as a certain number of kicks in a time period, because this approach has not been evaluated in the pregnant population as a whole (that is, "low-" and "high-risk" mothers) (Heazell & Frøen 2008). According to one perinatalogist:

> Probably the number of kicks in a given period isn't nearly as important as a mother sensing who her baby is, how her baby is, is there a change and if there is a change is that because of the baby or because of her anxiety. It's one more diagnostic clue worth a look at.
>
> *(Dr. Eric Knox, personal communication)*

No matter how the biophysical profile has turned out, if the baby's movement is different from what the parent has come to know, their health care provider may consider delivery. For example, a mother, with two previous losses at 32 weeks, was undertaking daily kick counts and biophysical profiles twice a week. The day after a perfect score in the baby's biophysical profile she returned because her baby was quieter than usual. The baby's status had changed overnight. The volume of amniotic fluid was markedly diminished from the previous day. Her baby was born alive that day. Without her careful attention to the baby and calling for help, based on technology alone this baby might also have died. The mother's knowledge of the baby's normal patterns was key; "the baby leads."

> *I learned a lot about my body in the process of the monitoring, about listening to the heartbeat, feeling the contractions and understanding what to do during them, and recognizing that they stimulate the baby's movements. It built some safety and trust in a totally different way.*

Attachment during expansion

It is normal for pregnant women to become more introspective as their body expands ready for birth; some parents are unable to focus on anything but the baby. However some parents may still be holding back attachment, consciously or subconsciously quashing those feelings because of their history. As one mother stated:

> *I looked in the mirror last week and realized I was 36 weeks pregnant and there was a baby inside me that I was about to have, something I had been denying would really happen.*

Helping the mother focus on the baby's patterns of movement is crucial. Braxton Hicks contractions leading to a "false alarm" for labor can be frustrating and upsetting for all parents but especially so for the bereaved. *I had a difficult time during the final two months. The multiple pregnancies had created an irritable uterus and I had five false alarms.*

Caring for oneself and the baby physically is very different than connecting to an unborn baby and explains why the concept of prenatal attachment is so much more than caregiving/caretaking (Walsh et al. 2013). To illustrate, consider Diane, 36 weeks into her subsequent pregnancy. She had been writing throughout the pregnancy about her on-going grief for her deceased daughter, together with descriptions of the physical aspects of the current pregnancy and her visits to the clinic; however, she had not written specifically to the son she was carrying. When asked why, she replied: *Everybody asks me about this pregnancy and baby but nobody asks me about Anna. I guess I write more to her because I don't want people to forget her.* While acknowledging her continued bond with and attachment to her daughter was important, it was not until she verbalized what her journaling was about that she realized she had not been engaging in a *relationship* with her unborn son. She had not fully grasped that she did not need to let go of her parenting relationship with her deceased daughter in order to love and be a mother to this new sibling too. This example illustrates two important points: first, when others do not acknowledge the deceased baby some parents feel they need to talk more about that child; second, without guidance in journaling, a parent may not necessarily be focused on what is most helpful for her attachment to the new baby (Lichtenthal & Cruess 2010).

Getting ready for the baby

Preparing to bring home a live baby can be difficult for many parents who still believe it may never happen. *I made no preparations until three days before the birth. I couldn't see the point because my baby probably wouldn't live anyway.* Most parents are reluctant to prepare a nursery. This is normal. *I refused to ever pack away another nursery so I didn't prepare or organize a thing.* Parents need to do what feels right for them. Sometimes an understanding family member might be able to help them prepare:

> *My mother shopped for clothes once he was born. He didn't suffer from lack of preparation at all!*

Other parents cautiously get ready:

> *I think I forced myself to do the room because she deserved it and she deserved her own room. I really was very conscious of not wanting her to grow up in the shadow of this but still have her know about him. He was her brother.*

The decision regarding whether or not to use the deceased baby's clothes and equipment can be quite painful, so it is helpful to discuss this with the parents. Some may purposefully purchase something because they had not bought anything for their previous baby:

> *Once I knew we were having a boy I actually bought a few blue outfits, although it was hard to do in case it was for nothing. I did it for two reasons—firstly, my daughter was nine weeks early and I didn't have a chance to prepare for her birth and, secondly, after Thomas' birth and death I felt that I was not able to do anything for him, so I needed to do something for this baby, even before his birth.*

One mother received a package of items her grandmother had made for her still-born son, together with a note saying, "These are gifts from Noah for his baby brother." It is a common practice for siblings to "give" their new baby brother or sister a present. This grandmother's actions thus seem a natural thing to do—honoring both babies.

> *I put a few special things away, along with her photo album. The rest of the baby gear I left for the new baby. I have put a few things away that were special gifts from Kirsty [deceased baby] to Adam [new baby].*

Meeting the baby face to face

Parents who have never experienced a loss appreciate how different children can be. When a baby dies, it is not so simple. Mental representation of the deceased baby is all that remains so separating the babies can be more complicated, especially if the gender is the same (O'Leary & Thorwick 2008). *I think the thing that might be the hardest for me, I realize this is a whole different baby and it's a boy.* While intellectually they know the baby is separate, emotionally they still struggle with wanting the deceased baby too. Other parents may have been expecting a particular gender as a result of the ultrasound only to give birth to a baby of the opposite gender (O'Leary & Thorwick 2008).

Accepting that this pregnancy is different is why I held off attaching for so long. I have a definite place in my life where he sits [the previous baby]. He [new baby] can't live in the shadow of him either.

Approaching birth

Many parents are very assertive, knowing what to ask for and insisting on what does and doesn't matter:

> *I felt I was in the position, I had suffered and wasn't able to bring any children into the world and felt that I'd earned the right to be direct, to be specific and to let them know what I needed.*

> *The birth plan was to induce the baby two weeks before her due date because of my stillborn daughter had gone four days over when she died and I wasn't going to go anywhere near my due date. That was something that I made very clear to everybody.*

However, some decisions are made from based on medical knowledge, such as timing of induction and mode of delivery. The doctor needs to be happy about both the baby's size and maturity and the readiness of the mother's body. Fetal testing drives health care decisions regarding why it is safe for the pregnancy to continue until labor begins on its own. In the US the 39-week "rule" can add a degree of complexity to a parental request for delivery. This rule, established in 2009, restricts induction of labor in the "early term" (weeks 37 and 38 of pregnancy) unless an accepted/approved "indication" is present (ACOG 2009). Even without the 39-week rule, parents should be aware that modern induction techniques are still very much like trying to push-start a car in the middle of a busy freeway. It is fine if all goes well and the car starts, but can cause all sorts of problems if it doesn't and may be one reason for the higher rate of esarean births today (Caughey et al. 2014). Whatever the decision, it is important that it be made together following a thorough discussion about the pros and cons. Parents need to be reminded that their care provider wants everything to turn out well too.

Understanding the emotional needs of the partner

As birth approaches this may be the first time that the partner becomes involved and may only then get in touch with suppressed fears. The partner can be scared and still be okay. Exploring the basis of fear is productive for both parents before labor begins. When this father was asked how he felt about the upcoming labor and birth, he replied, *I haven't let myself go down that road. It's so hard to see the end when we're just trying to get there.* Another father shares his excitement but confirms how long these pregnancies can feel:

> *I'm excited but it's a long ways between now and then when you've been through one before with a bad outcome. Nine months is a long time and you realize how much you are not in control of anything. I'll really be happy once the baby's born.*

Individual preparation is invaluable for helping parents be emotionally present for the new baby (O'Leary et al. 2012; Wright & Black 2013). Parents need to be encouraged to seek someone who can help them prepare (for example, a childbirth educator, early interventionist, public health nurse or perinatal nurse in the hospital). Many parents find simply acknowledging their fear helps them move forward in a more constructive way.

BOX 6.1

How professionals can assist during the expansion phase

The professional can:

- Recognize that parents may reach out for support as labor approaches and that anxiety may rise to a new level of intensity.
- Recognize that parents may want to rush through this phase, wanting the baby out while she is still alive.
- Understand that hoping is to risk re-experiencing the pain of loss.
- Remember that testing such as biophysical profiles and non-stress tests provides an opportunity to show the baby is safe and the pregnancy can continue until labor begins on its own.
- Provide reassurance by stating how she knows that it's safe to continue being pregnant and to let the baby grow more (for example, she can say, "It's hard to stay pregnant, isn't it?"
- Discern *why* parents ask the questions they do.
- Encourage parents to continue dialogue about the deceased baby to reassure them they needn't fear meeting this new baby who is a sibling.
- Recall with parents that, at some level, this baby has heard and knows the story of the past pregnancy/ies.
- Ask about the partner if they have had no involvement thus far.
- Recognize that partners may get in touch with their suppressed fears.
- Acknowledge the parents' fear: they can be scared and still be okay.
- Validate parents' feelings and accept that a sense of distrust is not a reflection on the provider or quality of care. These parents are naturally going to be scared.

To begin preparing for what seemed to me to be an impossible birth I first needed to acknowledge and talk about my fear with anyone safe who would listen; my support group, my birthing class instructor, my husband.

It is easy to say "trust your body and your unborn baby to provide reassurance," but helping parents do so isn't easy. One mother had attended the PAL support group weekly since week 16t. She acknowledged being woken at night with thoughts about how to trust the baby and allow the baby to be an individual. *[The care provider] would always say, "Listen to the baby, listen to the baby." It took a long time to be able to do that, to even know what that meant, but I finally did get there.* She put these feelings into verse in the last month of her pregnancy, speaking for herself and her unborn baby.

BOX 6.2

At last this baby and this mother

Hello baby, I'm glad you're here. Listen to my words, follow my lead, I have wonderful things to teach you.

Be strong baby. Bear the burden of my doubts and fears. They will lessen as we grow.

I'm ready to hold you close, to swallow the scent of your tiny head, to sing you songs about the moon and stars.

At last baby, enter this cold and crazy world.

We'll share our strength and courage and watch each other grow.

I love you.

Hello Mom. I'm glad you are listening to me.

I don't mind that you are afraid. I can help you with that.

I'm soon to be evicted from your warm and precious womb. I need help.

Your world is a cold and crazy place.

I'm ready to feel your fingers against my skin.

Hold me close, sing me songs.

At last Mom, listen to my heart, follow my lead.

For I have wonderful things to teach you. I love you.

Summary

The expansion phase is a time to reach out to parents who may have refused previous support. Anxiety may rise to a new intensity as parents approach labor and birth and meet a baby they may never have believed would be born alive. Parents will want to rush through this phase. Hoping a live baby will be born means to risk re-experiencing the pain of loss. They are naturally going to be scared and will not be relieved of that fear until a healthy baby is in their arms. They may feel sad and worry about meeting the baby for the first time because of conflicting emotions throughout the pregnancy. Parents need to be encouraged to focus on understanding that this new baby is a sibling to their deceased brother or sister. Some parents may not be able to be reassured and this is no reflection on the professional or quality of care.

7

PREPARATION FOR LABOR AND BIRTH

Life is new and yet it's a dangerous situation. For me, labor will always be a scary dangerous place psychologically.

Parents bring many fears into their subsequent labor and birth experience. Yet during workshops for those working in the childbearing area, many professionals have voiced a lack of awareness of the many difficulties these parents face. This chapter covers the issues parents face as they prepare for labor and the birth of their new baby. Preparing for the labor and birth can be an opportunity for support and healing. Therefore, this chapter outlines how to establish a birth class specifically for these parents, including suitable content and activities. Preparation for touring the birthing unit is covered and strategies for helping parents to cope with it are provided. The benefits of writing a birth plan are discussed and what kind of support may be useful for these parents during labor and birth.

The last weeks of expansion to birth

Three major questions guide the last weeks of pregnancy as women prepare for birth:

*   How can I learn to trust my body and my baby to give birth?
*   How can we create a safe place in which we can let go and give birth?
*   How will I love this baby when I want my other baby?

Increased fear and anxiety as birth approaches have been found to put these parents at risk for the symptoms of PTSD (Black et al. 2008; Räisänen et al. 2013), as well as a slower labor, increased rates of induced labor, instrumental delivery complications, and requests for cesarean section (Black et al. 2008; Crowther 1995; Robson et al. 2009; Walsh 2002). Fear of childbirth has also been found to be a predisposing factor for postpartum depression (Räisänen et al. 2013). While one study of women who had experienced a previous stillbirth found that they did not necessarily want a cesarean section (Robson et al. 2009), other studies suggest that Cesarean section was sometimes offered as a result of the shared desire of both the health care provider and parents to get the baby out before he died (Crowther1995).

Trust as parents prepare for birth

A less positive birth experience has been found to be associated with emergency Cesarean, instrumental vaginal birth, and dissatisfaction with medical care (Johansson 2012). Misconceptions and negative appraisals about reaction to a trauma have been found to be risk factors for the development and continuation of the symptoms of PTSD symptoms (Ehring et al. 2008).[1] Listening to parents describe their story of loss as they prepare for a new labor and birth cannot erase the pain but does provide a channel through which memories can be safely accessed and integrated into existing schemas (Brewin et al. 1996; Thomson & Downe 2010). Treating anxiety and fear of childbirth entails building a trusting relationship with the parents as they process their pain (Soliday & Tremblay 2013; Thomson & Downe 2010). Intervention around trauma does not need to be seen as formal therapy but can serve as a therapeutic function in the form of focused guidance and support specific to the family's situation (Dyregrov & Regel 2012).

Fathers may not appreciate how traumatic it will be to return to the scene of their loss but can have powerful memories of watching their partner go through a traumatic birth in addition to the death of their baby:

> *The horrible, the most traumatic memory I have of the last pregnancy was when they told us they were going to have to induce; the babies will be born today and they will die; how hard, how uncharted that was going to be. The final straw when I thought I was going to crack was when she was hemorrhaging; they couldn't get all the placenta out.*

> *My only experience with vaginal births was babies who died. I don't know what post-traumatic stress syndrome is but I think I've got it in regards to the birth of our twins. It isn't something that's with me all the time but when something reminds me of it, it kind of paralyzes me.*

Content of birth class

Whether through a formal class structure or individually, debriefing of the past birth is crucial to help both parents be more present for the new birth (Thomson & Down 2010). This can be especially helpful for a couple whose perceptions of what happened around their loss are not the same or the mother is in a new relationship. A special birth class with other bereaved parents spread over a three- to four-week period is ideal. This allows parents space and time to talk about what happened last time, helps tailor the class to the needs of each individual family, and is especially important for parents who have not experienced a specific intervention to help them deal with their grief and attachment issues.

Content is similar to any birth class but adapted to the needs of parents pregnant after loss. Parents must be given time to share their previous birth story, perhaps as they introduce themselves, and allowed to gradually unfold their story. This gives them an opportunity to process some of their pain before they feel at their most vulnerable when in active labor. Such a class may be the only place where they can do this work. As parents share the story of their previous loss, attention must be paid to words that may impact on the new experience. For instance, the mucous plug may contain some blood that might bring back memories of bleeding in the last labor. Nausea and vomiting are normal signs of transition, but may trigger memories of side effects from medication used to stimulate labor for a stillborn baby or pregnancy termination. It may be helpful for parents to know that an induction of labor for a stillborn baby can be much longer as the baby is unable to help descend during labor to move into the birth canal. Contractions can also feel very different when the baby is alive and able to help in the labor process. Responses during the needs assessment carried out in the first meeting will provide clues about parents' readiness and how much information they can absorb.

Professionals must constantly be cognizant of how these parents hear and interpret words and explanations of procedures (Parker & O'Leary 1989). Parents often raise questions about the circumstances of their previous loss, perhaps to try to comprehend what a placental abruption or "incompetent cervix" mean. The care provider must discern *why* parents ask the questions they do; they must listen with sensitivity and validate the parents' feelings. This may be the first opportunity for parents, especially the partner, to process and clearly understand the causes of the previous loss.

The parents' level of knowledge about the labor and birth process must be assessed. Some will have taken classes during their previous pregnancy, while others come with no background knowledge of labor and birth. The parents must be helped to identify the normal physiological changes of pregnancy not just the warning signs of an impending problem. Many couples report that discussing the assorted aches and pains of pregnancy helped them feel normal and reduced some of their anxiety. Displaying anatomy and physiology charts in an office or classroom setting to pique the interest of parents is common in a regular birthing class but this can sometimes overwhelm parents and cause flashbacks. For example, one father had to leave the room after seeing a poster of a baby's development in the second trimester due to flashbacks of his deceased twins, who died at 22 weeks.

As difficult as the pregnancy may have been, some mothers have voiced wanting to stay pregnant. They know the baby is safe now and fear what might happen in the postpartum period. Parents need guidance to help them separate the birth experience and deceased baby from the new baby. They need to be reassured that "the baby leads." While reviewing anatomy and physiology, the care provider can provide parents with information about the baby's development at each stage of pregnancy. For some parents, this might be the first time they allow themselves to acknowledge this baby as real and about to be born.

Watching a birth film

The educator must prepare parents to watch a birth film. This can trigger painful emotions and memories of loss. Some parents prefer to view a film in class, while others want to watch it more privately, alone with the educator. The visual load can be decreased by showing the parents several short clips and stopping to discuss content, share feelings or ask questions. Another strategy is to plan a specific focus for each clip. For example, the educator might preface a clip by saying, "In this section, I want you to notice the different comfort measures the partner and nurse are using to support the mother." Offering the option for parents to view a video alone at home is unwise as it can make old feelings and traumas resurface that one or both parents may need help dealing; also, one parent may prefer not to watch the video, causing conflict between them.

Breathing and relaxation

Teaching relaxation is crucial but can be very challenging. After working so hard to stay pregnant, parents now must shift their thinking toward relaxing and releasing the baby from the mother's body. Many parents have not relaxed during the entire pregnancy. A partner may have felt afraid to touch the woman's body since she became pregnant. One woman described her body as "frozen"; she felt unable to take deep breaths in case it harmed the baby. Another woman positioned herself on her left side when lying down throughout her pregnancy upon hearing that that position was better for the baby. During labor she refused to change position, stating, *It's the only way this baby knows how to stay alive.*

Most birth visualizations speak to the power of the woman's body to hold a baby and, when the time is right, to give birth. However, such visualization often does not work for parents pregnant after loss. Both the mother and her partner can have difficulty visualizing pregnancy as a safe place for the baby. One mother shared her feelings about a guided imagery written for parents who had not experienced a loss: *I was trying and trying to find that safe place within myself and it really upset me to figure out that I really didn't have a safe space. I couldn't find a safe place until she was born and I knew she was okay.*

Teaching relaxation, breathing, and effleurage[2] at the same time can be too much for these parents. It must be remembered that the anxiety and trauma of the previous loss is still felt within their bodies. Even while parents may be trying to pretend they are "just pregnant," they must be gently reminded that an unborn baby is already present. It is thus recommended that relaxation sessions begin by assessing parents' ability to relax by encouraging them to take several deep breaths. From there, the parents are helped to move on to feeling individual parts of their bodies—their faces, shoulders, arms, and legs. Gradually, as they relax, the parents should be guided to where the baby is situated and taken on an imaginary tour of the uterus. This stage has two goals in mind: (1) to help the parents discover all the ways in which the woman's body is nurturing and protecting the baby to help her develop trust in herself that she has been caring for the baby, and (2) to get to know the baby, maybe for the first time for some parents who have lived in their head, afraid to even think about what's going on in their or their partner's abdomen. The placenta can be described as a nice soft pillow for the baby, which also provides nourishment and helps her to grow. The amniotic fluid can also be visualized as a cushion protecting the baby from the outside world. The baby can be visualized as exploring the space, touching the mother's body, sensing her love and need to protect, hearing her voice and those of others around her (personnel communication, Lynnda Parker). This guided imagery can help parents visualize how the mother has already been a competent, caring parent during pregnancy to help the baby grow. Some mothers have reported falling asleep before they get to the uterus, a clue that they are not ready to go there. Both the mother and partner should be encouraged to practice this type of relaxation early in pregnancy because one study found that spiritually-based mantram (silently repeating a self-selected sacred word to redirect attention) taught in the last weeks of pregnancy did not help in preventing Cesarean births in their intervention group (Hunter et al. 2011). This suggests it is important to begin relaxation in the early stages of the pregnancy and not wait until the end.

BOX 7.1

Sample guided imagery

Settle back into your pillow/chair. Rest your head and body and let yourself begin to relax. Take one deep breath and then slowly breathe in … and out. Breathe slowly … and purposefully, as naturally as you can. Release your emotions slowly, bit by bit.

Think about the baby you are carrying now in your uterus. With each breath you take your baby is gently rocking up and down. She feels comfortable … warm … secure … rocking with each breath, hearing your heartbeat, feeling your worries and concerns, but knowing the worry relates to the baby who was here before; the baby you loved and wanted, but whose life with you was far too short.

This little person with you today has listened to your stories, has felt your pain, and knows your love is given cautiously, not because you don't love her, but because you love her so much. She feels deeply the protection you have given her during this pregnancy; your desire to make her feel safe.

Breathe in and out … visualizing this baby inside, loving you and all the other voices in the family that she hears. She is waiting to come out to show you her own unique personality and will help you believe again that life can be good and beautiful. Continue to breathe in and out at your own comfortable rate, letting go of your fear for this baby as far as possible.

You have nurtured and cared for yourself and this baby through all these long months. Now begin to allow your body to prepare for labor and birth. Let go of the tension ... let go of the fear. Let the contractions come when the baby is ready. Start slowly and build up your strength, opening your cervix and allowing this baby to come into your life. Let the children who came before celebrate with you this new life that will begin to heal your wounds and nurture your continued journey into parenting.

Touring the birthing area

The minimum preparation needed is touring the labor and birthing area where the mother will be giving birth. Parents often say they don't want to go there before they have to. Avoiding the space is not helpful and can hinder the learning process, leaving the parents vulnerable to the sudden unexpected occurrence of painful memories (Côté-Arsenault & O'Leary 2015; Shear 2012b). Returning to the space helps them prepare for the actual birth of their new baby.

> We haven't been in a delivery room for 11 months and to go back there, to give birth, all the feelings are just going to come back. It's going to be a very emotional time, very difficult.

A tour before active labor needs to be well supported, ideally in private with just one couple. This allows parents to raise questions, address issues in more depth, or raise new issues (Creedy et al. 2000). The sights, sounds, and smells of the hospital or clinic often trigger haunting painful memories, even symptoms of panic and post-traumatic stress. Touring helps familiarize parents with the equipment, sounds, and smells of the space, which may help prevent flashbacks during labor and birth. Flashbacks may cease when critical experiences are fully processed and integrated into personal narrative (Roos 2012). Remembering and touring helps parents think about ways in which they can have some control during labor, feel less fearful of re-experiencing their loss, identify triggers, and be more emotionally present for the birth of this baby. When parents learn what might cause flashbacks they are then more able to determine what they want and need, making the birthing space physically and emotionally specific to this birth.

For most parents, going back to the birthing area often marks the first time they have returned to the scene of their loss. Parents must thus be prepared for the flood of emotions and bodily sensations (Malkinson 2012; O'Leary et al. 2012) that will surface. Rational emotive body imagery (REBI) is a technique that is helpful for bereaved people who are using avoidance to try to circumvent the pain of an emotional experience (Malkinson 2012). The basis of this technique describes why touring and spending time in the birthing area is an important step toward feeling safe again. Going to a birthing room gives parents the opportunity to be guided in a safe setting to help process the distress of the previous painful birth in order to separate and re-script the space to welcome the new baby. This can help to actively call to memory the details of the physical space of their previous birth—the smells, the position of the bed, the materials and equipment. One couple remembered seeing their deceased daughter lying on a bedside table so requested not to have that in the room. Another couple recognized the same blanket their baby had been wrapped in when he died and brought another blanket for the new baby. Mothers should be encouraged to try different positions in the bed in the birthing room. Some will remember their position in the previous pregnancy and choose a different position for this birth. Care providers need to discuss who they want with them, and what they need.

> I brought a picture of our daughter who died to the hospital. It was important to me to include our daughter who isn't with us in our new family.

It must be remembered that the partner is often just as frightened as the mother, and yet still must support her. The partner should thus also accompany the mother on tour.

> For my husband, who was there during the first delivery, it was really frightening for him to go to the labor room. Going to the labor room really helped him with his fears. He was really nervous while we were there but at least he had a perspective; it's a different labor room, it looks different even though the equipment is similar and the bed is similar. He's beginning to feel more comfortable with it. And at least he knows. He's been there once before. It's not going to be a new place for him.

Parents who are birthing in the same hospital must be able to identify which room they were in before so as to be able to choose a different one for this baby:

> I didn't realize what an impact walking into that ward would have on me. I got goose bumps walking past the room where I delivered my stillborn son. In my birth plan, I requested a different room. The nursing staff was incredibly kind and very accommodating.

Even if planning a Cesarean birth, parents still benefit from touring the hospital ahead of time:

> It was good to go back to the hospital and put away those old ghosts. I used to just hate to even go by it. I would get such an awful feeling in the pit of my stomach. I had vowed I would never go back there. But now I needed to be there for this baby. When I went in there I saw the room I was in when we lost our daughter, in fact, it was right next door to the room they put me in this time. It was like a brick wall hitting me in the face and I broke out in a cold sweat. But now I'm glad I was able to do that. I will never forget what happened there, nor would I want to, but my feelings about the place are just put

in a quieter place. It was important for me to do that, to get it behind me. When it is time for the new baby to come I think I'll be more ready to go on.

Most parents want to use electronic fetal monitoring showing the baby's response to contractions. They must be shown how to navigate the cables and wires while retaining the benefits of movement. Other options that allow for monitoring and still laboring in a good position are a rocking chair or fit ball[3] close to the monitor. Some parents focus on the technology and emergency equipment for a sense of safety but this can remove the focus on the baby:

> *The thing I remember most about his delivery was watching his monitor to see if it would go above the safe line or below, his heartbeat. I was not completely unconcerned about my wife's health but obsessively watching that monitor. I wish that monitor hadn't been there because all you do is watch it and think about it. It was a long pregnancy, the labor was long, and I was really tired.*

Addressing fear and pain and considering medication

Parents pregnant after loss come to the labor and birth as highly fearful and anxious adults. Birth has been linked with death. Many women experienced births in which they believed they could have died or did almost die, so the partner fears this outcome as well. Teaching parents about medication involves more than just presenting information about drugs, dosages, and routes of administration. Parents benefit from someone helping them differentiate between feeling scared and experiencing physical pain and how one exacerbates the other (Van der Gucht & Lewis 2014). Likewise, partners who may feel too vulnerable to share how fearful they really are might encourage the mother to ask for pain medication, unable to cope with watching her in pain. The care provider needs to suggest to the parents ways in which to talk about their fears, not just the fear of physical pain, of ways of coping with emotion and fear that are separate to those for dealing with the physical pain of labor and birth. Women may say they need medication to manage their fear; for example, one mother related: *I didn't really need the epidural for pain. I got scared and took it out of fear, remembering pushing out my dead son.* Another woman chose to feel the pain to remind herself she really was having a baby. Sometimes, being able to give voice to their fear helps parents appreciate that, for them, fear is an accepted part of this birth experience.

Drawing up a birth plan

The depth of vulnerability these parents experience can be profound. It is difficult, and often impossible, for these parents to see themselves holding a live baby. Birth plans can be viewed as an unrealistic set of demands but are crucial for these parents. Significantly different from the mother's medical history on the chart, it is the parents' personal story, does not have to be elaborate, and is a tool for care providers to know who they are and what they feel they need for this birth. With a birth plan in place, parents also won't have to worry about saying the same thing over and over to respective shifts of nurses and it will help them approach birth with a greater sense of control and optimism. A flexible plan and caring care providers can go a long way toward increasing the parents' ability to cope while decreasing their level of stress.

BOX 7.2

Birth planning

Background information

What do they want the staff to know about *their* family that will help them during this birth experience (for example, history of previous loss and last birth experience, older siblings, how they cope with stress)?

History of this pregnancy

How the pregnancy has been for both parents (test results, incidents, fears, and concerns).

Labor and birth support

What will the mother and her partner need? Who do they want or not want with them?

Postpartum

Concerns about breastfeeding, siblings, anxiety, and so on.

It was very helpful to create a birth plan. It allowed us to work through the details of this birth with our doctor and other specialists. In the birth plan we had a section about the loss of our daughter. We also briefly described our fears and emotions surrounding this birth. This provided each care provider that we saw in the hospital with an understanding of our difficult circumstances. We didn't need to repeat our story to each new person. When they walked into our room they already had a sense of our situation.

Discussing support during the birth

The presence of an additional person to provide support for both parents can be extremely helpful, bearing in mind that the partner will be just as frightened as the mother. As one father explained: *There was no way for us to know ahead of time how we were going to handle the situation. We both ended up needing some support in different areas.* This mother felt that it was important to have another person present:

> *The subsequent pregnancy and labor and delivery is hell for the man too. Everybody focuses on the woman because they have to get her through it because of the safety of the child. So there's a lot more attention focused on you and not so much the man and I think that's very hard.*

Continuous emotional support during labor can be of particular benefit. If not a family member or friend can assume that role, the care provider can suggest using a doula. Doulas are women trained to provide continuous, one-on-one emotional support during the perinatal period and work alongside the medical team (Kozhimannil et al. 2014). Non-medical interventions during labor such as the provision of a doula may reduce the cesarean birth rate (Caughey et al. 2014). One study found that the odds of cesarean delivery for Medicaid beneficiaries were 40.9 percent lower for doula-supported births (Kozhimannil et al. 2013, 2014). Doulas can compliment medical care. For example, one Midwestern hospital[4] provides volunteer doulas who are called into the ER for parents who are experiencing a miscarriage. Some doulas also specialize in supporting families pregnant after a loss.

Parents also need to be prepared for pushing; this meant death is their last experience. Even though they can hardly wait to give birth, mothers often are afraid to let themselves push and release the baby. *When I was pushing I didn't want to push. I was afraid his lips were going to be blue. I was afraid there was going to be a dead baby again.*

Parents need to be reminded that a healthy baby plays an active role in labor. Most babies position themselves head down into the pelvis in the last weeks of pregnancy to prepare for birth. In labor the baby pushes and extends his body, working with each contraction to move into the birth canal. This visual image helps many mothers realize the baby is working with them. Comparetti (1981), a pediatric neurologist, found that babies who are compromised in utero cannot actively help in labor, which may explain why some mothers experience long, difficult labors that result in a cesearean birth.

Partners often report flashbacks during the pushing stage. The care provider needs to gently discuss how both parents are feeling and why the presence of another person to provide support for both parents can be helpful.

> *I was scared all the time. Once you've lost a child you can never rid yourself of that fear. When he was born I didn't look at him coming out. I didn't see him until the midwife lifted him up on my wife's chest. I was afraid to look and see that he would be dead.*
>
> *During the birth we had a scare where we lost the heartbeat on the external monitor and that's when I first started feeling some flashbacks to my son. Before that I was really calm and at ease, really good. Then I started feeling kind of trouble. When she was born I was crying tears of joy and after maybe 10 minutes after the birth I felt myself*

becoming angry with the people in the room because they were calling the baby a "she" and I felt myself attaching her to my son. I thought that it was a boy.

Another father had not participated during a home visit for birth preparation after the previous stillborn birth of a son, instead busying himself in a room close by. During the labor he was very quiet. When the baby was born, he engulfed him in his arms, sobbing. His fear throughout the pregnancy matched his wife's and provided an explanation for his behavior during the home visit. While too fearful to participate, he had nonetheless remained in hearing distance to gain the information he needed to.

After two previous losses, this mother could not believe she finally had a healthy baby born by cesarean:

> *When they push on your stomach and she pops out it seems like forever before you hear the cry. I remember thinking, oh God, what's taking so long? Don't tell me she's dead too. And then all of a sudden she cried and it was like oh … I couldn't believe it. And that was like a miracle. She was healthy and amazing.*

CASE STUDY

Sarah's birth

I went to the doctor at the 37-week mark. I felt that the baby was alive and we had made it so far, so why couldn't we bale out now? He was very understanding, recommending we have a CTG every couple of days until delivery. I went straight to the hospital and had a CTG, which was normal. I felt reassured by this and went home feeling much better.

When I went back at 38 weeks it took the baby 30 minutes to wake. Although the trace then looked okay, the midwives called the doctor in. He took one look and asked if I'd like to be induced that night. "YES" was the obvious and quick reply.

When we arrived at the hospital I was greeted by a midwife who had also had a stillbirth several years earlier. I knew that she would have a pretty good idea how I was feeling, I felt safe to cry with her. She did a CTG, then she examined me and said that she believed that I would probably give birth overnight.

Half an hour later, sure enough I started contracting. The contractions became stronger and stronger for a while but as the hours went by they began to fade and had weakened enough by 4 o'clock to allow me to sleep until morning. When the doctor came at 10 o'clock I was pretty keen to start the drip. I was 4 cm dilated so I felt I wouldn't need much syntocinon to go the rest of the way. Over the next few hours the contractions gradually became stronger again.

As I was breathing on the gas, hearing the same voices I heard a year ago, and in the same place, I had a sense of being in two places at once—one here and now and the other just as real, last year. I asked for the monitor to be turned up so I could hear the baby's heartbeat. Although that helped me differentiate between the different times between contractions, I could not hear it whilst having a contraction and so a deep sense of confusion continued. I kept on saying that it felt like last time, but neither the midwife nor Mike really had an understanding of just how lost I felt.

Time went on and I had another internal which still put me at 4 cm. It was hard to believe that I had made no progress when the birth felt so close. We decided to press on for another couple of hours.

But at 5.30 pm I was getting more and more distressed. The doctor came and examined me and said that I still hadn't dilated. I asked for a cesarean and he said I had taken the words right out of his mouth! Even though I had asked for a cesarean and knew it was the only option I had left, I panicked. As I was being prepared for surgery I slipped into a sense of unreality.

The anesthetist put in a spinal anesthetic which worked incredibly quickly, next thing I felt incredible pressure on the top of my uterus and Mike saying "It's a girl."

I felt only relief, no joy, no happiness, just the deepest sense of relief, like a massive weight had gone from my shoulders. As I listened to our newborn daughter crying loud angry cries, I wept tears of relief.

I had waited so long to hear those cries. I felt so privileged to hear them again but when she was wrapped up and passed to me all I could see was a frowning little face all covered with vernix (white creamy stuff). I immediately wondered if she was normal and quickly came to the conclusion that she was not. Relief became tinged with sadness. She was not normal. I looked at my gravely staring newborn and felt so sad.

I lay in recovery feeling shocked. I began to physically shake all over.

I asked the midwife if she felt Sarah was normal. She said "Yes" but somehow this didn't reassure me.

The children came, all so excited. The midwife asked Greg (10 year old) how he felt and he said his last baby sister had died. The midwife said she knew and it made this baby more special. Mom and Dad visited, there were tears from Mom and I joined in, of course. They said that as they passed the nurses' station they were struck at the contrast to last year. Nurses were all grinning from ear to ear. It seemed that everyone was happy that night except me.

Sarah came to me for a feed and the first thing I did was to check her from head to toe. There didn't seem to be any signs that she was abnormal. Gradually, over the next couple of days, I realized she was in fact normal and just because I couldn't believe our good luck at once again having a live healthy baby didn't mean it hadn't in fact happened. Still the joy and happiness did not come, just immense relief. A real sense of "Phew, we made it!"

Summary

This chapter has addressed helpful issues for parents preparing for labor and birth after a perinatal loss. Specific information on what both the mother and father may need, the use of a support person, such as a doula, facilitating a tour, helping them prepare a birth plan and parental feelings at the time of birth have been addressed. The next chapter moves into the immediate postpartum period.

Notes

1 Although this research was specific to vehicular accidents, we consider it is also transferable to parents who have experienced a perinatal loss.
2 A French word meaning "to skim" or "to touch lightly on," used during labor for effective pain relief and comfort.
3 www.birthsource.com/scripts/prodView.asp?idProduct=20.

8

"NEUROTIC" FITTING-TOGETHER PHASE

Birth–first six weeks of life

It's not that I didn't want this baby. I wanted both babies.

Smooth	Break-up	Sorting out	Inwardizing	Expansion	"Neurotic" fitting together
1	2	3	4	5	**6**
Egg	Fertilization–12 weeks	12–24 weeks	24–32 weeks	32 weeks–labor and birth	**1–4 weeks**

Although the term "neurotic" fitting together sounds daunting, most parents can easily identify with the overwhelming feelings it describes as they adjust from pregnancy to life postpartum. For parents who experienced a previous loss the normal sense of disequilibrium associated with the "neurotic" fitting together phase brings the joy of a healthy baby mixed with sadness about moving forward without the deceased baby (O'Leary 2005). *I think it made us even sadder for the loss of our daughter because we didn't really know what we didn't have until we had something else. Then it just felt empty.* Parents can be surprised to find grief remains. *I didn't think he would take away my grief but I didn't know he would magnify it.* Siblings may also experience renewed grief, realizing they are missing the deceased sibling too.

Initial feelings

Parents can be reassured that it is *normal* to still experience fears and anxieties that cannot be fully prepared for until they reach that point. This new baby fills a void left by the last baby but makes its own space. Parents are deeply aware someone is missing. The role of the professional is to continue helping parents understand that the new baby is a sibling to the deceased baby and they are parents to both babies (O'Leary 2007).

I have often said that Edward left a round hole in my heart. Although Samantha's birth helped to fill that hole she is a different person and is therefore a different shape and so she only partially fills it. She is a square peg in a round hole.

Parents need time to regain trust in the world again. If for any reason they need to leave their baby behind (for example, she is premature), this can trigger memories of leaving the hospital before with empty arms and they will need to process them.

Rebuilding trust: understanding the uniqueness of their newborn

The early postpartum period is pivotal for parents, especially for the mother's representation of sense of self; moving from trusting her body through the pregnancy to trusting she has a healthy baby. One mother said of her newborn son, *I see him but I don't feel him.* She needed guidance to risk attaching and seeing that he was really there.

One intervention to help parents trust that the baby is healthy and uniquely her own person is to demonstrate her newborn capabilities. Babies demonstrate six states of consciousness, from deep sleep to active alert, in order to regulate themselves (Nugent 2015; Pearson 2009, 2016) during the "neurotic" fitting together phase as they adjust from the inter-uterine environment to the outside world. Babies are adjusting to gravity, light, the feelings of their stomach being empty and full, how to eat, and sometimes learning a different suck from what they used in the uterus. Their range of vision, when held, is approximately the distance from the crook of their parent's elbow to the parent's face. During routine postpartum care or home visits, the care provider can point out how the baby is drawn to the parents' faces, now able to "see" the faces associated with the voices he heard in the uterus. Babies recognize their parents and siblings voices in comparison to those of strangers, and often do not startle upon hearing their siblings' loud voices, being already accustomed to them during pregnancy. Seeing and listening can be too much stimulation to take in so babies may avert their eyes briefly when alert if a parent is talking. This information provides a sensitive structured intervention to engage the baby in a relationship with the parents (Nicolson 2015; Pearson 2009, 2016) and individualizes the baby as his own person, uniquely different from the deceased sibling. It can be especially helpful for fathers who may have distanced themselves from the pregnancy, fearing another negative outcome. Parents learn that, just as during pregnancy, the baby continues to "lead" as they assume their parenting role.

Parents in "neurotic" fitting together

Parents move into the "neurotic" fitting together phase with the full realization they have survived the pregnancy. They may be surprised at how fearful they are about being able to take care of a healthy live baby. They may still be numb, having held their emotions tightly together throughout the pregnancy. Parents need to be reminded that many of their concerns are the same as those faced by all new parents: When is the baby hungry or just fussy? How do I help her learn to sleep? Is it okay to hold the baby all the time? "Normal" neonatal adjustment such as an elevated bilirubin or problems with breast feeding can cause a renewed and intensified fear and more anxiety than is the case for parents who have not experienced a loss.

Whilst they may want to hold themselves emotionally and perhaps even physically distant from their new baby (Warland et al. 2011b), parents benefit from understanding that their baby needs a protected nurturing environment, the social and emotional equivalent of the physical protection a fetus receives in the womb, during this period of brain growth (Lally 2014). Parents need to be reminded that this is the same baby they kept close during the pregnancy. During these weeks babies often prefer the "flexed position," which takes them back to the feeling of being in the uterus (Pearson 2016). This helps parents realize that they did know their baby before he was born. These parents, who had experienced many ultrasounds in their subsequent pregnancy, noted how their twin babies settle into the position they maintained inside the uterus:

> They were always head to head in the uterus because when I was in the hospital they would do ultrasounds every day so we could see them. Even when they'd move and change positions they were always head to head. They don't do it now [in their preschool years] but for a long time when they'd get really agitated they would lay down head to head and they would calm down.

Attachment during "neurotic" fitting together

> I couldn't believe she was really mine. I kept thinking someone would come and get her, as if I was babysitting or something.

This sense of unreality may lead to difficulty attaching. It may be hard for parents to feel attached to a baby who doesn't seem real and to believe all that went so horribly wrong last time has gone magically right this time. Thankfully most parents do quickly attach to their new baby and realize they love him with all of their hearts:

> Since James' birth I have felt an overwhelming sense of love for him. I did wonder before he was born if I would have trouble "bonding" with him, but this has not been a problem.

Changed people: trust in "neurotic" fitting together

It may also be hard for parents to trust and believe *they* are the ones who know their baby best and will be the only constant presence throughout his life. No matter how long it takes for the parent to feel a new sense of "normal," they will never stop being a parent to both their living children and those who have died.

> *After the birth of our baby we stopped at the cemetery on our way home from the hospital. We brought the new baby to our first baby's grave site. It was coming full circle for me. At the spot I laid my first baby to rest and said good-bye, we were welcoming a new baby and saying hello.*

They will always be changed parents. Some are able to see their changed view of life as a gift from their deceased baby:

> *If our first baby had lived, I know we would have been good parents. We would have done all the things we'd learned to do, but we would have done them with much less consciousness. Going through the deep traumatic loss of having our son come and leave so quickly made us more conscious human beings in this world, which allowed us to be different parents to the children who came after him than we could have been to him. I believe that's true.*

Other parents understand that the grief will remain, as it should; the deceased baby remains in the family. This dad explains:

> *We're not done yet. When you go through something like this you want to come to that end point, you want to finish it up because you don't want to sit there and grieve for six months, a year, or ten years. You want to find an end to it. And I guess I just don't think that's going to happen and I'm comfortable with that. Every day's a new day.*

Postpartum support group

> Comfort comes from knowing that people have made the same journey. And solace comes from understanding how others have learned to sing again.[1]

Many issues continue into the fourth trimester as parents begin the task of raising their child. For this reason, psychosocial intervention for parents who have suffered a loss should extend into the postpartum period (Vieten & Astin 2008). The first three months of life have been defined as the "phase of attachment readiness" (Mahler et al. 1973). Every parent needs time to adjust during these months, and that can be more the case with a subsequent baby. Attending a group to help with normal postpartum adjustment is important for any parents who have experienced a difficult pregnancy and may help in preventing postpartum depression (Hillman et al. 2010). It is important to assess a mother's feelings that may go beyond the normal disequilibrium of "neurotic" fitting together to check for signs of postpartum depression (Kim 2012).

Because of their history, these parents will continue to learn how to develop trust in the world. Like the PAL group, the postpartum group provides support and education about normal postpartum parenting issues after a loss and the baby's development. The group provides an opportunity to acknowledge and process fears while continuing to talk about the deceased baby, being supported by other parents who have walked the same path. Many themes seen in the PAL group can still be present, such as not trusting their ability to be a "good enough parent" and reflecting upon how they may be relating these feelings to the deceased baby. For example, one baby had not gained weight on his first pediatric visit and the mother was told to supplement breastfeeding with formula milk. She attended the group crying, and said: *My body couldn't keep my first baby alive and now my milk won't keep this baby alive.* She was encouraged by the group to continue breastfeeding. Over the next few weeks her baby grew appropriately without needing supplemental formula.

BOX 8.1

Interventions

The care provider needs to:

- Be sensitive to triggers for parental alarm, such as the baby's normal weight loss in the first few days.
- Take care not to offer general statements of reassurance because the parents may not trust them, just as in pregnancy.
- Demonstrate newborn competencies to support the baby's wellness.
- Remind parents that this baby is a sibling who will always miss the deceased baby too.
- Be aware that painful memories can resurface if the parents go home and the baby needs ongoing hospital care.
- Be sensitive to the fact that, if the baby is premature but healthy, the parents may not believe she will survive.
- Reassure parents that the normal postpartum period has both ups and downs.
- Help parents reframe protective parenting in a positive way.

The postpartum group I attended was a tremendous help to me in those early weeks and months. It was okay to cry and express my fresh feelings of grief for my daughter, and speak of my fears of losing my son. The weekly contact with other mothers and babies was always a favorite part of my week.

A PAL postpartum group supports people in their parenting role to the new baby, who needs them now, and to the deceased baby, while gently guiding them to seek further help from a qualified therapist if and when they need it. Facilitators need to be aware of their boundaries and know when to refer. Some parents will need to work through issues with a counselor. Others may be tired of being "in crisis" and just want to feel normal, even if they are still struggling.

> *At this point I was encouraged to seek professional help. This was useful in explaining about how the pregnancy had delayed my grief. I needed to talk and talk and talk. I was angry at everything, including the baby who had died. I was out of control.*

It is important to remember that previous loss does not necessarily presage disordered parenting in the years to come, or long-term psychological problems. One group of researchers (Turton et al. 2001) found that there was a significant improvement in families pregnant after loss at the postpartum assessment compared with the prenatal assessment, suggesting that, for many parents, pregnancy was a re-activating but self-limiting stressor. In general, we have found that parents rearing children after a loss are more intentional in their parenting (O'Leary & Warland 2012), as discussed in the next section.

BOX 8.2

One family's story of attachment focused prenatal intervention

This case illustrates the cycles of prenatal parenting as they appeared to one family as they moved through their subsequent pregnancy.

Linda and Paul's pregnancy followed a normal course and birthed their son Jacob at 42 weeks gestation. Within minutes of his birth, he was in distress. After 25 minutes of resuscitation, a chest x-ray confirmed a diaphragmatic hernia. He died four days later. Linda was in a profound state of grief but very much wanted to be pregnant again. Having heard about the subsequent pregnancy program, she came to see the parent–infant specialist shortly after the loss, wanting information on what the next pregnancy would be like for her, during the **smooth** phase. She was gently told that her grief for Jacob would always be there and a new pregnancy and baby wouldn't change those feelings. In fact, a new layer might surface. She wanted to know what kinds of feelings she might have so viewed the video, *After Loss: Journey of the Next Pregnancy* (1996). Although she wanted to believe that getting pregnant again would lessen her grief, she left understanding that it would still be with her when pregnancy occurred.

Four months after Jacob's death Linda became pregnant. She joined the PAL group when she was three weeks pregnant. She wept as she shared the disequilibrium of her feelings during the **break-up** phase. The simultaneous but conflicting emotions of joy at being pregnant, grief for Jacob, fear for this baby, and wanting Jacob back but knowing this was a different baby felt overwhelming to her. Others in the group validated her feelings and told her they were common and normal. This was important because many of her friends had been telling her to "just be happy that you're pregnant again." She left the group at eight weeks gestation as a result of her overwhelming feelings, only to return when she was 14 weeks pregnant. On re-entering, she said she hadn't been able to cope with her sense of anxiety when she listened to other people's stories of loss. She felt more stable now, during the **sorting**-**out** phase and was able to give to as well as receive from the other group members.

At 14 weeks, according to the schedule of the prenatal cycles, Linda and Paul spent time literally "sorting out" how they would cope in this pregnancy and handle the stress of their full-time jobs. They decided to have the triple-screen test,[2] hoping that it would give them some reassurance. Instead, the test suggested the possibility of having a child with Down's syndrome (Trisomy 21).[3]

During a developmental cycle of equilibrium, when parents should experience less anxiety, a crisis, such as hearing bad news, can push them back into the previous disequilibrium cycle before they are able to regroup and restabilize. This happened to Linda. She came to the group for support, sobbing and questioning what she and her partner should do. This situation was complicated by the fact that the son of one of the other couples had died as result of medical complications associated with Down's syndrome. They often shared how much they had not cared about his disability. Linda acknowledged how hard hearing about her struggle must be for them, as she openly discussed her choices, including termination, which compounded her grief for Jacob. The next week she returned, having decided that they would have an amniocentesis but would continue with the pregnancy no matter what the outcome. Within a week, they received the news that the baby boy they were carrying was normal. At this point, Paul also joined the group.

During the **inwardizing** phase, Linda worked very hard at trying to separate the new baby, calling Jacob the baby's big brother. She was reminded that her baby could hear and, at some level, understand her feelings. She was encouraged to journal these feelings. Because she was still more attached to Jacob, she began her journal writing to him, explaining that if he were alive he would be the center of her life; she found it was easier for her to write to Jacob about his little brother coming. She wrote about what a great big brother he would have been and that she would continue to love him even as she now worked at getting to know and love the new baby. When the baby's (fetal) movements became stronger, he began to draw her in. She slowly started writing more to the new baby about her fears and anxieties and describing what had happened to his brother, Jacob. Weekly non-stress tests were carried out during the last four weeks of the pregnancy for confirmation and reassurance regarding the baby's safety. She began to clearly articulate and demonstrate how she was parenting both children.

As they moved into the third trimester, the **expansion** phase, Linda began experiencing anxiety attacks. Her fear of the upcoming labor brought back all the memories surrounding Jacob's birth. To her and Paul, pushing a baby out meant death. She began to attend the one-hour weekly Body Works Class (guided imagery and relaxation), where she learned about the physiology of her panic attacks. This helped her develop relaxation skills and centered her focus on the new baby. She and Paul attended the special birth preparation class and began to plan for their new son's birth. Remembering that, in times of crisis people can't take in information, the childbirth educator used the birth class as another opportunity to help them process Jacob's labor and birth experience once again in order to help them focus and understand how this new baby's birth would be different.

Although they did not want to use medical intervention, Linda was fearful of going to term and asked to be induced at 38 weeks gestation. They were admitted to hospital and labor was induced using the standard pitocin protocol. They walked around in their street clothes using remote monitoring, but active labor never started. At the end of the day they decided to go home, having confirmed the baby was healthy and strong, and trusting it was safe to continue the pregnancy; they could wait until the baby was ready. Linda later described this time as "practice" in the hospital, allowing herself to let go of many fears for her own safety as well as the baby's. A week later they returned in active labor and birthed a healthy boy.

Linda and Paul joined the postpartum group when their new son Joshua was one week old. Here, parents could discuss all of the babies in their family. Now in the **"neurotic" fitting together** phase, they wept as they shared mixed feelings of joy about their healthy son and sadness as they faced the reality that Jacob was not with them. Over the following weeks, as they fell in love with Joshua, they expressed that their grief had deepened as they came to realize the full extent of their previous loss. They found the group a safe place in which to talk about the normal worries of all new parents similarly traumatized; that is, heightened concern for their baby's safety, fear of death, hyper-vigilance, and so on, which are exceptional to this population. Linda's thank-you note a few weeks postpartum validated the impact of the intervention on her parenting experience during both pregnancies:

> Being a part of the subsequent pregnancy support group has really helped me get through a difficult time in my life. Being able to figure out how to continue to hold Jacob close and be able to parent Joshua has been very important to me.... Thank you for getting to know Jacob and helping me to be a parent to Josh (starting in utero!).

As Attig (2002, p. 52) attests,

> As we relearn the world, we give lasting love for those who died a place within the larger context of our lives. No matter how important those who died and our love for them have been, we did not, nor do we, give our hearts to them alone. Not only must we struggle to let go of their physical presence and longing for their return, but we also need to let go of any singular, sometimes preoccupying, focus on them and their absence. We need to let go of loving only them to the exclusion of any others. ... We love those who died when we go on without them by our sides, with lasting love for them in our hearts and with our hearts open again to the wonders of life on earth.

BOX 8.3

Case study

This couple did not know the gender of their subsequent baby but felt sure it was a girl to follow the stillbirth of their full-term daughter. When a son was born, they were numb and speechless, unable to express any emotions. Minutes after the birth their four-year-old son entered the room to see his new baby and said, "He's supposed to be a girl!" the very thought his parents could not verbalize. After voicing his disappointment, the little boy embraced the baby and began to talk about how much he loved him. It was then the parents cried and embraced the baby too. The sibling's innocence expressed what everyone was feeling. Arriving home, they sat silently in the living room with the new baby in the car seat. The four-year-old child again calmly said what everyone was thinking: "Well, it's still not right. She's still not here." Someone was still missing.

The mother later shared that, as she watched her elder son walk into the room after the birth, she saw the shadow of a little girl walking in with him, her stillborn daughter now a toddler. While she and her husband, by choice, had used minimal support during the pregnancy, she attended the postpartum group for six months to work through her mixed emotions. She felt that her grief was deeper now than when her daughter had died. As she nursed her new son, she would think she was nursing her daughter. Her readiness to begin separating and individualizing her children did not surface until the postpartum period. Her story clearly illustrates how everyone travels the pregnancy after loss journey in different ways, accepting support and intervention only when ready.

Summary

This chapter has addressed the early postpartum needs of families after the birth of a healthy baby. It is important to "normalize" this period by helping parents understand that another layer of grief will surface because the deceased baby is still missing. Family members and friends will not necessarily understand why they continue to grieve and need acknowledgment of the deceased baby. Rebuilding trust in the world takes time, and follow-up into these parents' postpartum period is important.

Notes

1 www.azquotes.com/author/17714-Helen_Steiner_Rice.
2 Triple-screening measures alpha-fetoprotein (AFP), human chorionic gonadotropin (hCG), and estriol (uE3) in the woman's blood, to ascertain the likelihood of the baby having Down's syndrome, spina bifida, or anencephaly.
3 Down's syndrome is a condition in which a person has an extra chromosome 21.

9

LOSS IN A MULTI-FETAL PREGNANCY

This chapter addresses the complexity of loss during a multi-fetal pregnancy. Parents face intense grief for a deceased baby while continuing pregnancy with a living baby. Interventions to support parents as they hear the news, continue the pregnancy, and prepare for birth and early postpartum will be presented.

Relevant statistics

Assisted reproductive technology (ART) has increased the incidence of multiple pregnancies since the 1980s. Between 1–20 percent of these pregnancies result in three or more fetuses (Seoud et al. 1992), usually in the first trimester (the break-up phase).[1] Twin births rose by 70 percent between 1980 and 2004, and triplet or higher order multiple (HOM) births increased by more than 400 percent during the 1980s and 1990s (Martin et al. 2010). Single fetal demise occurs in 3.7–6.8 percent of all twin pregnancies; in identical twins, the remaining twin has a 12 percent risk of death compared to 4 percent in non-identical twins; and approximately 30 percent of twin pregnancies ultimately result in a singleton birth (Almog et al. 2010; Blickstein & Perlman 2013; Norwitz et al. 2005; Tummers et al. 2003). The death of a twin in the first trimester does not increase the risk for the co-twin but death in the second trimester or third trimester does increase the risk for the remaining twin (Morin & Lim 2011).

Single twin demise (vanishing twin syndrome) occurs in up to 6 percent of twin pregnancy and increases the risk of fetal mortality and rates of long-term handicap for the survivor, more so when the loss is after the first trimester (Hillman et al. 2010). A Scandinavian study suggests that 10.4 percent of all singletons following in vitro fertilization (IVF) are survivors of the vanishing twin syndrome (Pinborg et al. 2005). The live birth rate was higher in pregnancies associated with vanishing fetuses (Mansour et al. 2010). Pregnancies diagnosed with vanishing twin syndrome after IVF carry a higher rate of adverse obstetric outcomes in terms of preterm deliveries and lower birth weight, compared with IVF pregnancies that were originally singleton (Almog et al. 2010; Jauniaux et al. 2013). Others have found that the risk of maternal and fetal morbidity and mortality associated with assisted-reproduction twins is only increased in women with a pre-existing medical condition (Jauniaux et al. 2013).

The rate of perinatal mortality in triplet pregnancies is 13.8 percent, with this risk increasing dramatically with each additional fetus present (Newman & Luke 2000). The stillbirth rate for these babies is over twice that for singletons; they are also more at risk for preterm delivery and sudden infant death syndrome (SIDS) probably due to prematurity and low birth weight (Lisonkova et al. 2012). However, in the population of twin births, the stillbirth rate per gestational age is low, approximately 1 per 1,000 until 38 weeks, at which time it is increased to 7.0 per 1,000 twin births (Tang et al. 2014). Twins are five times and triplets are 15 times more likely to die within one month after birth (Little 2010). Stillbirth risk among twins is greater for identical (monochorionic diamniotic) twins as compared to non-identical (diamniotic dichorionic) twins. Twin–twin transfusion syndrome (TTTS) affects 10–15 percent of twin pregnancies with monochorionic diamniotic placentation (Mosquera et al. 2012). These twins have a fused placenta and the blood vessels between the twin placentas can be connected, which may result in one twin pumping blood to the other and subsequently being smaller. In this type of twinning, twin transfusion syndrome may occur with a much smaller (donor) twin and a larger (recipient) twin, with the potential for heart failure in the recipient. In addition, twins which are in a single sac (monochorionic monamniotic), without a dividing membrane, are at higher risk because the umbilical cords can become entangled.

When complications arise in a multiple pregnancy, parents face difficult decisions as the fates of these babies are linked (Malone et al. 1996). Their fears and anxieties are similar to those of parents pregnant after loss; often coping with grief and attachment simultaneously but sometimes not receiving equal sympathy (Hillman et al. 2010). Women (and their partners) can experience extreme anxiety over the remaining fetuses and have a significantly higher risk of depression (Leonard et al. 2006; Swanson et al. 2002), which should be monitored into the postpartum period (Hillman et al. 2010). That said, it is important to note that high rates of depression have also been found in twin pregnancies without demise (Benute et al. 2012b; Roca de Bes et al. 2008).

The death of a co-twin or triplet in pregnancy should be managed by close follow up and fetal testing; for example, biophysical profiles, at least weekly ultrasound observations, and observation of growth volume (Shek et al. 2014). In identical twins, the death of a co-twin may result in delivery, especially if the death occurs near term; if the death of the co-twin is preterm conservative management with fetal testing may be carried out or in some situations fetal blood transfusions may be given to the surviving twin (Gaziano, personal communication).

Providing emotional support and unique medical management for these parents is crucial. Three questions frequently verbalized by parents are: (1) how will

I know my other babies are safe; (2) how can I be happy for my surviving children when I am grieving for a deceased baby; and (3) will the loss of this baby affect my remaining babies?

Hearing the news

Parents conceiving through ART know through early ultrasounds during the break-up phase that one or more of their fertilized eggs may not develop and, indeed, are told to anticipate one "disappearing" (De De Pascalis et al. 2007). Others hear the news during a routine ultrasound during the sorting-out phase, when they may just be coming to terms with the reality that they are parents of multiples. Not well understood by parents or people in general is that the deceased baby remains in the uterus for the duration of the pregnancy, thus parents continue the pregnancy with both babies.

Learning of the loss can be especially difficult for the mother in the weeks before fetal movement is felt because she has no awareness that one baby has died. This mother was alone when she learned, during a routine ultrasound, that one twin had died. When the technician leaves (they are not allowed to give the news) to get a doctor, parents are left alone:

> She just did a quick scan. And I thought, "What?" It just threw me off like there was something in the first minute and a half. And she says, I'm going to be right back in one minute. Well, that's the danger of leaving the clock running on the monitor, you're watching for one minute. So one minute turns into ten and she came back with a physician, who says "We're not seeing any heart movement for twin A."

Sense of self as mother can be negatively affected. Another mother was not aware one twin had died until an ultrasound at 30 weeks and she immediately felt that the loss may be due to something she did:

> You feel guilty because you think, as non-rationally as you can possibly get, "What could I have done to bring this on?" I'm afraid of what the autopsy is going to say. Did I do something bad? So, was the bath too hot? Did I squash his head? I mean, what was in my control that I didn't do to prevent this from happening? So that's hard. I mean that brings up a lot of sadness. I don't really have words for this.

If parents did not want multiple babies, they can feel guilty that one has died. As one father said:

> When I discovered they were twins it just didn't fit in any of my intuitive reality. It just wasn't in our realm to have multiples. We went for an ultrasound and it was like, there's two! It was like fear coupled with feeling overwhelmed about having twins. I probably spent the first two to three weeks of the pregnancy just crying. So then you feel guilty because you think, on some level did you bring this on somehow because it just didn't fit. I was like, I don't want the attention. I just don't want that. I so wanted it to just

be like everybody else. I didn't want to stand out in any way. You deal with that. You get over it. You read books where some people actually say it's great because you get all this extra attention. It's like [sighs] maybe I'll get there. And then to have the demise.

Others mourn the loss of potential motherhood or fatherhood with multiple babies:

It was so hard because I was still carrying this healthy baby who was growing and thriving and then you had this other baby who had passed away. It was not only the loss but the loss of the twin thing.

The statement of the father below reflects research findings demonstrating that fathers in pregnancy after loss have no time to deal with their own feelings because they have to take care of the mother:

I was just worried about her not making it or something being wrong. I had no idea what was going on at that point. So that was the biggest worry for me. I'm not too sure how to characterize the loss of the child. I think partly because it's not over till it's over. It doesn't feel quite real. For me, it was painful but I'm not letting myself feel the totality of that pain because there's another child that is living. If we lost both children then I think we'd be in a real risky state.

The statement below is a potent example of why men can experience a delayed reaction to grief:

If I feel something I might not be able to stop it. Don't think about this. I have reflected on the thought of what could have been with two children. There is an odd sense of relief that the complexity of having twins versus having a single child, because I was handling a lot of the logistics. My wife was more in la, la land about how she was going to manage two kids. I was thinking, "Where are they going to sleep?" It just changed the dynamics. It's not a happy relief; it's not like "Oh, this is great." Rather, this is okay, this changes, simplifies things. There hasn't been a lot of time to reflect.

Continuing the pregnancy

After the initial shock parents need professionals who will provide guidance in coping with their conflicting feelings of grief for one baby while carrying a living baby (De Pascalis et al. 2007). Some parents fear attaching to the baby who is still alive. Until they feel consistent fetal movement, parents will need frequent follow-ups to check the heartbeat and gather concrete information confirming that the other baby is safe:

There's nothing you can do for twin A so you start to rally round twin B. You put your energy towards there but it comes with a lot of pain, because you start to feel like I messed up before [crying] so how can I stop that this time? That's the hard part.

On learning that the death of one twin was not caused by twin–twin transfusion, one father felt some reassurance but was still worried:

> *We had a little higher level of confidence that [surviving twin] was going to be healthy for the rest of the pregnancy but then we were walking on egg shells about everything else, like is she going to pass away and we aren't going to know anything about it because it was such a shock to us that we had healthy babies and then all of a sudden one was dead. So what's going to happen to the healthy twin or could the death of one baby cause issues for the other?*

As with parents pregnant after loss, the attention paid to fetal movement also changes. *With my first pregnancy it was "Oh a kick count, here and there," but now every time there was decreased movement I was really paranoid about that.* Due to the risks regarding loss in multi-fetal pregnancies the surviving baby's wellbeing "leads the way" and is monitored closely. Parents remain anxious until the surviving baby is born alive and rely on technology to confirm all is well:

> *We were very paranoid. I was going in weekly for ultrasounds to monitor to make sure our surviving baby was doing well. I found it very reassuring.*

The continued bond/attachment-based intervention becomes a guide to help parents embrace their role with both babies. During the inwardizing phase of prenatal parenting (22–32 weeks), intervention focuses on helping parents learn ways in which to trust the surviving baby will remain healthy. They need to be shown how to monitor patterns in the baby's cycle of sleeping/wakefulness and instructed to make contact immediately when they recognize a change in those patterns. They also need to be given information on how the mother's body is protecting and nurturing the surviving baby's development, which means being able to understand the meaning of their baby's clinical data: proper size for age implies wellness, amniotic fluid volume indicates good blood flow and kidney function, acceleration of fetal heart rate with movement reflects appropriate brain regulatory function.

Future ultrasound examinations will be difficult. Just as with parents pregnant after loss, these parents need to see the heartbeat first:

> *The first couple of ultrasounds were really hard because it brought back all the memories of that ultrasound where we found out her sister had died and there were no signs before that. You try not to take the pregnancy for granted but every little sign she was doing well was reassuring.*

It is important to ask parents if they want to see the deceased baby on subsequent ultrasounds. Some will and others will refuse. Respecting the parents' wishes on this subject is crucial:

I remember the ultrasound tech asking me at one of the first ultrasounds after she had died if I wanted to see her. She asked with an expression and tone that was similar to what you'd use if you were asking someone to see a wretched car wreck or disaster. I remember thinking, "Of course I want to see her. This was my baby." I had to ask a couple of times after that, but it then became part of the usual scan.

Regardless of the situation, the behavior and medical needs of the remaining baby continue.

I was 31 weeks on Tuesday and it's part of the monitoring because Dr. G said there's not a hundred other women who have had my experience. I said, what are the statistics? What do you do? It's a hostile environment now because there's the sloughing off tissue…. Can all the fluid and the decay, I mean basically it's a decomposing entity, can that back up into that cord and cause problems with twin B. Is the membrane permeable enough where there's a transfer of this healthy alive fluid, and this sloughing off coagulated fluid? What are the dangers for twin B? And Dr. G said, we'll basically monitor you for that. On Wednesday when I go back they'll look at that pathway and see the flow of blood because it's unknown what happens. You know it's a greater concern because if there's a vascular problem for one and they're identical, the chance of it being a vascular problem for B exists. That's where it is day by day. You think, what is going to happen because you just don't know. I say to my husband, I come in here and I can go to a cesarian delivery today, just because they get concerned. If I don't score at least an eight then it's just a concern; a four means I'm going under. So it's really minute by minute as far as getting twin B out alive.

In spite of technology providing objective data, parents still do not completely trust that all is well for the baby. They still worry, especially if previously told that everything was fine and then learning at the next appointment that one baby has died:

On Wednesday I had a biophysical profile and when [the technician] did an ultrasound on Tuesday [the following week] and looked at the edema around the head and between the ribs and on the skin, she said this looks like he's been gone for five, six days. That also blows my mind, because it's like what was Saturday night with all that activity? What was I feeling? Was that all twin B, and now twin B feels totally different than that experience. He could have been dead since Wednesday night? So it's like, could she be wrong? Could it have accelerated at that rapid rate? And what's causing the acceleration at that rapid rate? Where do you find solace? You're intuitively tuned in, listened and felt like things were okay or that they know what they are talking about. There's no way I could have prevented this because there was no really clear indicators for me. I left on a Wednesday, they did a biophysical profile, they got an eight, I went out the door and so…

Managing grief and attachment

Regardless of the gestational age at which the baby died, it is common for parents to ask how they can continue the pregnancy and be happy for the surviving baby or babies. Grief for the deceased baby remains and should not be dismissed. This means that parents need guidance on how to manage grief alongside their attachment to the baby or babies still alive. Parents can begin to build memories by starting a journal that contains ultrasound pictures of all the babies. As discussed during the "sorting out phase" in Chapter 4, journaling helps with healing by putting words to their feelings of grief and attachment and offers a way to "tell the story" with the surviving baby or babies when they are older. This helps parents understand that their grief can be shared with the surviving baby or babies while they also develop an attachment relationship with them. Bringing the conversation to the forefront lets the parent lead the way in how much information they may want to take in. One mother, remembering how connected her twin boys had been, did want more information:

> I feel like there are a lot of things I want to ask them [the health care provider]. How does it feel being in there next to this body? And what is his consciousness of this body that's just kind of dissolving around him, not around him, but right next to him? I mean I have an ultrasound where one has their arm around the other one. So you feel like saying, I know there was this connection.

Other parents shared what they believed was grief in their surviving two unborn boys of a triplet pregnancy when fetal growth restriction caused the loss of one at 28 weeks gestation. The two surviving boys showed no heart rate variability during the following three days. On day three, the baby lying closest to his deceased brother turned away, finishing the pregnancy with his surviving sibling until they were born at 34 weeks. The parents commented that they believed *they were grieving with us.*

The above couple attended the PAL group for the remainder of the pregnancy and returned two years later when they were pregnant with twin girls, both of whom survived. They gained much information over their three-year involvement with the prenatal parenting program and had come to an understanding that the surviving children may want more information at a later date. David Chamberlain (1998, 2013), one of the founders of the Association of Prenatal and Perinatal Psychology and Health, suggests that some children are able to articulate their pregnancy and birth stories between the ages of three and five. For example, when the child lying closest to his deceased brother was three he asked his mother, "Did Sawyer die because I didn't give him enough room? I remember crawling up under your ribs to give him more room." His mother also remembered feeling him under her ribs and reassured her three year old that he did not cause his brother's death—Sawyer was sick. She respected that, at some level, her three year old carried the memory of his brother's loss. Such accounts of young children remembering the events and feelings that occur around pregnancy and birth have been confirmed by others (Phillips 2013).

Preparing for birth

In the expansion phase until birth the health care providers continue to monitor the surviving babies frequently by carrying out biophysical profiles to determine the best time to give birth. Although many twins can be born vaginally, the majority of multiple births are by cesarean section. Collaborative studies on twins found planned cesarean delivery did not significantly decrease or increase the risk of fetal or neonatal death or serious neonatal morbidity, as compared with planned vaginal delivery (Barret et al. 2013). Care providers may be surprised to hear a mother express not wanting the pregnancy to end. This may seem strange for someone who has spent weeks worrying about the safety of the surviving baby; however, birth ends the physical connection with the deceased baby. This fact should be processed with parents before the actual birth.

Birth preparation should minimally involve a tour of where parents will give birth. They also need assistance in writing a birth plan that reflects the needs of all the babies, both living and dead. Babies who die after 14 weeks gestation usually have some resemblance of a baby. In clinical practice we have even been able to get foot and hand prints of these tiny babies. Parents can ask if this is possible. A nurse who has had experience with infant death is often more skilled at helping with this request. Regardless, no matter how small, it is helpful for parents to have visual evidence that there was a baby. Some babies will be reabsorbed in the placenta. The Ancient Greeks called them "paper babies" because they were as thin as paper but still visible on the wall of the placenta.

Discussing the parents' wishes for the deceased baby is an important part of birth planning. Do they want to see the deceased baby? If possible, do they want pictures of the babies together? If the loss was before 15 weeks it is likely the deceased babies will be reabsorbed so parents may want to consider cremating the placenta.

If the birth will be early the parents need to make decisions regarding who will go with the babies to the neotal intensive care unit (NICU) or special care and who might be a support person to stay with the mother and the deceased baby. The care provider should enquire about spiritual support and whether they want other family members to see all the babies. It is rare for parents to want an older sibling to see a baby who has died before 20 weeks gestation but occasionally this may be requested. One family let their six-year-old daughter see her deceased twin sister, at 16 weeks gestation, lying in a small basket wrapped in a hanky that had belonged to her deceased grandmother.

The birth is extremely emotional. As this father prepared for the birth of two surviving boys, he shared:

> My biggest fear approaching the birth was not knowing what was going to happen, not knowing how I would act emotionally to the situation. What happened was two opposite emotions: the joy at the birth of my two living sons and the sadness of my third son's death sort of cancelled each other out.

It is not unusual for parents to initially request more time with the deceased baby after the birth. This is the only time they will have. Now in the "neurotic" fitting together phase, this couple describe the time spent with their deceased twin. *We were able to hold her, we had a little ceremony, took pictures and footprints, that was really helpful.* It is appropriate to have the surviving baby in the room too and for parents to verbally share their sadness. The deceased baby will always be missed, the living child/children will always be from a multi-fetal pregnancy and this should be reflected on the birth certificate. Parents who were not able to see their deceased baby have expressed regret about not having those memories.

Postpartum parenting

In the "neurotic" fitting together phase, the full impact of the loss is felt. The joyous event of a surviving twin's birth can cause grief to be more intense as parents realize what they have missed in not having all the babies (Hillman et al. 2010) just as found in parents pregnant after loss. Demonstrating newborn capabilities, as discussed in Chapter 8 regarding the postpartum period for parents pregnant after loss, makes parents aware of the competencies of their healthy surviving baby or babies. Going home without all their children brings another layer of grief.

Keeping the twin/triplet relationship alive

Respecting the experience of the intrauterine loss and knowing how to support the surviving baby or babies twin relationship are important. Letting the parent lead the way, the care provider needs to gently and carefully acknowledge to the parent that the twin may also be feeling the loss of his sibling. Surviving children need to claim their twin relationship and are thankful if their parents are able to show them photographs validating it. Research with adult surviving twins found that, if they don't know the story, surviving children may sense that there was something odd or hidden about their birth (Haydon 2008, 2011). This vagueness can be more troublesome to the surviving child than a proper knowledge of the loss of a sibling (Hayden 2008; Lewis 1987).

Maintaining a connection with a deceased sibling is not a new concept in other cultures. The belief of some African tribes is that the spirit of the dead twin must be preserved in order to ensure the wholeness of the survivor (Leroy et al. 2002). Yoruba twins from Nigeria carry a wooden image representing their dead twin around their neck or waist, which is said to provide company for the survivor and a refuge for the spirit of the dead twin.

Most parents understandably worry about the impact of loss on the surviving baby. Research on the impact of the mother's emotions on the unborn child suggests it is plausible that the physiological responses to grief and mourning may affect the uterine environment. The twin relationship in the womb is the first relationship for the womb twin survivor (Hayton 2014). At some level we cannot quantify, the surviving baby shared the innate sense of physical proximity within the uterus and was also exposed to the emotional turmoil and physical grief of the parents. Adult survivors of multi-fetal loss suggest that they have never known life without partners and find this deeply disturbing (Barron 1996; Hayden 2008, 2011).

While some may argue that the sadness this mother senses in her remaining twin daughter is a reflection of her own emotions, it is nonetheless important to honor those feelings:

> *It's challenging every day just because of the fact I see her grow and talk, do everything. I have that constant day to day reminder, of which I'm thankful for, I'm thankful that I didn't lose her also, but it's very hard. I see her in the bathtub playing and I get sad because her sister should be here playing with her, fighting over the wash cloth, sitting down playing with toys. It just makes me feel sad because I think she feels sad and I can sense that sometimes.*

In an unpublished retrospective study on the effect of the death of a member of a set of premature multiples, statistically and clinically significant changes were found in the physiological parameters of the survivors (Pitts 2000). The most frequent life-threatening complications documented in the surviving infants surrounding the death of their sibling were sepsis, intraventricular hemorrhage, high incidence of hyperglycemia, and hypotension (ibid).

Many of the surviving babies are born prematurely, thus requiring early intervention services. As parents move from the medical setting to the community, it is helpful for professionals to have a history of the high risk pregnancy from the perspective of the parents' experience. The trauma they have experienced can provide clues to guide intervention. Early childhood professionals often think they shouldn't bring up the topic but most parents appreciate that their deceased babies are acknowledged as missing members of their family. If that is not the case, parents will generally make that known.

The following early intervention professional shares how she approaches parents:

> *I used to be very fearful of opening this can of worms for fear of not knowing how to respond and [it's] a difficult thing to have parents share during a home visit. Then I realized how critical it was and how parents wanted to tell their story. So now the first time we meet a family, we go out as a team and open the door to that. We always ask the family, what would you like to tell us about your story? We know it's a great question because parents are very grateful, are very articulate and they are very forthcoming. It gives us an opportunity to know much more than we ever could, what they've been through and where they might be at. It's been surprising to us that parents are more forthcoming than not. They tell us more than we ever would expect and they welcome that. The parents will actually bring out photo albums; sometimes that doesn't come [until] after a few weeks but some parents will show you that right away. They really do want to introduce you to their family and where they've been. I don't think a lot of people ask them [about] their story; certainly pediatricians don't have a lot of time. I always say to parents the first session is a "getting to know you session"; what you want to share and what we can offer you.*

By asking parents to tell their story, professionals gain information that will help them provide the right services for them. The simple statement allows parents to have control over how much information they might want to share. This is important not only for parents of surviving babies but also for those who have been through a difficult pregnancy such as birthing a preterm baby or a baby born with special needs.

Summary

This chapter has addressed the complex issues parents encounter when they experience a loss within a multi-fetal pregnancy. It has described ways in which to help parents deal with the complex process of mourning the loss of one or more babies while continuing the pregnancy and attaching to and parenting the surviving unborn babies. The prenatal parenting relationship-based intervention is also a helpful guide for parents who know one baby may die at birth or shortly after. In both situations, parents need information on how to make meaning of their continued bond to the deceased baby while attaching to the surviving baby or babies.

CASE STUDY

This case summarizes the chapter content. Particularly significant are the mother's "intuition" that something wasn't right, the parents' fears being dismissed by care providers, and how this couple consciously parented their daughter before she died.

The 20-week ultrasound revealed to these parents that they were having twins and they described the moment "as one of the most joy-filled days of our life." Switching their care from a midwife to an obstetric gynecologist, they had a level-two ultrasound[2] at 24 weeks where they learned that baby A looked great but baby B was about half the size of baby A and there was only a 10 percent chance that she would make it. The mother remembered naïvely thinking, *She's just a little small. She's moving; her heart is beating; she looked great a few weeks ago. She'll be fine.* She went on to say, *I was carrying this little baby girl fighting for life and they were telling me that she probably wasn't going to make it.* They were referred to a specialist, not sure if they would lose one or both babies, deliver early, or have a child with severe developmental delays and medical issues. Knowing baby B would not make it and that she could hear, they showered her with parenting. *We sang, played fun and loving music, danced, rubbed my belly and tried to comfort her in any way that we could. It was important to us that she felt loved.* By the next appointment baby B had died.

> *I will never forget the image of her still little heart, next to her sister's healthy beating heart. I hoped that her short life was filled with love and she knew nothing other than comfort, love, joy, and peace.*

Told that Baby A should continue to grow and develop normally, the parents asked what would happen to baby B and were informed that she would "get reabsorbed." They continued weekly reassuring ultrasounds and non-stress tests and saw baby B every week for the rest of the pregnancy.

> She was getting more crowded as baby A grew to be full term, but she was still very prominent. You could see all of her little bones and parts. Even though she was no longer alive, I wanted to make sure that she was "comfortable" and looked okay. It was also helpful to see where she was so I could rub her and talk to her as well. It was sweet to see baby A's head so near hers and comforting to think of her dying so close to her sister.

The birth plan included doing something small to celebrate the short life of baby B, but the parents were told, "there won't be much left of her." This didn't feel right to the mother but because she felt *overwhelmed [she] had given up on listening to [her] intuition, just wanting to trust what the doctors were telling [her].*

Baby Lynnea's birth went smoothly; in fact, the parents barely made it to the hospital in time and she was born following just two pushes. A midwife was reassuring amidst the chaos, exactly what was needed because of their fear of the unknown. The mother said, *It was such a relief to hold this perfect, beautiful, pink, crying healthy baby after we were so close to losing her. We had lost her sister in the same uterus.* The obstetrician noticed a small white spot about the size of a quarter on the placenta and said, "This must be twin B." The mother intuitively felt that this couldn't be but both parents nodded agreeably. Experiencing extreme cramping in the night, the mother mentioned it to the nurse but was told to toughen up. The mother then passed a few pieces of tissue and was reassured by the nurse that expelling clots was normal. At around 6 a.m., the mother went to the bathroom and felt something huge passing out onto the floor. *To my shock I saw a huge mass about the size of a football. At first I thought that I was hemorrhaging, but there was not an excessive amount of blood. The first thing that I saw was a perfect tiny little arm and little perfect fingers. I knew that it was my precious twin B. I just stood there frozen and remember feeling so sad and awful that she had landed on the bathroom floor.* Her husband notified the nurse, who came in immediately. The mother continued:

> They cleaned Isabelle up and brought her back. She was pretty macerated from being inside so long, but she was fully formed, including hair and fingernails. We kept her in a blanket near us, had a nice ceremony and spent the day honoring her until they took her the next day.
>
> A special nurse that deals specifically with loss talked about Isabelle in the present tense, handling her as if she had been born alive. There was such

a sense of closure, so helpful in dealing with the grief and pain. One of the most painful moments was when we had to hand her over for the last time, knowing that an autopsy would be performed and she would then be cremated. No matter how small, there is nothing quite as shattering as realising that you will never hold your child again. The bittersweet part was holding our precious, healthy baby girl in our arms, which was comforting but almost magnified the pain. We cherished her all that much more, but there was always that nagging emptiness in the back of our minds that was aching to be holding two healthy, baby girls.

Notes

1 Medical content in this chapter summarized by Dr. Emmanuel Gaziano
2 A level-two ultrasound is similar to a standard ultrasound but more detailed.

10

FETAL REDUCTION IN MULTI-FETAL PREGNANCIES

Loss in a multi-fetal pregnancy can occur by choice when parents are pregnant with too many babies or one baby is extremely ill. This chapter addresses loss in these situations. These parents also need guided intervention on their prenatal parenting relationship as they struggle with grief and attachment simultaneously. Supporting parents as they make decisions, saying goodbye to one or more babies, continuing the pregnancy, and preparing for birth and postpartum issues will be covered.

Tesch (2007) summarized that, regardless of parents' choices, four key points are important to keep in mind when working with parents who choose multi-fetal pregnancy reduction (MFPR): (1) it is not about whether parents should make the choice—it is about supporting them through the choice they have made; (2) it means understanding that it is less about statistical outcomes and more about emotions; (3) it is about assessing the strength and resiliency of parents and connecting them with sources of support; and (4) it is about empathy and non-judgment.

Infertility overview

The struggles can begin long before conception, especially if the inability to conceive has already depleted parents' emotional reserves and placed a stress on their relationship. Once conception occurs the stress of infertility appears insignificant in light of the news that they are carrying multiple fetuses. Parents spiral through the emotional trauma of making the decision to undergo MFPR, having the procedure, continuing with the pregnancy, and preparing for the birth of their surviving babies. It is through the process of parents telling their story that others can begin to understand what undergoing MFPR means.

Although prenatal testing and selective termination are more clinically normalized, open discussion surrounding the procedure remains taboo (Thachuk 2007). Depending on cultural and religious beliefs, positions vary on abortion but influence both the grieving process and those involved in the act of making the decision, as well as the attitude of society towards them (Little 2010; Korenromp et al. 2005, 2007; McCoyd, 2007, 2009, 2013). Parents might feel that the only way to avoid the potential hostility and unsupportive responses of family members and friends is to share only with those who they know will endorse or understand their decision (Britt & Evans 2007). Grieving can be accompanied by intense guilt for those who regard abortion as "murder," and further intensified by social stigma and religious views (Gordon et al. 2007; Korenromp et al. 2007; Young & Papadatou 1997). This conflict makes getting support more difficult at a time when parents most need it and counselors and church workers need to recognize this.

The Christian faith provides little written information specific to fetal reduction. In contrast, the Islamic faith recognizes high order multiple pregnancies as dangerous and unnatural and has a provision for parents to make this choice (Angelfire 2004). In one study, women who identified themselves as Jewish found the decision to undergo MFPR less morally taxing, as Jewish law places the value of the life of the mother before that of an unborn fetus thus allowing rabbis to give parents the spiritual permission to make this choice (Eisenberg 2004).

Multi-fetal pregnancy reduction

Multiple births are often glamorized but in reality a twin, triplet, or higher-order pregnancy is complex and risky. Parents who experience multi-fetal pregnancy through reproductive technology may have already endured several years of treatment failure or pregnancy loss during what should normally be the smooth phase of prenatal parenting (Little 2010). Women may enter this phase fearing that their bodies are unreliable and both parents fear that the pregnancy may not lead to a happy conclusion.

The most common form of MFPR is the trans-abdominal procedure, performed when parents find themselves with too many babies. Families terminate one or more of the fetuses to increase the chance of a successful outcome for those remaining (ibid). An ultrasound is necessary before the procedure to determine which fetuses are most accessible (Evans & Britt 2008; Evans et al. 2005) and is generally carried out during the break-up phase of prenatal parenting. Viewed by the maternity care provider as an option to increase the odds for a successful outcome, it is not a medical procedure like having an appendix removed. Health care providers can utilize terminology such as "fetus" and "embryo" to soften the blow but parents know it is their baby. One mother describes her conflict thus: *It's so hard because I had a connection to the babies as soon as I found out I was pregnant.*

Children from a multi-fetal pregnancy have a higher risk of neurologic impairment, including cerebral palsy (ASRM[1] 2006; Lee et al. 2006). Some parents learn during the break-up or sorting-out phases of prenatal parenting that one or more of the babies may have abnormalities. Parents have almost no time to celebrate their newly diagnosed multiple pregnancy before they are told they need to consider MFPR (Collopy 2004; McLean 2013; Wegner 2015). From the perspective of

ASR/MFPR, the disequilibrium of the break-up phase is intensified. Parents who receive information in the sorting-out phase are pushed back into disequilibrium, going from not being able to get pregnant to being pregnant with too many babies or a very sick baby. Parents become increasingly overwhelmed as result of news of yet another complication:

> At our first ultrasound we saw one embryo. The next week the ultrasound showed two and I said, "Oh gosh, twins." The next week we saw three embryos and I thought, "We need to stop having ultrasounds!"

Making the decision

Because reductions are performed within a certain gestational period, many women are forced to wait and often not offered support during these days. As one mother states, *Making the decision was hard. I was so tired of being in limbo, I didn't think I could be pregnant with triplets another month.* As they wait they vacillate between feeling it is the right decision and wanting another alternative. The decision can be complicated by the fact that they may be choosing to remove a healthy baby. They fantasize desperately about ways in which they can avoid making the choice (Culling 2013). Choice seems outlandish as there is no winning solution; parents must simply face the task of making the choice that will result in the fewest losses. Ambivalence can be a recurring emotional state for women in this position (Tesch 2007):

> When I was deciding, I was wavering between twins or one. I studied the research and thought the statistics were better for one, but I knew there were no guarantees.
>
> It's hard not to think of this as gambling, weighing the odds of one decision over another. Problem is I have never been a gambler.

In Tesch's (2007) study, all the mothers made the decision by weighing the risks and benefits and, in their minds, the risk of carrying multiples was far too great. Many base their decision to reduce on their fear of losing all the babies or what is best for their family:

> We needed to do it or we would lose the whole pregnancy.
>
> Deciding to keep all three of them, it's not the best solution. I've experienced the NICU and what premature babies face, how their brains develop. I've seen kids with all sorts of problems. I just can't, I can't do that.

Mothers undergoing MFPR report feelings of grief, accompanied by intense sadness, stress (Little 2010; Maifeld et al. 2003; Porreco et al. 1995; Wang & Chao 2006; Wegner 2015) and extreme anxiety regarding the remaining fetuses (Leonard & Denton 2006; Sutcliff & Derom 2006; Swanson et al. 2002). They also face a significantly higher risk of depression. The grief of mothers is reportedly more intense and more expressive than that of fathers (Schwab 1996; Wheeler 2001). It is not uncommon for women to pray for a miscarriage (McCoyd 2007) or for their own life to end to save them from having to "make" the choice (Tesch 2007). *For several weeks I prayed that the pregnancy would end spontaneously and when that didn't seem to be happening, I wished I would die.* These feelings, although alarmingly suicidal in nature, appear to be common and just part of how women process this experience. *I didn't really want to kill myself, I just wished something, anything would happen so I wouldn't have to make the choice.*

Experiencing the procedure

Scheduling the appointment delivers another emotional blow. One mother described being asked to book her appointment for the reduction under a different name to protect her privacy. Another described her "shock and horror" when she realized her medical insurance did not cover abortion: *It actually didn't seem like an abortion to me, it seemed like a reduction. I can't believe I didn't put those two things together, she [the insurance agent on the phone] said abortion and I said but I'm still pregnant and started to cry.*

As has been discussed in earlier chapters regarding parents pregnant after loss, the simplest sight, smell, or sound can trigger a traumatic memory of being in the room, on the table, and at the moment of the child's death as the result of a decision they made. The bleep of the heartbeats slowly fades into silence, signifying for some in that room a successful procedure, but for others the end of a dream:

> There I am in this darkened room, lying on a table with my stomach, with all this brown stuff on it, the smell of iodine, lying in this freezing cold room; the air was cranked. The curtains were closed and I could feel the glow of the ultrasound screen, the reddish/greenish, snowy kind of image. The doctor's obnoxious manner, his bald head, and the smell of that room, they just stay with me, I could not get out.
>
> I watched them do the ultrasound and saw the babies for the last time, and as soon as they began prepping my stomach I looked away, just looked at the ceiling and started crying. But I didn't move, knowing that if I moved it could hurt all of the babies.

One mother described the comfort she gained from singing to her babies the night before her reduction, behavior that speaks to deep love for all her babies:

> I just kept taking baths with the lights out just singing to my babies, just knowing that it would be the last time I would be with them all [crying]. I had a special song that I sang.

Continuing with the pregnancy

After the procedure parents are expected to return to their normal lives and stay focused on the goal, a successful outcome for this pregnancy. But as they leave, their deceased baby (or babies) remains alongside the living one/s, causing enduring complicated issues; they experience guilt and grief that they often cannot share. *Every day, you think about what is inside you, there is life inside you and there is death inside you.* Those who do try to give support, often say, "Be happy you still have a living baby." *It isn't very consoling to hear that you still have a healthy baby in the midst of grieving the loss of the others. It is not like they are replaceable, babies I mean.*

Success and failure are measured in gestational milestones unique to the individual experience. One woman described feeling able to relax after she reached the 22-week mark because her doctor had told her that most miscarriages related to MFPR happened between 18–22 weeks. Another woman waited until week 24 in her pregnancy—the age of viability. Still another could not see even 35 weeks as successful because anything short of full term was a failure.

Unfortunately, "medical curiosity" can surround MFPR. Doctors, nurses, and ultrasound technicians can all be fascinated by the learning opportunity provided by someone who has undergone MFPR. Parents should be informed they have a right to privacy and to refuse some requests if they feel something is being done for non-medical reasons regarding their case. A mother who reduced her quadruplet pregnancy to twins recalls feeling *like a freak on display*. She described many situations in which either the medical staff failed to read her chart beforehand or were just curious to see what a reduced pregnancy looked like:

> *A doctor examining me claimed that he was not able to find the second heartbeat and suggested we go in and take a look. He took me into one of the ultrasound rooms but I just sort of felt like he wanted to see the other babies. A lot of the time it just felt like some of the ultrasound techs and that doctor in particular were interested in what was left of the other babies. At my ultrasound the next week, the ultrasound tech didn't read my chart so when she was scanning she said, oh my goodness, I think that two of the babies have died. I just said I know that. That was sort of upsetting and it happened a couple of times.*

Martha[2] (described in Wegner 2015) learned she was pregnant with twins during her first ultrasound at 13 weeks gestation, a boy and a girl. At the same time, she was given the news that her daughter had Down's syndrome and severe hydrops, the latter condition meaning she would likely die in utero or at birth. Subsequent ultrasounds showed a heart defect and fluid filling her lungs, which meant that, as she developed in the womb, she would produce too much amniotic fluid. The loss of both babies was a real possibility. In Martha's previous pregnancy, with her healthy three year old, she had barely made it to term so was already at risk for preterm labor. *Based on her very slim chances of survival, and the very real threat her presence caused to the survival of her brother, we opted for selective reduction, a decision no parent should ever have to make* (ibid, p. 6).

Told to go on as if she now had a "normal" singleton pregnancy, Martha was confused:

> *Soon after the death of the baby my midwife assured me, "Everything can be normal now. There is no reason to believe this dead fetus will cause any problems for*

> *the pregnancy. In fact, we can proceed as if this is just a normal pregnancy." I was so relieved. No more decisions. No more anguish.*

Initially believing the worst was behind her, Martha's feelings did not match those of a "normal" pregnancy. She was not feeling relieved and struggled with sadness, anxiety, and anger; feelings the health care provider led her to believe she shouldn't or wouldn't have. She sought help in trying to understand why she could not stop crying or be happy for the surviving baby:

> *After a long, tearful talk with this woman, I asked, "When will I finally stop feeling as if I'm carrying twins?" She answered quietly, "Never. You are carrying twins."*
>
> *We had experienced a death in the family. I realized the only way I was going to get through this was to acknowledge it. It was not a normal single pregnancy. We had seen this baby on ultrasound. She looked to us just like her brother, bouncing and kicking in the water around her.... I decided to reclaim the truth. I was carrying twins. One was living; one was dead. This was and is our child.*

Claiming parenthood for the deceased baby as a member of the family is important for parents who go through MFPR. Learning she was still carrying twins validated her feeling of grief as legitimate and normal. She needed to grieve for her loss and claim her child, not the loss of a "genetic abnormality."

> *As part of our process of reclaiming the truth, we decided to name the baby who had died. She was, after all, our baby, and deserved a name. We chose Laura. John and I always loved that name, just as we would always love this baby.*

Joe and his wife Joy (pseudonyms) were pregnant with triplets who died at 22 weeks gestation, apparently as the result of an infection following the placement of a cervical cerclage.[3] Joy described vomiting throughout the pregnancy: *The triplet pregnancy was just a nightmare 24 hours a day until they were delivered.*

In the smooth phase, as they prepared for another round of IVF, Joy was adamant she would not carry triplets again, because she was not willing to lose all of them. They discussed reducing if this happened because she had no confidence in her body's ability to carry three babies:

> *I processed a lot of it before I got pregnant. I met with an ethicist, talked it through with him, someone from my religious perspective who does a lot of medical esthetics. I told Joe, I think we need to make this decision before we even try to get pregnant again, which is that I won't have triplets again. I can't. I had my sort of justifications and reasons for thinking why reduction would be better than risking triplets again. And he really agreed with that and talked it through.*

Joe understood her reasoning but made an emotional plea to not reduce, praying they would not have to make the decision: *I really understood where she was at with it. She wasn't being callous or dismissive about it.*

Two years after their loss they conceived following reproductive assistance, and were again pregnant with triplets. In the break–up phase of prenatal parenting they were taken back to how the last pregnancy ended; feeling the same kind of stress and anxiety, getting bad news from the medical people, and having to make hard decisions:

> We did the ultrasound at six weeks gestation and we could see three of them in there but the tech. didn't really want to talk about it too much. And the doctor tried to down-play the third one. "Well, it doesn't look good. We're not sure about this." So it was just, go in there feeling, for me, anxious and the physical feeling of it's already beyond our control, taken out of our hands. We didn't want to relive what happened the last time. We tried triplets before and we would have better odds reducing to twins but emotionally it felt completely wrong. We spent the last two years caring about those triplets, trying to make sense of their deaths, recognizing them as individuals, with individual lives and so forth and suddenly to turn around and be like, well this B or C has got to go. That felt really wrong to me. It just felt like an instance where technology has really gone on too far ahead of where we are at as human beings. To even be thinking of that would not even occur to anybody prior to technology.
>
> But Joe doesn't process things deeply until he's actually in the situation. And I do both. I do it ahead of time and I do it at the time. So I think it was traumatic for him at a really different level because he kept thinking, and he said it recently in the last couple of weeks, like maybe you could have handled triplets.

Joe shared his feelings about those weeks:

> It was hard and painful for her. She ultimately just related, this is what it is. We have to do what I can. That was the low point and what can you say? It's a horrible decision to make and I'm okay with why we did it and from that point she improved. Her nausea got better within a day or two. Also the second trimester she started feeling better. The similarities between the first and second pregnancy stopped. This is a different path that we're now on and the decision started lessening the fear of just what had happened before.

They also experienced complications due to their conservative faith community. People were happy for them but Joe and Joy couldn't tell anyone the truth about the pregnancy so they had to pretend:

> Our whole world is considered to be Evangelical, which complicated the decision that much farther. Just the rigidity of pro-life things that I live in and work in makes it, I don't know how I could talk about it, it is just so much part of abortion. So that whole religious thing made it very, very hard.

During the sorting-out phase Joy viewed the pregnancy as hypothetical, waking up at night and thinking *Am I still pregnant? Did this last through the night?* If she was around other pregnant people, she would think:

> *Well, I'm not really pregnant the way you are. I'm sort of, I might be pregnant. I might be having a baby. We talked to them as people, as babies but very conditionally, like if it happens, if they live, if things work out.*

Both parents struggled with emotional cushioning, holding back feelings of embracing the pregnancy and baby, while also wanting to believe all would be well (Côté-Arsenault & Donato, 2011)

> *If they died we would have been devastated and would have said, you can't control how much you want a pregnancy or how much you love a fetus. We both sort of pretend that we don't pretend that we didn't love them. But at some level we know that wasn't true.*

When Joy passed 18 weeks gestation she realized that if this pregnancy ended they were going to hold and see visible babies:

> *We started talking about names at that point. I'm going to deliver these babies one way or another and however it is they need to have names and be part of our family as opposed to, I don't think we would have done that if we would have miscarried earlier.*

As they moved into the inwardizing phase they felt more confident in handling the pregnancy. Joy fully embraced the babies' personhood:

> *There's also a sense in which the more they move it starts to feel, it might or might not work out. I felt like I'm not going to say to a two year old, you may or may not become an adult so I'm not going to take you seriously until you prove yourself. You take a person seriously from where they're at, at the time. The more alive they seemed the more I felt like I owed them my whole heart. I should put my whole heart into this. Because they're doing the best they can. But I think it was 24, 25 weeks when I said to Joe, "I'm just putting my whole heart into this. I'm just going to, [crying], I'm not hedging my bets and talking badly about it. I'm going to believe it's going to happen."*

They began to believe they were going to take home babies even though Joe continued to worry. His comment below calls attention to research suggesting that bereaved parents are prone to more health issues later on in life (Li et al. 2003, 2005).

> *I have a stress level that I'm just so used to and feel like my general health and well-being is gone. But overall the experience is …. breathe a sigh of relief that she's 24 weeks and there's no reason why she can't get to 36 and be happy to induce at that point. The babies seem to be thriving and doing well at what they do.*

Some parents go on as if they became pregnant with a certain number of fetuses while others want to continue honoring the deceased baby. Joe asked if he could see the deceased baby during one of the next ultrasounds but was dismissed by the doctor who said, "What's there to see. You are pregnant with twins." This compounded his sorrow.

The birth: expansion to "neurotic" fitting together

As parents move into the last weeks of pregnancy they will need guidance on how to prepare for the birth, such as touring the birthing area and the NICU/special care nursery in case one or more of their babies may be admitted and considering who will be their extra source of support. Just as found with parents of a surviving twin, birth signifies the end of the relationship they had with all their babies:

> And then all of a sudden, boom, this was over and as soon as they sewed me up there was no longer this connection with this triplet. He is literally gone from my life. At least when he was inside of me I could grieve., I remember just sitting up at night and rocking my arms and saying, I'm sorry that I have done this to you, this ghost baby, that was no longer going to be a part of me anymore. I now wish I could have buried him or something, no one even told me that I could and it made me angry.

Parents also need to process whether they wish to see their deceased babies or, if reabsorbed, take the placenta to bury at their place of choice. Some mothers felt they missed an opportunity to say goodbye:

> I was offered an opportunity to see the other babies. At the time I was shocked by this and turned it down. I wish they had given me information so I could have made a choice.

> I wanted to prepare myself. After talking with women in the group I contacted our local cremation society and they took care of things. The state where I lived issued death certificates for fetal deaths after 18 weeks, mine died at 23. I put them on my contact list for delivery and they handled it. I hated to have to think about that, it was sad, but I needed to be responsible and take care of it.

> I got to spend a few hours with her and they took pictures. I am now glad I have them … I have her ashes. I just can't imagine not having her with me. Our plan is, the first parent that dies, which ever one of us that will be, will be combined with her ashes. We are going to put them in the ocean when the last parent alive feels comfortable enough to do that, to say goodbye. That way she will always be a part of us.

Martha was told throughout labor not to have hope, that Laura would have been reabsorbed because she died at 15 weeks gestation. The medical staff were wrong. After her healthy brother was born, Laura was brought in to her:

> A few hours later I asked to see Laura. They had put her body into a little crib. She weighed 2.2 ounces and was 3½ inches long. I held her in my hands. She was

perfectly formed. She had arms, legs, fingers, ribs. I wondered, "Who would you have looked like?"

(Wegner 2015, p. 10)

Signing the birth certificate is another milestone for these parents. Are they parents of multiples or do they wish to list based on the number of babies born alive? Martha was adamant Laura needed to be claimed:

Before I left the hospital the nurse sent down the birth certificate for David. On it was checked "single birth." I sent it back unsigned. It was a twin pregnancy and it would be listed as that. This was my first time advocating for my unborn daughter.

The presence of healthy babies, while a celebration, is also a constant reminder of other missing children. Leaving the hospital with healthy babies does not change the fact that there is still a missing baby in the family:

As we left the hospital I couldn't shake the nagging ache that while I was taking David home with me, I was leaving Laura behind. It felt like the beginning of two separate journeys. How could I take one with me and leave the other?

Most parents need reassurance that their baby did have a disability in order to know they made the right choice. Parents who are struggling with these feelings need encouragement to get more information, as indeed this mother did:

After David's birth I was a little shell-shocked. I was filled with remorse and nagging doubts as to why Laura had died. Was she really that sick? Maybe we had made a mistake. A friend suggested I obtain my medical records and call Dr. Nelson who had been there when she died … reading the reports was painful but strangely reassuring. Laura had been very sick. Her condition was laid out for me in black and white. I read these records many times, so I could know what had ailed my daughter, and why death was inevitable for her.

(Wegner 2015, p. 10)

Other parents want the records for the surviving children when they are older:

A year after she died, I requested her medical records. I just wanted her notes, mainly nurse's notes. I wanted the records about when she ate, when she peed; it helped validate her for me, it proved she existed.

Parenting after the loss

Parenting after MFPR is best described as a journey. A journey of making meaning out of this unspeakable loss and forging a parent–child relationship with both the surviving baby or babies and those who have died. As with parents who birth a healthy baby after a previous loss, parents struggle with a new layer of grief as they watch the surviving child grow:

> *The more I loved David, the more I missed Laura. He was so precious and sweet, I yearned to have another one just like him. Each day my increasing joy and love for him made me realize how much I had lost when his twin sister died. I told myself that when I could finally hold David in my arms everything would be all right. The pain would go away. I would be able to put Laura's death behind me. I was wrong.... The pain continues.*
>
> (Wegner 2015, p. 12)

Others will not necessarily understand that parents will continue to grieve, wanting them to be happy for the surviving baby. But parents continue seeing their role as a parent to their deceased baby; a role that they feel goes virtually unrecognized by anyone other than themselves:

> *The majority of people had no idea the depth of pain a loss like this causes. For some, it's a matter of "out of sight, out of mind." Others believe one should just "get on with it." Pick yourself up by the bootstraps, stop feeling sorry for yourself, and move on with your life. After all, I had one healthy baby to love, wasn't that enough?*

This speaks to the dilemma faced by parents and the reality that they will never be the same again:

> *Sometimes I get this desperate feeling that I want to go back and change the course of time. Not that I don't have you two because you are the light of my life, but that I never had to make the choice. It has changed me forever.*

Changed relationships

The extent to which parents are able to see and understand the relationships that are changed forever is dependent on where they are in their journey. The focus of taking care of a new baby often prevents them from seeing the big picture:

> *For the first couple of years I didn't have time for the grief. Maybe it was too scary, maybe it was too big, maybe I just had too many other things to do.*

Marriages are challenged, some survive, some fail, and others are described as "hanging in limbo" waiting for the grief to subside:

> *Just to understand what my husband was feeling. He had absolutely no connection. We just grieve in such different ways. He doesn't understand. If only I could understand him, it might have helped.*

Some marriages are "stronger after their loss," attributed to understanding that grief was different for their partners:

> *With the reduction, it wasn't an issue for him, it was harder for me. Maybe it is because he didn't carry them. He definitely feels the loss of the twins, he just keeps it to himself and that's okay.*

Relationships with family members and friends can also be affected; some can not share the truth about their choice. Parents encounter mixed reactions: for some, the support and love they need; for others, harsh judgment from loved ones who do not understand or accept their decision, or provide support. Searching for support without judgment, some families turn to cyberspace and a web-based selected reduction support group[4] where it feels more comfortable to share this loss.

> *Friends would come by and give their condolences about the triplet and how it was up with God. I was like, I don't even want to talk about this because you don't even know what really happened.*
>
> *My mom, who used to be a midwife, totally understood. She said we were totally doing the right thing.*
>
> *My grandmother, who is a Catholic, told me that she believed the two babies I reduced were in purgatory and I was going to hell. She said the other two were in purgatory too because they hadn't been baptized.*

Probably the most significant relationship that is impacted by the MFPR decision is the one between the mother and the surviving children as she begins to bond with them and to feel joy in the face of guilt, shame, and grief:

> *The day my son rolled over for the first time was bittersweet. I was so excited and then so sad. My heart begins to ache for what could have been for my daughter. His firsts really cause me to remember all the pain and heartache of the last year. I don't regret my decision, it's just that we had planned for twins for 20 whole weeks and now there is only one.*

They also anticipate every developmental milestone, looking for "healthy outcomes" to prove their decision was worth it. Even outcomes that fall short of "healthy" meet this same need:

> *When I see my little girl and know that she is healthy and happy, I know we got what we wished for. I know we did the right thing.*
>
> *Having one struggling made me think what if I had three boys really struggling. His difficulties helped me let go of my "what if's."*

Moving forward: building memories

Healing, moving forward with grief and finding ways to honor the children as still part of the family in concrete ways, is an important step that professionals need to help parents make. People know they must move forward. But just as there is a difference between curing and healing in disease, so there is a difference between being stuck in grief and honoring one's parenting role, continued bond with and attachment to a child no longer physically in their family.

> I've started on my journey to heal. It will be long but hopefully by the time you make this journey yourself [speaking to her two surviving children] I can be a strength and support for you. I have decided to have a memorial service for your brothers and sisters. It will allow me to embrace them in death just as I embrace you two in life. I have also decided to have a memorial stone made and place it at the cabin. It will always be a place we go to. It will be passed down to you two and your cousins someday. There will always be love and a sense of family there.

Other parents seek a place or object that they can see, touch, or visit:

> I bought a memorial brick and put it in the garden. I also contributed to a quilt square for a quilt that is hanging inside the hospital and it gives me a … I don't have a grave, but it was the hospital that they were all born at so it gives me a place to go.

> I was just looking for some kind of connection to all the babies. I was at an Irish import store and in Ireland the trinity is really big. There are these three circles that start and they spiral, spirals that are the druid representation of death but also the circle of life. The beginning, middle, and end; of life and family, and then the end. I flipped it over and read the back and I thought wow, this is something I could use to memorialize the triplet. I used to look at it and feel sad but now I look at it and I see compassion, empathy, and forgiveness.

The day before they baptized David, Martha held a memorial service and buried Laura's ashes in the roots of the tree planted in her memory:

> The tree has helped immeasurably, giving us a place to go when we need to remember Laura. We put flowers at its base on the anniversary of her death. We put a red ribbon on the tree and sang for her on Christmas Day. The tree is small, but strong and beautiful, and seems to be the perfect object for receiving our grief.
>
> (Wegner 2015, p. 14)

Sheri[1] wrote a journal so that her living children would understand the story of who they are in relationship to what happened during their pregnancy. In order to get through her experience she had to believe in a supreme being:

*I have given your brothers and sisters the chance to live a peaceful life in God's hands…
I hope you listen to my prayers which tell you all I love you. I know we will make it
through all of this. You will all be our guardian angels. I hope you have had the chance
to meet your brothers or sisters who preceded you. I will see you again someday. I know
that the souls of [names five children] are in heaven and have been for some time but
in my body you were all with me. You were mine.*

When to share the story with surviving children

When or whether to disclose the fetal reduction becomes another ethical dilemma
(Little 2010). One study that included 28 mothers and nine fathers (seven of whom
were partners to the mother) found that only four women got advice on whether
to tell their children, and this was sought out by the parent rather than offered by
their health care provider (France et al. 2013). When advice was given, it was to
share the information at a developmentally appropriate level but without giving
details on how to do so.

*I am not sure we'll tell our daughter. If we do, we'll say that we couldn't have carried
three. They made a sacrifice out of love for her. I still don't know if we will tell her.*

What do survivors remember? One can never underestimate what cannot be proven
quantitatively. Some mothers farther along in their journey believe that their children already know. One mother recalled an event that happened as her family was
celebrating Mothers' Day:

*We were all at the dinner table and the boys had made me a nice meal. It was really nice.
I have six chairs at our table; I have had six chairs forever but there are still only five of us.
It was in the middle of dinner and I was enjoying my dinner and it got kind of quiet. My
son, the one who had the most difficulty after the birth and still struggles with some developmental stuff, umm looked over and he had difficulty talking anyway. He struggles with
his apraxia. He usually just says stuff to be part of the conversation. He looked over at the
empty chair and asked where is the other boy. It was so bizarre. My husband and I are
like dead silent and just kept eating. Stuff like that makes me wonder what they know.*

Infant massage intervention with fathers was found to be beneficial in reducing
paternal stress (Cheng et al. 2011). Martha worried about her husband's attachment
to David so gave him a gift certificate to attend an infant massage class. Being in
the group alongside other babies seemed to bring back a deep cellular memory for
David. As noted by Phillips in regards to infant memory (2013, p. 67), "the perceptions and interpretations are sometimes skewed, but the vividness and accuracy of
specific details and events are often astounding,"

*When David was four months old, John took him to an infant massage class one even-
ing. John came home very frustrated. "All David did was cry. I've never heard him cry so*

hard. I couldn't do a thing to comfort him." I told him I would join him the next week to see if I could help. Again, during that second class, David cried; a high pitched, loud, inconsolable cry. The instructor pulled us aside. "I've been doing this for a long time," she said, "I know this kind of cry. It's called a 'release cry.'" It sometimes happens as a baby is being massaged. That's why it sounds so different from his other cries. That's why you're not able to console him. He needs to release his pain."

(Wegner 2015, p. 15)

Children at a very young age understand the emotions and feelings going on in the household. Martha was encouraged to tell her three-and-a-half-year-old daughter about the loss of Laura because she needed to understand why her mother was crying all the time. Martha also realized Christine needed to claim Laura as a sister, an important member of the family:

I had just received a bill for amniocentesis performed on twins, and I was crying. Although I felt unprepared to tell her the sad truth, I struggled as best I could to explain that mommy was carrying twins, that one of them had died, and that I was really sad. I tried to express optimism that the other baby would be just fine. She said nothing, and quickly returned to her play. It wasn't until a few hours later that the questions started: "Why did the baby have to die? Does that mean God won't take care of me either? It isn't fair, I really wanted two babies." It seems that out of the mouths of babes come our deepest thoughts. I answered as best I could which was mostly to say, "No, that doesn't mean God won't take care of you."

(Wegner 2015, p. 7)

Older siblings can feel a fierce sense of loyalty and love for the missing baby and help parents heal with their openness and honesty:

My best friend, Mary, stopped by to visit me and David soon after his birth. No one mentioned Laura. As she [Mary] was leaving, Christine [the big sister] said, 'You know, we had a baby that died. She was David's twin sister. Her name was Laura, and we feel very sad about that."

(Wegner 2015, p. 14)

Sheri received supportive intervention, both individually with a bereavement counselor and through participating in a pregnancy after loss group. Like the other group members, she was also grieving and attaching simultaneously during her pregnancy. From the beginning she knew the surviving babies were part of the experience of their sibling's reduction and, at some level, already knew the story. She lives her life around the belief that her other children are the guardian angels who are watching over them all. As preschool children, her daughter drew pictures of her siblings as angels watching over the family and her son drew a heart at the front door, his father without a mouth, and what appears to be a stick figure holding up the house. There are also five angles to the house, not four as one would normally draw. Sheri

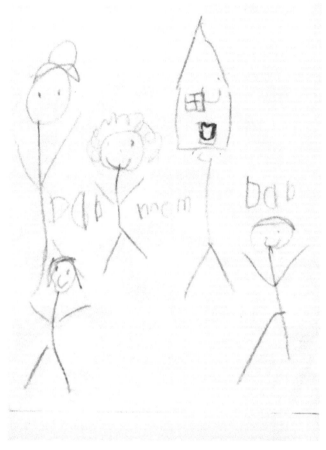

FIGURE 10.1

believes the figure holding up the house represents all the people who supported her through the pregnancy. The father's face lacking a mouth she interpreted as his difficulty in talking about the experience.

Her daughter has given permission to share the two poems she wrote about her siblings in a school assignment when she was 16. The content in both poems is based on her family's faith/belief system as a source of comfort (Thompson et al. 2011).

BOX 10.1

Septuplets

It's been 16 years since the last time we were all together.
   I have so many questions for all of you. Do Jessica and Blake look like me?

Which two of you are identical? How is our older sibling? But … the biggest question is have you thought about how you would tell our story? Because how does one understand these series of events that happened to our mother for her to only have twins. Because I can't help but wonder what if someone told me what I have said a thousand times. "I am a survivor of septuplets."

Jessica's poem is separate as she was the last to die, at 16 weeks gestation, and was born two hours before the cesarean birth of the twins. She was wrapped in a small outfit and held by her father. This speaks to the strength of this mother's ability to not only heal but also provide a foundation from which her children can understand trauma, truth, and love; messages her children will carry throughout their lives.

BOX 10.2

Jessica

She holds his hand and asks why, "Why do I have to go with you?
    Where is my mom?" He grabs her hand and looks at her with the answer in his face.
    A face filled with forgiveness and reassurance. He knows what it's like to be taken from his family on earth and brought to this new place. Four other angels begin to walk towards their sister with the same questions. All five hold hands as they stand in a line looking down at their feet through the clouds. Below sit a brother and sister playing with their mom. This family is theirs, a family only watched from above.
    Smiling they wave while whispering to their mother loving words for her to one day hear.

Case study

BOX 10.3

Sheri's[5] story

Note the love and protection Sheri shows to her deceased babies, interwoven into their family life, and her respect for Courtney and Nathan's emotional understanding of what happened. She is aware that many parents are not able to openly share their experiences and thus wrote her dissertation on this topic.

One year after marriage we began the rollercoaster ride of infertility, entering the smooth phase of prenatal parenting. Referred to an obstetric gynecologist who "did fertility" at my local clinic, I was prescribed Clomid. We became pregnant on our first dose but my body didn't recognize the pregnancy and I miscarried. This was followed by five more cycles, three "diagnostic procedures," and zero luck. Each month I would tell random people that I was pregnant and each month be devastated. Finally coming to terms with my infertility, I accepted referral to an infertility specialist and realized I needed to seek therapy to cope. The therapist helped me through my journey of pregnancy, loss, and the birth of my surviving children. During the pregnancy, she conducted phone sessions, often giving me longer than an hour. She was the first person who allowed me to feel my sadness and wasn't trying to fix or pretend it wasn't there, especially after the loss, when "everyone" wanted to just move on with a normal pregnancy.

The first meeting with the infertility specialist found that my hormones were "off" and I was prescribed medication to reduce my testosterone level. I was given the option to try Clomid again or to move to injectable fertility drugs. Choosing the injectable option, we completed our first cycle with the addition of IUI [intrauterine insemination], where my husband's semen was injected directly into my uterus through a catheter. After nine months of infertility treatment, the quest to become pregnant became an obsession for me. It changed my personality, impacted my ability to regulate my moods, and placed a strain on my marriage. Our first cycle failed but our second was a charm.

The morning I drove to the doctor for the pregnancy test, I was vomiting all the way. Not getting my hopes up, I instead chose to think it was somehow related to the crazy amount of hormones I had been taking. After 21 needle pokes to attempt a blood draw, the test confirmed that I was pregnant. The hCG numbers were "higher than expected," which could indicate multiples.[6] An ultrasound scheduled the following week placed me at four weeks post-conception. I was finally in the break-up phase, full force!

At the first three ultrasounds four gestational sacs were present; however, we were told that the chances were slim that they would all develop into viable fetuses. We left that appointment feeling a mixture of fear and sadness. If they were all viable, we would be faced with a decision about having quadruplets; if they didn't, we would have another loss. At the fourth ultrasound, scheduled the following week with our first prenatal checkup, they found one heartbeat. My husband asked what the chances were that there would be more than one baby and was told they were slim. I was prescribed prenatal vitamins and then scheduled for another ultrasound the following week.

We arrived at the fourth ultrasound, nervous that we had lost the baby as I was spotting almost daily. Instead this ultrasound showed the presence of multiple heartbeats. The nurse and ultrasound technician began counting and recounting; one, two, three, four, five…. One went to find a doctor, who came in and examined the screen. She counted, one, two, three, four, five … six. The room was quiet and all I could do was cry, knowing what this meant. My husband, still in a daze, asked "What next?" Apparently, I would need to speak to the doctor to discuss my options but reduction was recommended. She said I would be provided with the name of a physician who performed the procedure. We went home and cried. We had talked about this before we began treatment, agreed that we would undergo a reduction with anything higher than triplets, but never truly believed we would have to make this choice. It seemed so easy "before" but now just seemed so unfair. The next appointment resulted in few answers and we were given the number of a perinatologist who performed reductions. I went home, called to set up the appointment, and waited for the doctor to call. At the time of my decision, no one had successfully carried seven babies to a viable age. Bobbi McCaughey delivered septuplets that November and the issue of MFPR became front and center.

Then we told our family. Knowing that this was a controversial decision and having already experienced close friends offering an opinion on what they would choose, we quickly learned there was a great deal of judgment and shame associated with this decision. We asked our parents to respect our right to determine who we would tell and when. My parents respected our wishes and supported our decision. In contrast, my husband's parents struggled with their religious beliefs and our choice and arrived the next evening to "talk about it." My husband was not home. My mother-in-law told me she felt that I was killing my babies, she didn't agree with the decision, while my father-in-law talked about the financial obligations of having seven children—both clearly inappropriate conversations. I defended my decision but knew they were passing judgment. On another occasion, my mother-in-law asked me if abortion rights activists picketed my doctor's office. I reminded her that my doctor did reductions not abortions. She then told others about our decision. It felt like she was making it about her and that it was "interesting." Family and friends talked about us behind our back or told us what choice they would have made, none of which was helpful or supportive. That year, we got five Christmas cards. People stopped coming over or inviting us to family activities. I was on bed rest and couldn't attend, but they stopped inviting my husband too.

Three weeks later, my husband and I found ourselves sitting in the office of the doctor who would perform our reduction. She did an exam, explained the procedure, answered our questions, and suggested that we do another ultrasound to see "if Mother Nature" had taken care of the problem. We walked over to the hospital for the ultrasound, the first of many appointments at the hospital we would become so familiar with. As we watched the screen, and prayed that there would be one or two heartbeats, that God would be kind, we heard her begin counting, one, two, three, four, five, six … seven. She could now see a set of identical twins in addition to the other five fetuses, which presented a new problem. The identical set was sitting close to my cervix but needed to be reduced as the complications associated with identical twins decreased our chances of a successful outcome. She said that we should go home and schedule our first reduction in one week.

The day of the reduction, 10 weeks along in my pregnancy, we arrived at the hospital at 5 a.m. They said that the procedure was scheduled before clinic hours for our benefit but it felt as though we were booked so early because there was something secretive or shameful about our decision. After all, we were feeling a sense of shame. We were escorted into the room and the lights were dimmed. The doctor explained that she would be inserting a needle through my abdominal wall, into my uterus and then into the heart sac of the fetus. She would reduce two today and two in two weeks' time. My husband sat at my head, the ultrasound technician at the foot of the table, and the doctor on my right. She gave me the options of turning away for the procedure or watching the screen. I decided that, as a mother, I needed to watch the screen and felt it was necessary to be present in the final moments of my children's lives that I was choosing to end. As the needle entered my abdominal wall, my husband got up and left the room. I waited for him to share my pain and sorrow, to somehow make this day easier, but he never returned. Later, he told me that the needle made him feel faint and he couldn't watch. I didn't get to leave that room and pretend that it was not happening. I don't think I have ever been able to leave that room because, as I write my story, I am taken back in time. I can see the room, smell the smells, and hear the sounds of the ultrasound recording the slowing of their heartbeats and then the silence, signaling a successful reduction and the death of my children. For the second reduction, scheduled at 12 weeks, I asked my parents to come because I just couldn't do that alone. My mom stood by my side, never leaving or looking away, helping to reassure me that I would survive this day, that I would not have to do this alone, because my husband's absence made me feel so alone.

I was told to rest for a few days and then given the clearance to go to our cabin for Labor Day weekend. This was the first and the last time I would be able to go to my parents' home for the next eight months. That weekend, Princess Diana died in a tragic car accident. I apparently was having contractions, which I didn't recognize as I had never been pregnant and they didn't hurt. I woke up that Tuesday morning bleeding red blood. I went in immediately to the doctor who told me that due to a complication of the reductions, one of the remaining fetuses had died. I now needed to be on full bed rest. At 3 a.m. approximately a week later, my waters broke. The fear and despair I felt knowing that another one of my babies had died was overwhelming. I called the emergency number of my OBGYN as my care had been returned to him after the reductions and told I would now be a "normal triplet pregnancy." I was instructed to go back to bed because there was nothing they could do at 12 weeks. I hung up and phoned the on-call service for the perinatology practice where my reduction had been carried out. They told me to come to the hospital—the first of many middle of the night trips to the hospital. The next day the doctor did an ultrasound and confirmed that the two surviving babies were healthy and growing, and that the water I lost must have been embryotic fluid from the triplet. I transferred my care to the perinatology practice and was sent home with an appointment scheduled for three weeks' time, when I would be at 15 weeks gestation. All of these events occurred before I was halfway through the sorting-out phase of prenatal parenting.

For the next three weeks, I cramped, bled, and worried but was told that this was normal and to drink water and rest. My parents came to my next appointment and we met my husband there. The doctor did a routine ultrasound in the office to check on the remaining babies. As she scanned the reduced fetuses, she noticed what she thought was movement in the triplet. Just as a precaution, she said that we should go to the hospital for an ultrasound. The doctor confirmed that there was a heartbeat in the triplet; however, the embryotic sac had ruptured at 12 weeks and the baby's chance of survival was low. He also said that the chance of losing the entire pregnancy was extremely high and recommended that we reduce the triplet immediately. He added that if by chance we did carry the baby to a viable age, the lungs would not develop and it would most likely die at birth. We made the only choice we could: another reduction was scheduled.

I knew that my baby could hear at 15 weeks and that she knew that we were making this choice. That night I remember lying in my bed, talking to her and the other two, trying to justify my decision and to let her know how much she was loved. My husband, overwhelmed by the whole experience, would say that he felt scared, sad, and helpless and had taken to sleeping in the next room, partially because I was sick 24 hours a day and partially because it was just easier. I felt alone, abandoned, and left to "do this on my own." The next day we went to the hospital at 5 a.m., into the same room, and watched another one of my babies die. But this time she looked more like a human than a fetus, and as the needle approached, she reached out to touch it. I watched the screen until the blip went silent and the doctor left the room. I got up, dressed, and went home.

After this reduction, I met Joann who ran the PAL groups and provided one on one support for mothers who had experienced or were experiencing high-risk pregnancies. She called the day after the reduction; the second person with whom I could talk openly about my feelings. She didn't try to convince me to be happy or change the subject. She met me at my next appointment and invited me to attend the weekly PAL group. We attended one meeting but it felt weird. These women had experienced a loss in a previous pregnancy and I had experienced loss in my current pregnancy. Hearing their stories increased my anxiety and doubts that my babies would survive. I then attended a group where we did guided imagery and relaxation activities with Joann and her colleague, Lynnda Parker. This group felt more comfortable because we didn't have to talk about grief and loss. Joann met me at every appointment, called often, was present for my delivery, and supported me after the birth.

Still in the sorting-out phase of prenatal parenting, I had weekly visits and was monitored closely. My days consisted of watching the clock and count-ing time until I was 24 weeks, just hoping to get to 34 weeks. At 18 weeks I began having contractions. I knew what they were this time and called my husband to ask him to bring me to the hospital. He was frustrated and felt that I was over-reacting as we had just been to the doctor the day before; however, I knew that something wasn't right. We agreed that he would take me in when he was done with work. I was admitted to the hospital with pre-term labor. The doctor said there was little he could do at 18 weeks but he would try administering medication in the hope of stopping the contractions and I should prepare to be hospitalized from this point on. After 24 hours of being contraction free, I was sent home on an over-the-counter magnesium supplement. After the hospitalization, in-home services began; first weekly and then twice weekly. The facilitator of the group called weekly to check in to see how I was doing.

At 20 weeks, we had a level two ultrasound where we would hopefully be able to determine the gender of the babies. I had heard the heartbeats multiple times and knew that there were two very different heart rates. The ultrasound confirmed that we were having boy/girl twins, who then became referred to as Courtney and Nathan.

After I reached 24 weeks, now in the inwardizing phase, something changed for me and I was able to embrace the pregnancy. I still didn't trust that I would have "live" babies, but I was able to begin planning for their delivery. I wrote my birth plan and decided what to do with the remains of the other babies, toured the NICU and special care nursery, and planned for what might/could happen. It gave me a sense of control over what was happening.

At 31 weeks, Courtney stopped growing so delivery at 34 weeks was rec-ommended. An amniocentesis was scheduled and doctors reviewed delivery options. Courtney presented breech and doctors feared that she would not descend if I delivered vaginally. Nathan was head down so I was given the option to deliver him vaginally and then do a C-section for Courtney. I chose the C-section, partly because the thought of doing both seemed like a lot of work and partly because if they surgically removed the babies they could get them out where they needed to be quickly and I felt that would be the safest.

By 32 weeks, entering the expansion phase, my blood pressure had risen and the in-home nurse was concerned. The medical staff determined that I should go in to the hospital to be evaluated and I waited for my husband to come home. My mother, who happened to be visiting (she came every two weeks to clean, grocery shop, and makes meals for us), went to the hospital with us. The nurse had explained the risks associated with pre-eclampsia and how dangerous they could be for my health. I remember thinking that I had worked too hard to lose the babies now and asking my husband what decision he would make if he had to choose between me and the babies. He said me. At the time, I thought he didn't care as much about the babies as I did. The answer for me was clearly to save the children. Later, I understood that was an impossible choice for him to make. He was fearful of coming home from the hospital with no wife and no children.

I was hospitalized, monitored throughout the night, and administered medication to prepare for a preterm birth. The next morning Nathan's waters broke. I did not go into labor for nine more days but the babies were healthy. At 33 weeks and 5 days, I began to have contractions early in the morning and they continued throughout the day. I was not dilating so the doctors were hoping that they could do the amniocentesis the next day. However, at 2 p.m., I passed the triplet who had died at 15 weeks (Jessica), born looking like a baby and approximately 4 inches long. The nurse dressed her in a gown and let us spend the day with her. My husband held her in the palm of his hand. It was sad, hard, and a bit scary but I feel that Jessica prepared us for how small Courtney and Nathan would be. The nurse also called the doctors, advocated for me to deliver that day due to the emotional strain, and worked an extra shift to stay for their births. Courtney and Nathan were born crying and alive, breathing on their own. I have forgotten the nurse's name after all these years but I can still see her face and feel deep appreciation for how much she cared and her willingness to be part of my journey.

Now in the "neurotic" fitting together phase, being discharged from the hospital was difficult. The intense grief and sadness I felt walking out of the hospital room caught me by surprise. This was the last place in which I had had all my babies with me. I would be leaving five behind. Joann's office was across the hall so I walked over to get her. I felt so sad and such intense grief and loss. No one understood because I would soon be leaving the hospital with two living babies. We went back into the room and took pictures of the last place in which I had had all my babies. I should be grateful and happy but I wasn't. Holding the opposing feelings of grief and joy is complicated, but I was able to leave and move to the hotel room; my home for the next four weeks. I was grateful for the stay in the hospital because my home was not the last place they were all with me; the loss was associated with the hospital.

We arrived home on an unusually warm gray day in February. My other babies were sent to the pathology lab for 30 days to examine the reason why my placenta had failed to nourish the two remaining, and then sent to the Cremation Society where they were placed in a container. We thought about burying them at the cemetery or at our cabin, but the nagging thought of what would happen if we moved house or sold the cabin always entered my mind. I finally decided to keep them at the house with the request that, when I die, they be buried with me.

Everyone wanted to come and visit. I limited visitors, saying that no one could come until cold and flu season was over, but in reality it was because I couldn't bear to put on my happy face and pretend that I wasn't sad. My mother-in-law told me to "get over it." My mother felt that I didn't have time to be sad because I needed to care for my babies. I suffered with what I now know was post-partum depression but was afraid to say anything for fear of being seen as ungrateful or a bad mother. I didn't sleep because they didn't sleep. The first night they came home from the hospital and I placed them in the quiet dark room, they screamed. I felt like a failure when I could not console them. I didn't consider that they had experienced multiple traumas too, that they had been born into the world early, not yet able to regulate the sensory experiences of the outside world.

Over that year, I worked to move forward. I joined ECFE (Early Childhood Family Education) and met other moms in the community; went to the library, the book store and scheduled play dates like normal moms. I learned who I could share my story with and who I could not. Along the way, I found small ways to heal. The year my children were born *The Next Place*[7] was published, and reading it brought me peace and comfort. I found the children's book *Baby Angels*[8] about baby angels watching over an infant and keeping her safe. The story featured five angels, just like my own five lost babies. I read this book to Courtney and Nathan and this helped me heal.

As they grew and became verbal, there were signs that they too knew their story but I had never given words to it for them. Courtney used to ask me to tell her "how the doctors chose her." When playing house, Courtney would introduce me to her "family" saying "This is my new family. My old family is dead." When they were about 3 ½ we talked about their birth story. I told them they were part of a septuplet pregnancy and had five other brothers and sisters. Courtney asked me if I loved them and Nathan asked me if I was sad and then they went to their room to play. Over the years we have talked more about the details of their story based on their developmental readiness to comprehend the information. They know the truth and have also had to learn when to share and when to keep it a secret. Courtney talks about it more often than her brother. In her graduation pictures, she wore a necklace with the number 7 on it. We came across it shopping. It's funny how we have happened upon items, experiences, and people throughout our journey that have helped us to created meaning from our experience.

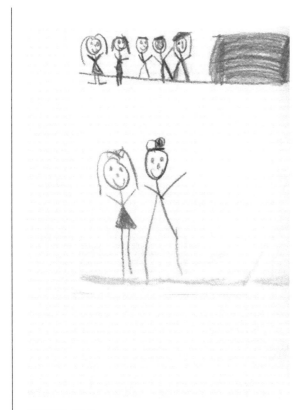

FIGURE 10.2

Summary

This chapter has addressed the complexity of loss in multi-fetal pregnancy when the loss was by choice. Although parents may be at different places on their journey and perhaps on slightly different paths, they share a common destination. They seek forgiveness, to make peace with their spirituality, their children, and their choice but understand it must first come from within. They are unsure of where, when, or even if their journey will end but understand that finding the meaning in the journey is far more important than reaching the final destination.

These stories illustrate the importance of receiving supportive care as they address their parental feelings during the decision-making process, continuing the pregnancy, experiencing birth, and moving forward to raise their living children. These stories are told from the perspectives of the mothers; only one father is represented. Further research with fathers is clearly needed. Parents need a place in which to tell their story and to process with caring professionals when and how to tell it to their surviving children. The issue is not about whether MFPR is right or wrong; that is for the individual making the choice to decide. The issue is how to best understand and support parents who choose to undergo MFPR.

11

HEART-BREAKING CHOICES

Elective termination as a result of a genetic abnormality in one's baby is an extremely political topic yet little has been explored from the parents' perspective. While personal stories have been written by parents who choose to continue their pregnancy (Grady & O'Leary 1993; Kuebelbeck 2003; Kuebelbeck & Davis 2011), this chapter explores the experience of parents who made a different decision: ending the pregnancy of their much wanted baby.[1] This choice can mean parents feel judged and unwelcome in infant loss support groups. In spite of societal views in regard to fetal reduction and termination, the prenatal parenting model of intervention can be a useful guide to help parents make meaning of their attachment relationship and continued bond to their baby when they make this painful decision.

Incidence of termination

It is estimated that 40 percent of women in the US will have at least one abortion in their lifetime (Henshaw 1998). The euphemistic medical terms "elective termination of pregnancy" and "selective reduction" shield parents and health care providers alike from this quandary resulting from advances in perinatal technology. Genetic counseling is not routinely offered by perinatal clinics at routine 18–20-week appointments to confirm dates (McCoyd 2007) and so parents are often naïve at the beginning of a "routine ultrasound" (McCoyd 2009).

The increase in prenatal screening and testing has resulted in detecting an ever-widening range of fetal abnormalities (Bourguignon et al. 1999). There is an expectation that women feel grateful for technology, tempered with a sense of reassurance that all is well; however, technology can also bring life-changing news leading to disillusionment (McCoyd 2009, 2010). The medicalization of human fertility contributes to the illusion of omnipotence within reproductive health care, which is difficult to reconcile when things go wrong (Earle et al. 2008). In McCoyd's

(2013) study, fewer than half of the mothers had discussed the possibility of a fetal anomaly with the father of the baby and fewer than a third with anyone else, indicating a relatively high level of denial or lack of preparation for this outcome.

The advent of ultrasound technology, assisted conception, and amniocentesis means the personhood of an unborn baby and discovery of its gender occurs for many parents at an earlier gestational age (Sell-Smith & Lax 2013). In one sense, medical technology has created as many problems as it has solved (McCoyd 2009). Learning their baby has a genetic disorder interrupts parents' fantasies of the hoped-for child (Bourguignon et al. 1999; Collopy 2004; Côté-Arsenault & Denney-Koelsch 2011; Côté-Arsenault et al. 2015; Culling 2013; Grady & O'Leary 1993; McCoyd 2009). The diagnosis is not only traumatic but also in direct conflict with parents' myths and expectations when they arrive for an ultrasound (Culling 2013; McCoyd 2013; Sutan & Miskam 2012). Parents are faced with the choice of becoming bereaved parents or parents to a child with a disability and often significant health problems in a society where funding for support services can be limited (McCoyd 2007; Parish & Cloud 2006; Parish et al. 2012). Health care providers are often uncomfortable when seeing a baby with abnormalities and, without intention, may lean toward termination (Earle et al. 2008). It is important that providers refrain from making assumptions regarding parents' likelihood of terminating based on factors such as maternal age, gestational age, type of procedure, or ultrasound result (Hawkins et al. 2013).

The decision to terminate a baby with a genetic abnormality is a painful one and never taken lightly (Brady et al. 2008; Culling 2013; Geerinck-Vercammen & Kanhai 2003; Grady & O'Leary 1993; McCoyd 2007, 2009, 2010). Regardless of the severity of the diagnosis, pregnancy termination is an emotionally challenging experience influenced by many personal, social, cultural, political, and psychological factors (Hawkins et al. 2013; Sell-Smith & Lax 2013). While presented as a medical decision by health care providers, families view decisions through the lens of being a parent (Culling 2013). Some parents face the decision within a tight timeframe due to the narrow window of gestational age during which terminations can be performed safely and reliably (McCoyd 2013). The ambivalent societal messages and political climate surrounding choice in the US strongly influence the emotional responses of women and their partners, causing many to suffer in silence. Women and their partners may be influenced by the generally negative attitudes toward abortion, increasing their sense of guilt and often discouraging open discussion of feelings, all of which complicate the grieving process (Gordon et al. 2007). Parents' ability to receive the empathy and support they desperately need is thus compromised (McCoyd 2007), their sense of guilt may continue long after the pregnancy has ended (Benute et al. 2012a), and their parenting status remains unvalidated (Grady & O'Leary 1993). Parents are rarely able to share how their baby died, and, fearing the reactions of other people, often choose to say they had a miscarriage (Thachuk 2007). Termination for a young mother can be viewed as a positive solution to the "problem" of teenage pregnancy, further complicating grief (Brady et al. 2008). In the case of elective abortion without a known disability, grief is almost inevitable, with intensity found to be related to the length of pregnancy (Little 2010; Korenromp et al. 2007; Peppers & Knapp 1980). Although they were assessed only four months after termination, one study found that 44 percent of men and women demonstrated symptoms of depression and PTSD (Korenromp et al. 2007).

Cultural considerations

Positions on abortion vary depending on the cultural and religious beliefs of the parents. However, they influence both the grieving process of those involved in making the decision and societal attitudes towards them (Little 2010; Korenromp et al. 2005, 2007; McCoyd 2009, 2013). In Brazil, termination of a lethally malformed fetus is possible only after judicial authorization (Diniz 2007). For Malayan Muslims, termination is dependent on husband and family approval (Sutan & Miskam 2012).

In some countries, such as Malaysia, maternal prenatal diagnosis is not a routine practice except for couples who have experienced a previous perinatal death or abnormal fetus (ibid). In India (Amarapurkar 2010) and China, ultrasounds are often done to screen for gender, both countries preferring boys.[2] By ethnicity, the highest termination rates have been observed in Asian and Asian Indian populations, followed closely by Caucasian populations; rates are lower in Filipino and Hispanic populations (Hawkins et al. 2013).

It is important to view the definition of personhood for a deceased fetus through cultural and societal lenses (Sell-Smith & Lax 2013). According to Shari'ah law, the soul (*Ruh*) enters the fetus at 120 days (four months) from conception. The abortion of a fetus within the first 120 days is approved within the Islamic community if it is affected by an incurable disability that can result in a miserable life for the child and family.[3] For Japanese mothers who choose to abort, the family still respects that child's life (as they consider the fetus to already have a soul) by honoring them in special places set aside with Jizu statues, the Buddhist protector of the souls of children.[4] Statues of Jizo can sometimes be seen wearing tiny children's clothing or bibs and parents place toys beside the Jizo statue to invoke his protection of their dead child.

Unlike the Japanese culture that provides a place to honor the personhood of babies, many countries have no forum to address parents' grief following a termination, and little understanding that they need to make sense of their feeling of still being parents (Thachuk 2007; Wegner-Hay 1999). Prenatal intervention at the earliest point in care may reduce symptoms of negative mental health (Miesnik et al. 2015) and help parents respectfully say goodbye to their baby.

Hearing the news and making the decision

No one expects statistics relating to having a baby with problems to apply to them or that they will ever need to make a decision to terminate a wanted baby. Most parents hear that something is wrong during a routine ultrasound, usually in the sorting-out phase of prenatal parenting, following the words, "Let's look at your baby." Learning that a very much wanted baby has a genetic problem or syndrome is a devastating experience for parents (Hawkins et al. 2013). It is not uncommon for a care provider to switch from the word "baby" to "fetus." One screening test often leads to others for more specific validation. Continued visualization makes the baby more real, further validating parenting feelings. Parents see a baby, not a disability. For many couples this is the first time something "bad" has happened and they want to believe that the technology and doctors are wrong (McCoyd 2007; Sutan & Miskam 2012) or assume that medical technology will be able to fix the problem:

> I was in a state of shock when I received the first report that there was something wrong with our baby. I tried to convince myself that the doctor was wrong, they were not reading the ultrasound pictures correctly and the next appointment would show everything to be fine. It did not turn out that way. The news was worse; two abnormalities were evident with our baby. The doctors were very solemn and discussed the options we had for our baby and the pregnancy. An amniocentesis was performed that day. Another ultrasound was scheduled for two weeks later to get a better look at the baby.

This father recalls his sense of hope as he and his partner anticipated their first baby:

> When we first began trying to have children, we spent a lot of time with the "what ifs," all the horrible things that could go wrong, never really thinking that they could happen to you. Hoping you don't have to face those situations.

At a routine ultrasound, however, as his worst fears were about to be confirmed, he correctly read the technician's body language. Looking for reassurance, the silence only enhanced his fear:

> Then you see the smile fade from the nurse's face. She doesn't say anything, then goes to get the doctor. … You're not sure what was supposed to happen, but you're pretty sure that that wasn't it. The nurse comes back in with the doctor. He's not smiling. He doesn't say anything, just studies the ultrasound machine. That's when things start to fall apart. You keep telling yourself you can handle whatever happens. Your only concern is for the health of your baby. You'll do whatever it takes. After several minutes you nervously ask, "Is everything alright," hoping for a reassuring "yes."

His daughter's multiple problems left this father with a stark choice (Grady & O'Leary 1993; McCoyd 2007). Choice is mixed with confusion, helplessness, and hopelessness; whether to bring a child into the world who will suffer (as no parent would wish) or to let her die (Korenromp et al. 2007). Below are some examples of parents' reactions:

> The doctors tell you there's nothing you could have done, nothing you can do. You simply must choose. And what choice do you have? Will you have the opportunity to do something noble? Unfortunately, no. You must choose between a lifetime of pain and

suffering, and a lifetime of heartache. Does it matter which one you choose? Yes, and perhaps no. You will have to make a decision that you can't live with, and then be forced to live with it. Whatever decision you make, people will criticize you.

After days and long nights of agonizing, we finally made the decision to end the pregnancy. This decision was so heart wrenching. How could I let this much wanted and dearly loved baby go? I loved you from the very moment I knew you were with me. That love deepened as I saw you move on the ultrasound. I loved you when I felt you move inside me. … Our decision was borne out of our love for you. In the end, that is what it all came down to.

In a review of the literature addressing decision making after a diagnosis, one study identified the role of significant psychosocial factors, including: perceptions of disability; perceptions of the burden for parents and family members; and likely support from friends, family, and the religious community (Choi et al. 2012; Korenromp et al. 2007). Many parents make the choice to let their children with a disability go peacefully without undue suffering after birth (Culling 2013; Gawron et al. 2013; Grady & O'Leary 1993; McCoyd 2007; McEwen 2013).

Choosing to birth early can be a wise option for some parents. In essence, when the diagnosis is fatal, circumstances have taken the decision regarding whether the baby will live or die out of their hands. The only outcome is death; not if, but when. Other family concerns might need to take precedence over the longer life of an unborn baby:

When originally faced with the decision to continue or terminate my pregnancy, I concentrated mostly on three things: how I felt I could deal with a baby with severe physical defects; how the attention required of this baby would take a way from my two-year-old son and our marriage; and what life could possibly be like for a baby with these defects. Knowing how life can be so very difficult when you are "normal," I knew our baby would be at a severe disadvantage.

During this difficult time parents need guidance and ample time to discuss the best options for their family. For some mothers, birthing early is precipitated by their health being compromised. This mother had rising blood pressure and polyhydramnios[5] in the seventh month of her pregnancy, which would have required complete bed rest. Since the baby would die at birth whatever happened, it became apparent that her living children needed her care and concern more.

Arrested parenting behaviors have been described in association with a baby diagnosed with a lethal abnormality (Côté-Arsenault & Denney-Koelsch 2011). This was not the case for the parents below, however. They were very aware of their unborn baby's personhood:

Tonight we cried together in each other's arms. The three of us cried for you and you cried for us. Our hearts are so heavy. There are no words.

Just as found with parents who continue their pregnancy (Kuebelbeck & Davis 2011), this mother struggled with her baby's inevitable death. Two days before ending her pregnancy, she wrote;

> *Our hopes, dreams and desires for you and for us have been derailed by one quirky chromosome. Our hearts are breaking and our future together will no longer be [what] we dreamed of with you. I cannot fully face the reality of your imminent death.... I want to hold you in my womb forever ... to keep you safe from harm, to protect you from the harsh realities of this world, to defend you against death.*

Spending last precious moments with the baby are remembered by another mother, as she acknowledges her love and his personhood:

> *I remember the night before I was induced; I just didn't want to go to sleep because I kind of thought this was as much as I was going to know this baby alive.*

Over 40 when she conceived for the first time, only to learn her much wanted son had a genetic abnormality incompatible with life, as she embraces him she begins the process of saying goodbye with love, a situation also encountered by McCoyd (2007):

> *I was thinking of you. Not sad thoughts, just what you have meant to me, and how I am so lucky to be your mother. ... You are a gift to me and to your Daddy. ... Thank you for coming to us, sweet little boy. Nothing can separate us from you. I love you today and I will always love you.*

Spiritual considerations

Religion and spiritual beliefs have been found to help parents relay their fears and more freely discuss concerns (Seth et al. 2011). Some parents coped by believing in a higher power; that the child has a spiritual existence in the present to help them through the experience (Cowchock et al. 2011; McCoyd 2009; Rosenblatt 2000a). For others, religion can complicate parents' choice if there is no support from their family members. Below are comments from two families:

> *Being Catholic, "terminating" our pregnancy would not be acceptable. However, the feeling that "terminating" was the right thing to do for our baby, preventing any further suffering, overrode our religious beliefs. We discussed this with both of our parents, who unanimously supported our decisions. I believe that God will not judge us for the choice we made. I think God knows how we agonized over making the decision and it was not an easy one. I believe this entire event is all part of a plan, perhaps a learning tool for life itself so we can help others in similar situations. It also shows how precious life is and to appreciate healthy babies much more.*

> *A counselor baptized you and I tried to imagine the loving arms of an angel waiting to welcome you, to hold you until I could be with you again.*

For families who do not have a religious belief, the following spiritually-based text can be helpful.

BOX 11.1

Spirituality and loss

We never own our children. They come to us briefly and leave a mark upon our heart that is always remembered. When parents are faced with returning their child to the creative life that formed her, they need special strength and wisdom to move through this experience.

The decision parents are confronting or have confronted is probably the most difficult of their lives. They may know what they want to do and believe the course of action they chose is the best one, the most loving approach to take. Or the parents may experience an impossible dilemma, not knowing which way they should go and what the right thing to do is. Birthing early feels just as wrong as continuing the pregnancy. There is pain, loss, guilt, and crisis no matter which way the parents decide.

Because of the technology today, many babies are born who might never have been born before. This very technology gives parents choices they never had to make before. Guilt attends any significant loss, especially where one has had a choice. There is no guilt-free or loss-free decision that can be made. At this moment the parents may have a hurt so deep and inconsolable that it is unbearable. Comfort is far off; acceptance or even peace seem impossible. Yet the striving for that goal will not stop. The questions that have no answers keep coming. All the words seem empty as the parents search for some sense to it all.

Parents will have a hard time coming to terms with the end of their baby's life. Parents have expressed that this can be even more difficult when they were unable to see the baby. While some may feel paralyzed or numbed by the pain, others experience a flood of feelings ranging from emptiness to rage. Getting in touch with anger can be most useful in mobilizing toward healing. Sometimes it is helpful to have parents vent feelings by writing about them. They may use writing in a ritualized or ceremonial way to help define or dissipate their feelings. Others seek support from their spiritual leader, family, and friends.

Whatever the parents' spiritual history, there can be no question that conception is a miracle. Their baby is a spiritual being and can never be separated from creation. There is evidence of conscious communication even at the earliest stage of prenatal development without language but with a heart connection. Parents need to be encouraged to talk to their baby as they would any loved one ready to depart on a great adventure. They can send messages about the time they have shared and the vision they have for this spirit who has come to them for a brief time. This child returns to familiar enfolding love quickly and quietly through death's door.

No one else can really say what will work for another. Parents will need to find their own way. They can find peace as they seek it; not in forgetting, but in remembering their unity with life and their child. Healing is a process of enfoldment that will bring a sense of peace. It will not be easy and it will take time.

Support from health care professionals

How these families are cared for during this extremely difficult time is dependent on the education, experience, and level of skill of professionals and their ability to provide compassionate, integrated, skilled, and non-judgmental care (Nicholson et al. 2010; Simmons et al. 2006). In a qualitative study with 45 nurses dealing with reproductive failure in the UK, Bolton (2005) found that some regarded this part of their role as tainted, "dirty work." The attitude of staff can help or hinder healing as the memory of the care they received during the termination is embedded in parents' minds. For example, birthing their son diagnosed with Potter's syndrome (which results from too little amniotic fluid) at 22 weeks gestation, a condition often fatal at birth, these parents hoped he would be born alive so that they could have some precious seconds with him. Instead he was stillborn. The mother sensed the doctor seemed relieved:

> *One of the most disturbing things for me was in the birth. I felt like the doctor who delivered him seemed so relieved he was dead. We knew he could live for a little bit. I will never forget that she seemed relieved that he was dead. It was her tone of voice, "He's dead." I don't know if she really felt that way but it was what I heard. I felt her discomfort around the whole situation. I think it would have been more uncomfortable for her if he had been born alive and then died.*

In contrast these parents had a caring physician who knew how much their baby with a neurological condition meant to them. At the birth, the physician cradled the deceased baby and said to them, *Oh look. You had a baby. You had a baby girl. Do you want to hold her?* As the parents wept, a nurse wrapped the baby in a tiny blanket and gave her to the mother, with the father close by. The personhood of this baby girl was acknowledged by giving her a name, sharing her brief life with her older siblings, and burying her remains with her grandparents.

Case 1

Dorothy and Mark, married a year, anxiously awaited their first ultrasound at 22 weeks gestation in hope of discovering the gender of their first baby. Twelve years later, they still remember the words spoken to them:

> *We brought in a video tape of the whole ultrasound. We still have that video tape. And he typed in, "It's a boy." Then he must have gone to the head and noticed the*

> *hydrocephalus; we couldn't tell what was on the ultrasound. He saw that and didn't say anything. Then he went to the spine and saw the spina bifida, and didn't say anything. He just left the room and said, "I'll be back." He came back a few minutes later and we didn't know what was going on. He asked me to get dressed and go into this waiting room. We sat in that room for about a half hour before the doctor was able to come in.*

Mark shares his memories of the day:

> *I often tell people it was the best day and the worst day of my life. The best part of that day was waiting to go into that ultrasound with him at 22 weeks. I was so excited; I couldn't wait. Got out of work, went in, the technician had gone over all the different things, was taping it, and he said, "Do you want to find out if it's a boy or a girl?" and we said, "Of course." And we found out that it was a boy. So for me, it was just crazy! I've never felt those kinds of emotions before. Up to that point it was the best I've ever felt in my life. And then shortly thereafter came the worst I've ever felt in my life. I went from the highest to the lowest in a matter of about 15 minutes. The technician turned off the video machine, paused for a second, and then said that he had to go speak to the doctor.*

Receiving support when they make the decision to terminate is important in the parents' healing process (Choi et al. 2012; Culling 2013). Dorothy and Mark were able to reach out to their parents. *We drove to our home town to meet with our parents, to have them, not help us make the decision, but be supportive. We just couldn't do that on our own.*

In some health care settings, if the staff have strong religious beliefs or receive a lack of support from colleagues the situation can be made more difficult for the parents (Marshall et al. 1994; Mayers et al. 2005). After making the decision to induce labor, Dorothy and Mark ran into another barrier that made an already painful experience more so:

> *Then they said we don't know if induction is a possibility because the nurses don't have to participate in this if they don't want to. So we'll have to see if there are nurses on staff who are willing to do that. So here we have to make this real hard decision and then we call with our decision and they might not be able to do that after all.*

In the end, they were able to induce the birth of the baby, giving them and the grandparents the opportunity to hold him. As found by others (France et al. 2013), the outward signs of the disability provided reassurance for the father. *Some of the outward symptoms of spina bifida were actually comforting to see so that we knew we had made the right decision.* Mark remembers his wife's reaction after the birth, and the helpfulness of the information they received from the counselor before it:

> *I'll never forget, ever, that night after our son was delivered and passed. He was born with a heartbeat and actually lived for quite a while. It was late at night and they had*

taken him away. The whole family had gone and I was lying in bed next to her and she turned to me and she smiled and said, "Everything's going to be alright.'"She knew that what she went through was the right thing to do; she felt peaceful enough to smile and comfort me! And I'm the one who's supposed to be comforting her. She was more educated about the process that she was going to go through and the counselor helped her a great deal.

Mark also experienced the unnatural feelings reported by other parents whose baby has died. Rather than bringing a baby home, he had to plan a funeral. *It was a crazy time, to actually go to a funeral home and pick out a casket. We'd just been married a year. What in the world had happened to me? How did I go from everything's terrific to wow.*

Continued bond and attachment: building memories

According to Leon (1990), pregnancy creates a mother and father and this is true regardless of the outcome (O'Leary et al. 2012). Actually, it is not uncommon for some parents to try not to attach to the baby until after the birth (Côté-Arsenault et al. 2015). *To deal with the decision, I felt I had to disassociate myself from the baby. This changed after the birth, when we realized the depth of our loss.* Rosenblatt (2000a) states that parents continue to have a relationship with their deceased child. The bereaved parents' problem, pain, or embodied memories are not removed by the baby's death. The identity of being a parent does not stop and parents do not just "move on."

It is important that parents rely on external sources of help (McCoyd, 2007). This couple had three days to prepare. They relied on their faith and community of caring friends as they took time to say goodbye to their son and honor their continued bond with and deep attachment to this much wanted baby:

> *We are so thankful for this time to prepare. How could we possibly walk through these days without you? How could we honor your life and death without this time together? How will we even when death comes? Hugs, sighs, tears, tears, tears. How long will we cry, oh Lord? How many nights will end and days begin with salty tears? Will there ever be respite from this grief?*
>
> *Your life in the womb will be over soon. Your life in this world will be over soon. Your life in our hearts will never end. We love you, sweet baby boy. We will always love you. You will always be a part of us and we a part of you.*

Finding ways for parents to say goodbye to the baby before the termination is an important step in making meaning of their continued bond/attachment relationship. Most babies with a severe disability hear by the second trimester. When parents are open to information, gently pointing this out lets parents know that the unborn baby has been part of the experience, felt their love, emotional struggle, desperation, and helplessness. This becomes important when they enter a subsequent pregnancy as some feel they don't deserve the opportunity to attach to a new baby. Integrating the competencies of the new baby and talking about the deceased baby knowing them as parents, helps them understand that the deceased baby is still part of their family. Parents who make the painful decision to terminate their baby suffer the same grief as parents whose baby dies spontaneously (Brier 2008; Cowchock et al. 2009; Culling 2013; Grady & O'Leary 1993) and need the same support.

Case 2

Sarah terminated her much wanted second son after hearing he had Down's syndrome.[6] She painfully processed her journey by attending the genetic loss support group. Intellectually, she understood her choice but in her profound grief could not forgive herself. She felt she had no right to honor her baby and build memories, a common thought among such parents (McIlwraith 2013). She cried, remembering the termination and sharing how she wailed in grief. She turned to the facilitator and asked; "Do you think the baby felt pain?" The facilitator gently replied, "I think he was wailing with you because he had to leave." The love and connection between this mother and her baby's personhood was important for her to understand. At some level, the baby understood the choice she and her husband made.

Her healing began when another couple returned to the group as guests. They brought their baby book of memories made by the father, and shared all the ways in which they were able to memorialize the daughter they had terminated. The book was kept openly in their home so that their other children could also know about their sister. This made Sarah realize that she could honor her baby and her identity as his mother. On the anniversary of what would have been her son's birth she spent the weekend alone writing about the previous months. As described by Sell-Smith and Lax (2013), she wrote about holding on to the few memories she had, including the positive pregnancy tests and ultrasound pictures. She poured out her love and how she had been looking forward to being his mother. She gathered together the medical correspondence, ultrasound pictures, letter reporting the diagnosis, and information regarding the termination and put it all into a baby book for her son. She began to weave her baby into the fabric of her parenthood (Cote-Arsenault 2003) and her healing in moving forward began.

It is important for parents to understand that they have a right to memorialize their baby and to create a place for her in the family (ibid). Parents have done a variety of things to honor the short life of a missing baby in the family. Some volunteer in special olympic events, others buy a piece of jewelry that is a symbol for their baby. But, just as there is a difference between curing and healing in disease, so is there a difference in being stuck in grief and honoring parents' continued bond with and attachment to a child no longer physically in their family.

Case 3

While everyone's "road map" is different, this case is a profound example of the long-term impact of making the decision to terminate and the subsequent healing that can occur when a parent is ready. This mother suffered the loss of a planned and much wanted baby at 16 weeks gestation after previously terminating two other babies at this gestational point. The hospital social worker spent the day gently encouraging her to see and hold this little baby, returning three times. On the last attempt, the mother agreed. The baby was brought to her dressed in a gown and wrapped in a beautiful blanket. The mother held the baby and began to howl, rocking back and forth in her grief for 30 minutes. When she finally stopped, she looked at the social worker and said, *How is this different?* The very wise social worker simply replied, *Because you're different.*

Support from others

People survive this tragedy in different ways. Many parents are fortunate to come through the experience through the support of family and friends (Choi et al. 2013). Some do not ask for help because of the circumstances of their loss while others learn they have many people in their lives to depend on, something they did not know they had or needed until the loss of their child. Some see this as one of the gifts the child gives them. This mother wrote of her despair coupled with the realization of the gift her son had revealed to her:

> As I felt myself slipping, drowning in despair, I felt terror at my inability to care for myself. It was then that I began to feel an invisible safety net surround me. I felt the love and care of so many people—friends, family, professionals, and other parents—who all helped me when I could no longer bear the weight alone. I learned in a very profound way that I am not alone.

Parents will appreciate when friends and family acknowledge the ongoing presence of their deceased baby and their parenthood. As one mother shares:

> Earlier this morning the house was quiet.… The phone didn't ring. No one came to the door. We felt abandoned. New questions haunted me. … Are we just a flash of tragedy that arrested their attention for a moment? Has everyone who said they loved us already moved on with their lives? Around 11 a.m. the phone began to ring. Guests began to arrive. Flowers were delivered. You are here! Not just real to us, but real to all who love us.

The following parents had a very different experience after terminating their baby. They were alone in a state far from their family when they learned that their 20-week baby had multiple problems. The father remembers how the doctor told them the tragic news, saying they had a lot of decisions to make, and then *washed his hands of us.* They were sent to an abortion clinic to end the pregnancy and given no other guidance. In spite of having a two-year-old child at home, they had difficulty finding someone to come to help:

We had to basically beg people because I needed somebody to come and help with [our daughter]. I think because it happened in another state it was easier for people here to act as if it had never happened.

They were not given the option of keeping the baby's remains and did not think to ask for them until it was too late. They moved back to their home state within weeks of the loss and held a memorial service, hoping others would acknowledge their daughter and the pain of their loss. The father expressed his feelings in a poem.

BOX 11.2

We are heavy with you[6]

We are heavy with you
Though lighter for your loss
It's been years since we missed you,
Before you went across
Yet still we weep

There's an emptiness in our lives
Sorrow fills our hearts
And full too, our eyes with tears
Leaving emptiness, despite the fullness of our parts
Your name is all we keep
You're part of our lives each day
The part that hurts like a knife

We try to fill the void
That's filling up our life
And yet, remember you, too
We've discovered an infinite love
For our children in our heart
Yet, infinite as well, the pain for you
And being kept apart
We will always miss and love you.

We waited three months to have a memorial service and everybody was like, "Why, why are you having one?" And we felt we needed to. Everybody came but, again, nobody talks about it at all.

In spite of their two year old talking about her baby sister, the inability of the mother's family to share the loss was painful to the parents:

[She would talk] about how we had just been to the cemetery and she was running about and putting flowers. And the whole room just went quiet. They just didn't know what to say. She would just talk about how I have a sister in heaven and nobody would talk back.

Looking back on this couple's family history, the mother had been a subsequent child herself, born 12 months after the loss of a 10-month-old brother who died of bacterial meningitis. As she grew up there were no pictures of this deceased brother in the house and, after his death, the family moved to seven different houses until she was born in the house her parents still live in today.

This story illustrates the potential impact on a family when a deceased child is not recognized or memorialized in any way. The intergenerational fall out and inability to help an adult child when they experience their own loss of a child can be profound. Assessing the history of parents in regard to losses in their own families is therefore important in understanding how to help with their grief.

Moving on in a complicated world

Veninga (1985) describes six characteristics of a crisis. It hits suddenly, without warning, it threatens security, its resolution is unpredictable, it presents dilemmas and it erodes self-confidence. A difficult experience helps us redefine our values. All of these characteristics define what these parents have been through. The stories reflect experiences unique to each family yet with a common shared theme: turmoil, deep soul-searching, and pain as the decision to terminate is made, and the ongoing parenting relationship with a baby who is no longer physically there but is very much spiritually present. Sandelowski and Barroso (2005) suggest that guidelines for professionals dealing with stillbirth can be adapted for parents ending a pregnancy as a result of serious fetal abnormality; paradoxically, however, the involuntary nature of this outcome sets parents who chose to terminate a baby with a fetal abnormality apart both from those who experience a spontaneous loss and those who electively terminate because they do not want a pregnancy at that point in their lives.

Responding to an unexpected diagnosis in pregnancy is about parenting precious babies (Culling 2013). In working with these parents it is important to understand that, after birth, they mourn not a fetus with a genetic abnormality but a lost baby (Grady & O'Leary 1993; Hunt et al. 2009; Statham, 2002). They need guidance and support during the decision-making process and afterwards, as they begin making meaning from the experience and thereby healing (Hunt et al. 2009; Korenromp et al. 2007). Unfortunately, few agencies exist to provide such support. An exception is New Zealand, where some special units do offer this care and compassion to grieving parents, in Wellington and Christchurch (Culling 2013).

The stories described in this section reflect the lived experience of parents facing a decision that no parent should ever be asked to make, in a society that typically does not understand the significance and impact of genetic termination of pregnancy. Roughly 39 percent of the world's population live in countries with highly restrictive laws governing abortion (Center for Reproductive Rights, n.d.). Because of the political climate surrounding termination, it is very difficult for families to get the support and help they may need to process their grief and manage ongoing parenting. In the US, it is currently extremely difficult, if not impossible, for parents to birth a baby with a genetic abnormality in a hospital setting because hospitals fear being labeled "abortion" advocate centers. "The ideologically and religiously motivated backlash against abortion is increasingly resorting to misrepresentations and avoidance of public health evidence, and is undermining human rights standards applicable in this context" (Finer & Fine 2013, p. 587). Mothers sent to an abortion clinic are denied the possibility of gaining memorials such as foot and hand prints, leaving them with only the ultrasound pictures if they know to ask for them.

Korenromp et al. (2007, p. 714–715) identify four key points to keep in mind when working with parents who experience either a fetal reduction or termination: (1) both partners have to be equally involved in counseling. Both are parents of the child, the choice not to continue the pregnancy is their joint decision, and both suffer psychological distress. The fact that partner support is an important determinant for coping underlines this. (2) Parents who show evidence of high levels of doubt during the decision-making process may benefit from psychological assistance. (3) Parents should be informed that needing time to come to terms with the event is normal. This might have an impact on sick leave, ability to concentrate on other activities, general well-being, and their relationship. (4) The availability of contact groups and/or psychological support should be mentioned in every pre-termination counseling session.

Summary

This chapter has addressed the complex issues parents face following diagnosis of fetal anomaly and having to make the decision to end their pregnancy. Little is written on this topic from a parenting perspective, either for parents going through the experience or professionals working with them in order to guide their healing. These stories show that the decision is sacred and never taken lightly by parents. These parents saw the personhood of the unborn baby just as clearly as those who chose to carry a baby with genetic problems to term. The stories also reflect the parents' love for their baby and show that their grief is no different than that of parents who experience a spontaneous loss except for the added component of needing to make the choice.

Regardless of personal views on termination, it is important for professionals to remember that it is the parents' decision to make. Professionals can help by following the lead of the parents. Agreeing with the parents' decision is not necessary but professionals must nonetheless be non-judgmental, respectful of their role as parents, and responsive to the grief they carry. The continued bond and attachment theory-based intervention can be useful in helping parents make meaning of their experience and to respectfully say goodbye to their much wanted baby.

Notes

1 All the parents received genetic counseling during the decision-making process. After the birth they attended an infant loss group specific to this population. Quotations are shared but the names, ages, and other identifying information were changed to protect the privacy of participants.
2 See more at: http://www.dharmacrafts.com/2ITM015/DharmaCrafts-Meditation-Supplies.html#sthash.gaMwmgjl.dpuf.
3 http://www.zawaj.com/articles/abortion_permitted_when.html.
4 (http://www.onmarkproductions.com/html/jizo1.shtml).
5 A medical condition describing an excess of fluid in the amniotic sac surrounding the baby.
6 Reproduced with the kind permission of the poet, Darrell Peterson.

12

OFFERING A THERAPEUTIC EDUCATIONAL SUPPORT GROUP

Parents of deceased babies have the same needs as anyone who suffers a loss: to confront reality, receive emotional support, and engage in healing and growth. A major challenge of grief work is coming to terms with a loss while honoring and holding on to the meanings, memories, investments, and identities connected to the deceased (Neimeyer et al. 2014; Rosenblatt 1996). This chapter explores face-to-face support groups, and discusses how infant loss and pregnancy after loss are similar but also uniquely different.

Why bereavement support?

Despite much positive feedback from grief group participants, there is scant knowledge regarding why some people benefit from participation while others do not; empirical evidence on the positive impact on mental or physical health measures of support groups is likewise meager (Currier et al. 2008). That said, the availability of a support group at the time of loss and during the pregnancy that follows can be an important resource because, although most people come to terms with bereavement over time, the risk of succumbing to health disorders is greater in bereaved verses non-bereaved individuals (Song et al. 2010; Stroebe et al. 2007). Meaning integration following loss also contributes to the prediction of mental and physical health outcomes when demographic background of the mourner, their level of complicated grief, and circumstances of the death are accounted for (Holland et al. 2014).

Online PAL groups can also be helpful (Carlson et al. 2012), and an online magazine is available[1]; little research has been carried out on these resources, however. Gold et al. (2011) reported that some women can feel a strong sense of support and community from participating in these types of group. A study examining the efficacy of an internet-based cognitive behavioral therapy program for mothers after pregnancy loss found that participants in their experimental group showed significant improvements in posttraumatic stress, grief, depression, and overall mental health, but not in anxiety or somatization (Kersting et al. 2011).

Disagreement is evident in the literature regarding the efficacy of support groups and who might benefit because the majority of people do not need formal intervention to help them cope with their grief (Neimeyer & Currier 2009). Psychological counseling has generally been found to be beneficial in reducing anxiety for women pregnant again following a miscarriage (Nikcevic et al. 2007). In the realm of professional therapy, a meta-analysis of 23 randomized controlled studies found that the average participant in grief therapy was better off than only 55 percent of bereaved persons who received no treatment (Neimeyer 2000).

Most bereaved parents would be identified as experiencing uncomplicated grief, defined as "an emotional reaction to bereavement, falling within expected norms" (Stroebe et al. 2001, p. 6). For parents who have experienced the loss of a child, group support can be useful as a means of validating grief, offering suggestions for coping, and providing hope (McKeon Pesek 2002). Access to adequate social support has been suggested to be essential in enabling successful cognitive processing and re-alignment of information following a traumatic event (Brewin et al. 1996; Prati & Pietrantoni 2009; Tedeschi & Calhoun 2004).

Support groups in general are open-ended, taking members at any time, and attendance optional (McKeon & Pesek 2002; Umphrey & Cacciatore 2011). Before inviting parents to join a group they need to be given information on the purpose, structure, organization, meeting frequency, and number of participants, including whether fathers/partners are welcome. Parents generally also want to know about the background of the facilitator, the positive and negative aspects of attendance, and if the group has a religious affiliation (Dyregrov et al. 2013b, 2014a). A negative aspect of group attendance is hearing about all the ways in which babies can die; parents may experience emotional responses parallel to those of the person describing their loss (Creedy et al. 2000). All losses are different but the focus of both infant loss and PAL groups is to support parents' continued bond with their deceased baby while they also learn how to move forward; professionals need to understand how difficult it can be to find a new identity of self as parent (Neimeyer et al. 2014).

At the time of loss

> Emotional expression of grief is painful but also natural and necessary, as moving through grief is how parents move toward healing.
>
> *Deborah Davis (2016, p. xi)*

A perinatal loss support group exists to help parents work toward positive resolution of grief, as well as to provide information, education, and resources in a safe environment with people in similar circumstances (Gordon 2007; Littman et al. 2009; McKeon Pesek 2002). While maintaining memories of and a connection to their deceased baby (Carlson et al. 2012), the support group also offers a place in which to process the trauma of their loss, which may impede healing. Dyregrov and Regel

(2012) argue for more proactive early intervention for traumatic events that have the potential to lead to extreme psychic distress, PTSD, or complicated grief reactions. Traumatized individuals cannot embrace the process of grieving until they are given the opportunity to process the primal emotions associated with trauma and make new meaning of their life experience (van der Kolk 1994).

Grief can be overwhelming, making it difficult for parents to reach out for help or know what they need. In one focus group study of participants in support groups for various types of loss, the parents who had suffered the loss of a baby reported wanting information given to them at the hospital (Dyregrov et al. 2013b). However, the Dyregrov study also found that the optimal time to invite someone to enter a support group is 6–12 months after their loss. They suggest this timescale allows time to overcome the initial shock, trauma, and anger. There is currently little research to suggest when to reach out to perinatally bereaved parents but 6–12 months can be a long period if their grief is marginalized by others who want them to recover sooner than they are ready for; parents need to seek help if this happens (Umphrey & Cacciatore 2011). This suggests that information about the support group should be given in written form at the time of the death and parents told that they can refer to it later. If a hospital employs a member of staff to work with bereaved parents, that person can remind parents about the group during periodic follow-up calls over the first year.

Dyregrov and Regel (2014b) feel that watchful waiting may not be beneficial for this population, especially for parents with other children. In a misguided attempt to protect their children, parents may make themselves emotionally unavailable rather than seeking advice from a support group regarding how best to support them (Crenshaw 2002; O'Leary 2007). A connection with a couple to share how their other children are coping when a baby sibling dies can help normalize feelings for other parents whose children may be reacting similiarly (Cacciatore 2007; Neimeyer 2014).

One of the benefits of being with others is that, until they attend a support group, parents do not necessarily understand that their feelings are a normal response to what they have experienced. Parents find they are not alone, a key therapeutic factor contributing to the potency of the group experience (Yalom 2005). Another benefit is that it provides a place to freely talk about their deceased baby. One mother shares:

> *I always felt like it was my time with Emma; that I was doing something special with her, talking about her with other people. That was a great experience, being with other people that had been through a similar experience at different stages. In some aspects I felt like I was able to help and in other aspects people were able to help me.*

Support groups also help parents see each other's progress. Meeting others who manage to live with grief provides hope to others that they can do the same (Dyregrov et al. 2011). A sense of hope can help parents transcend the psychological impact of emotionally and spiritually devastating circumstances (Roscignol et al. 2012). A week after the loss of their son one couple attended the infant loss group, and the husband said, *We didn't get to bring him home so we needed something to do.* Hope began for his wife after she listened to another woman in the group:

> *The woman with the scrap book, I remember thinking, if I ever get there that would be amazing. She was six months out and they were trying to get pregnant again and we were just trying to wrap our heads around what happened. She was in the same career as me and I remember talking to her. Okay, it is possible; there is something beyond where I felt we were stuck. For me it was like, this is manageable. You can get through it.*

Discussion in an infant loss group almost always includes when parents might be ready to try again. Once pregnant, mixing parents pregnant after loss with the newly bereaved may be traumatizing for the latter as the needs of these two groups are uniquely different.

The pregnancy that follows loss

The purpose of a PAL group is not to revisit loss but rather for parents to learn ways in which to empower and advocate for themselves and the new baby and to gain mastery of their lives (Wiggins 2012). Health care providers may say, "They don't need to go back to that grief," not understanding that it is already there. Such paternalistic intervention (presuming what is "best" for others, as defined by Attig 2001) has been found to be destructive and may impede healing for some (Toller 2005). Such remarks fail to respect autonomy, compound helplessness, delay relearning, and postpone parents' ability to reshape and redirect their lives. What both parents and providers need to hear is that the focus of a PAL group is *this pregnancy and this unborn baby*, while also acknowledging that there will be discussion about the deceased baby too.

We have found that parents pregnant after loss and their unborn babies benefit enormously from an educational support group when it is grounded in a theoretical framework that utilizes the continued bond and attachment theory. Unborn babies need parents who are aware of their presence and individuality (O'Leary & Gaziano 2011; O'Leary et al. 2006b). The focus of the support group is helping parents find ways to control what they can control and let go of what they can not. Fear and anxiety are framed as normal parenting behaviors for the safety of the new baby. This framework also supports the meaning-reconstruction theory whereby intervention is a process of facilitating parents as they re-author their life story following the trauma of loss into a more coherent and purposeful narrative (Neimeyer et al. 2002).

Joining

It is sometimes difficult to determine whether parents are ready to engage in the conflicting feelings that are common in a pregnancy after loss. It is not unusual to hear parents say that if they let go of their emotions they may never stop crying. Although it may be tempting to try to comfort, solve, or be sympathetic, it is important to support parents in their struggle and not short-circuit the constructive processing of trauma and loss. If parents initially say they aren't ready, details of the support group can be offered at a later date. The facilitator needs to stress to reluctant parents that the goal of the group is to help normalize feelings that others in their social network may not understand (Dyregrov & Regel 2015a). *Everybody else tells you you're crazy. It's normal to have these worries.*

Just as in an infant loss group, parents can be reluctant to participate in a PAL group, fearing secondary trauma (Rando 2000) as a result of hearing about the many ways in which babies can die. One father explained: *I don't know why or how sitting in a room with a bunch of people who have had a tragedy like ours and hearing their story is actually going to help me deal with anything.* Most alumni of our PAL group say that the benefits to themselves and their unborn babies far outweighed their fear. They also report that learning about ways in which babies die empowered them to ask more questions, giving them information on how to protect their unborn baby.

If the mother has a new partner, attending a group can help that person begin to understand that her fears and anxiety are normal in light of her past experience. For example, Tracy was a single mother when her daughter was stillborn. Her new partner was part of the group as she processed her sense of guilt that she did not pay attention to the fetal movements of the child who died and her difficulty in sharing with him her excitement about the new baby:

> *I don't tell him that much but it's really difficult for me to be pregnant every day because she was my little girl. I mean with her, I didn't think about her being born and with this one it's like, even if I'm forcing myself, because I'm still stuck in the, well is this one going to be born alive?*

Rather than therapy, the support group offers an attachment-focused intervention. According to Yalom (1970), "the crucial task is not to uncover, to piece together, and to understand the past, but to use the past for the help it offers in understanding (and changing) the individual's mode of relating to others in the present" (pp. 148–149). The pregnancy provides an opportunity for integrating the loss at a new level; for understanding that parental grief, even though it may seem enduring, is not necessarily unresolved or complicated grief. When past stories not processed (that is, parents are unable to separate one baby from another) are part of future stories, grief work must be included regardless of time constraints because later in life this grief can resurface when parents least expect it (O'Leary et al. 2012). Parents do not realize what they need until they join:

> *No need to explain feelings. I couldn't have made it through that pregnancy without the group. Nobody else knows how you feel except these people.*

This is true for fathers too:

> *I had a lot of fears and anxieties that I wasn't aware of. I got involved because she said, "I need you to be there." My initial reaction was "Why? I'm not the one who's pregnant. I think I'm okay." I realized [after going] I had a lot of fears of my own.*

Group composition

A PAL group is defined by the length of the pregnancy, is thus open-ended, and parents can join at any point. While some have cautioned that a group comprised of members at different stages in their grief can be too complex (Galinsky & Schopler 1994), this can actually be a strength. Veninga (1985) writes that it is important to have at least one person who will stand by, support, and give a sense of hope to someone who is overcome by their tragic experience. Parents farther into their pregnancies become that source of support to others and are role models. They provide encouragement and hope to those in earlier stages of pregnancy, who, in turn, often show the "older" members the extent of their progress. As in an infant loss group (Umphrey & Cacciatore 2011), parents gain confidence from each other and share the story of the deceased baby while learning ways in which to know their new unborn baby and cope with anxieties, social issues, family and work situations. Parents learn from each other how to ask for what they need from their care providers who may not understand the dynamics of a pregnancy after loss.

> *It taught me that I could ask for what I needed to feel reassured and comfortable with the progress of my pregnancy. If only I'd known more in my first pregnancy.*
>
> *I think one of the best ways to relieve the stress was to share our feelings with each other, whether in group or at home, to help deflate that big emotional balloon.*

Structure

Each group session begins with introductions. Members of longer standing tell their stories, weeks of pregnancy, and give a synopsis of their loss(es). By this time the newcomers feel less unique; they are part of a group of people who know and understand their concerns and share as much of their story as they choose. This check-in information helps participants and the facilitator keep track of the group's assorted pregnancies and approaching anniversaries of events associated with their loss(es).

Rather than focusing on specific topics, the parents lead the discussion. The mix of subjects will vary from week to week. Parents take turns sharing events, milestones and setbacks since the previous meeting. Doctor visits, ultrasound examinations, feeling fetal movements for the first time, trips to the hospital fearing lack of movement or preterm labor, unkind or inappropriate comments from others, or any other relevant topic stimulates lively discussion in this open and safe environment.

Asking broad, unstructured questions allows parents to tell their stories with minimal constraints, inviting them to be informants. Stories have been found to add coherence to events and help people comprehend a "new normal" (Cacciatore 2007; Keesee et al. 2008, p. 95).

The facilitator needs to maintain a focus on the developmental stages of the unborn babies present in the room. Reporting the events of the week allows the facilitator to become the voice of the unborn babies, to share their competencies and teach about fetal movement, uterine contractions, preventive care, and health care options—all while revisiting the competencies of the deceased babies. Parents learn that the new baby is already aware of the outside environment and the deceased baby also knew their voices and felt their love. This helps parents reconstruct their sense of security (and role of self as parent), not by relinquishing but by re-emphasizing attachment; their back story (Neimeyer & Thompson 2014) provides a sense of continuity between the life they had with the deceased baby and the life they now are developing with the baby in this new pregnancy. *Outside of the group I couldn't talk about him. The grief resurfaced in some surprising ways.*

Rebuilding trust

In the book, *The Sacred Tree* (Bopp et al. 1989), it is said that people need a gathering place where they can feel protected and safe enough to discuss their most private concerns; this may be the only place where their rawest emotions can be released As members demonstrate vulnerability, the group becomes a place where actions are normalized, painful feelings recognized, and parents give and receive support from each other (Dyregrov et al. 2014a; Umphrey & Cacciatore 2011). New bonds and a sense of community are formed. Everyone in the group understands the difficulty of anniversary dates and discusses ways in which to establish some control of those days by planning what they might do to honor the deceased baby. Parents who haven't planned an anniversary day often say they are overwhelmed with grief they hadn't expected.

Tears can be a healthy release and don't always need to be fixed. Crying is accepted as normal by participants (Umphrey & Cacciatore 2011, p. 95). The group setting may be the only place where parents can really cry. Health care providers can be guilty of trying to cheer up parents and often pride themselves on keeping people happy. Facilitators must be aware that tears may upset some members of the group. For this reason, it is helpful for two people to facilitate each meeting to observe all group members. Facilitators need to be comfortable with tears and able to accept the strong emotions that sessions may stir in themselves as well as in the parents:

> *It was the only in-person place I ever had to pour my heart out.*
>
> *It gave me great peace of mind … a weekly place to have personal contact … sit and cry if you need to, or laugh.*

Lesbian parents

The experiences of bereaved lesbian parents are more similar to those of het-erosexual bereaved mothers than different (Cacciatore & Raffo 2011). Although Cacciatore and Raffo's study found that lesbians were hesitant to fully disclose their identity, in our clinical practice one couple found caring support that was beneficial:

> I was very nervous to tell people how afraid I was being pregnant again. One thing that was different was to ask for help. This was hard because I had to talk about my relationship. On top of worrying abut my feelings after our daughter died, I worried about whether I would be accepted because I am lesbian. My partner and I decided we just had to be "out" so we could get the support we needed through such a high anxiety time. After the first couple of support group meetings I felt fine. Everyone was very open and we all shared a common thread of having our babies die. It was no different for us as lesbians—we still had the same feelings that other members had. I felt so supported through the next pregnancy. I don't know how I would have made it through without the help of group members, professional staff, and the wonderful caring and sharing we did. I still keep in touch with members of the group for support in raising our daughter.

Guidance

A key aspect of bereavement is the impact of the loss on the self-organization of the bereaved person (Adolfsson 2010; Lee et al. 2013). Constructive cognitive processing of a loss or trauma in a supportive environment fosters self-disclosure (Tedeschi & Calhoun 2004). Facilitators need to listen to how loss has affected group members' sense of self as parent. When there is no known cause for a loss (for example, spon-taneous miscarriage or unexplained stillbirth) women tend to believe they played a role (Warland et al. 2015). If the pregnancy was high risk because of a condition suffered by the mother, she will need more support from the group, and her health care provider must help her understand what is being done to keep her baby safe so that she can trust her body as a safe place for the baby to grow in. The facilitator must listen and listen again until they understand what the parents are really saying and can thus discern what they need. As described by Kauffman (2012) in relation to mirroring, through holding and bearing witness to their feelings the facilitator can transform the pain of the previous loss to help members create a new sense of self as parent for this new baby. By listening to what is spoken and unspoken the facilitator learns what further education and support the parents may need, includ-ing when they may need a referral to therapy.

Rather than being intent on promoting certain changes in the parents, the facili-tator is most effective when listening allows them to be changed by the parents' experience (Calhoun & Tedeshi 2001). Attention must be paid to how parents ver-balize their grief and struggle in attaching "overtly and in the shadows, verbally and between the lines, silently through speech, in words and actions" (Kauffman 2012, p. 12). For example, Mark attended the group with his wife only sporadically. I (JOL) had been at the birth of their previous son and vividly remember his focus on caring for his wife through the labor, birth, and postpartum as their son died in their arms. When asked how he was doing in this new pregnancy, he would glare and say "Fine." Mark chose not to share his feelings even though, from his wife's previous discussions and his body language, it was apparent he was carrying a lot of pain. My role became one of waiting until he was ready, which came 10 years later when he agreed to be interviewed on the experience of parenting after loss:

> *Even though I attended, I kept it inside. I tried to let it out, I really did. It wouldn't come out. My brain just wouldn't let it come out. In many ways this whole process was controlled by something in my brain saying, 'You know what, you're not ready for this. Just what you went through, I'm going to let you be exposed to it but emotionally you're not ready to deal with it."*

While open to whatever emerges, the discussion is always focused on how the past may be affecting the unborn baby in the present and providing clues as to how to support parents now. Guidance involves finding a positive cognitive reconstruction (Boyraz et al. 2010). Processing their words from the developmental framework of parenting during pregnancy is important; such as reminding parents how hard they tried to seek help for their deceased baby if they were dismissed by their provider and that at some level the baby sensed their struggle. To help parents open up the facilitator can ask questions such as, "What was going on at this point in your previous pregnancy which ended in loss?" or "What do you think is the impact of your words and feelings about the pregnancy on the baby within?" This approach uses an early intervention model of purposefully structured support (Dyregrov & Regal 2012) while also supporting their parenting to the deceased baby.

Parents attend as unique people and find a commonality. Rather than confronting a parent's resistance to giving up grieving, the facilitator should empathize with and support them, thereby creating an opportunity for self-reorganization. When feelings are reframed as parenting behaviors (grief for one baby and fear of attaching to the new baby) both are recognized as expressions of loving parents. Within the support group setting parents can renew their self-confidence, self-esteem, and self-identity. The group participants and the facilitator are catalysts to the mourning process, playing an active, central role in labeling the feelings of mourning and grief as parenting behaviors. In helping parents find meaningful ways to remember the deceased baby, the other group members also get to know him as part of their family too. One father expressed this really well: *Everyone in this room knows Francis [his deceased son] is part of their family.*

The baby leads

A PAL support group can easily devolve into just another bereavement group if it is not based on a specific framework for understanding the issues associated with pregnancy after loss. This is one reason why mixing together parents who have suffered an infant loss and parents pregnant after loss in one group is not helpful. When parents become pregnant they need to risk attaching to the unborn baby while maintaining their connection to and memories of the previous baby. It takes a lot of work to differentiate one baby from another and trust the new baby will be born alive. Parents need guided facilitation from a person who is skilled at identifying both the developmental stages of the unborn baby and her parents. This is pivotal in helping parents differentiate their babies and take on the emotional journey of this subsequent pregnancy:

> *The support group I attended helped me advocate for myself and ask my doctor for more reassurance and a second ultrasound.*
>
> *The group also helped me to start thinking about our son-to-be as a separate person, while still letting me honor my daughter's memory, and to speak openly about the grief I was still feeling so strongly.*

Assessment of the group's progress

Group progress can be ascertained when the discussion is evenly distributed around the room. There can be a lot of emotion in the room. People may be crying or laughing but there is rarely a flat, stiff, empty kind of feeling. Above all, there is a sense of caring, of sharing a common bond that is often not understood outside the group setting.

The facilitator's role

In the Jewish ritual of "Sitting Shiva" an emotionally protective setting is established, providing a sense of psychological safety for participants (Iimber-Black 2004). The usefulness of a support group depends on the skills and abilities of its facilitator (McKeonPesek 2002). A facilitator should be empathic, have distance from their own loss if they have experienced one (Dyregov et al. 2013), and understand how a PAL group is different than an infant loss group. The facilitator brackets all subjectivity in order to provide emotional space for whatever needs surface for each parent. This helps parents explore and test out feelings that others in the larger society are neither able to listen to nor understand.

Facilitators are empathic listeners (Kauffman 2012) who guide and reflect parents' feelings while educating and intervening in crises. They need to be non-judgmental with a clear understanding of each unborn baby's development and each parent's stage of prenatal parenting. The facilitator needs to be aware of their personal comfort level when dealing with grief and loss so that their "own needs, anxieties and defenses do not close off pathways of receptivity" (ibid p. 14). The needs and responses of individuals and the health of the total group are crucial. The facilitator ensures the group remains a safe place and each participant who wants to speak has time to do so. A facilitator can neither recommend care nor criticize care in the current or past pregnancy.

If the parent is having difficulty, the facilitator may ask after group if he or she would like to meet outside of group time. They may sense that a couple is coping with other marital issues but recognize that they need to get through the pregnancy before they are ready to address other emotional and psychological issues under the surface. Rather than seeing a support group as a form of therapy, MacKinnon et al. (2014) refer to meaning-based group counseling that provides educational intervention on the altered developmental tasks of prenatal parenting. Facilitators need to know their boundaries and when to refer when an issue is beyond their scope of practice. One father was clear he did not want therapy:

> *I was looking for somebody to talk [to] who isn't going to diagnose me, who isn't going to tell me that it's okay to cry … I know it's okay to have those feelings. If I didn't have those feelings that's when I'd need to go to somebody and say something's wrong with me.*

Parents want and need consistency. As much as possible the facilitator should remain the same week to week. Rotating facilitators is counterproductive for parents who are trying to learn to trust themselves. The facilitator should be mindful of each group member, observe their behavior, be comfortable with anxiety as normal behavior in pregnancy after loss … and let go. Wanting people to be farther ahead than they are or trying to push them forward can be difficult to resist. The facilitator must consciously accept that the unborn baby's developmental process will carry parents through when they are ready, not the facilitator. Facilitators also need to listen for the clues parents give about unresolved trauma from the last experience (Engelkemeyer & Marwit 2009; Gudmundsdottir & Chesla 2006). The ability to reflect parents' words helps them clarify their needs (Neilsen-Gatti et al. 2011) and supports healing.

It is always best to have two facilitators, so that they can monitor group dynamics more closely, support each other, and debrief after each session. When there is only one facilitator, that individual carries the burden of attending to the person who is speaking while also trying to monitor the impact of the discussion on other group members. Caution should also be used in determining who might facilitate a group. Health care providers are trained in diagnosis and treatment and may not necessarily be the best people to provide the emotional support parents need (Parkes 2002). A facilitator does not need personal experience of loss to be effective. In fact, having experienced a loss could be detrimental if the facilitator does not guard their boundaries carefully. From an ethical perspective, a helpful rule to follow when considering sharing personal experiences is to evaluate the purpose of a particular story (is it perhaps to make the facilitator feel better?) or consider whether there is another way to address the issue. That said, a parent volunteer from a former group can be a valuable resource. This person represents "survival" of a successful subsequent pregnancy and can make suggestions and comments that a professional can not. The volunteer also understands parents' fear and sense of reservation regarding joining a group and, with permission from the parent to the referring professional, can make phone calls to invite new people to the group.

Ultimately, the background of the facilitator may be less important than the ability to follow the parents' process, stay with them in their stories, provide factual clinical information, and be open to discovery. Collaborating with professionals such as child life specialists, childbirth educators, social workers, or family educators can be an important component of meeting the needs of these parents. Regardless of the facilitator's background their role is to provide the holding environment and understand continued bond and attachment theories as the foundation of the intervention whereby "the baby leads the way."

BOX 12.1

Qualities needed by a facilitator when working with people who are suffering[2]

- Presence
- Heart-centeredness
- Compassion
- Humility
- Ability to embrace silence
- Ability to provide a sacred space
- Honor
- Strength to bear witness without comment
- Ability to serve, not fix
- Ability to listen not teach.

Confidentiality

Absolute confidentiality is critical within a support group. When new parents join, the ground rule "What is said in group stays in group" is reiterated. This especially applies to reporting back to health care providers. Even when physicians ask specifically about how a group member is doing, the issues discussed by a parent during a group session should never be reported without that person's consent. Instead, parents should be allowed to share information about how to ask questions and seek answers directly from their health care provider. The group's power lies in the group process, not in the facilitators.

Group closure

Bowman (1995) stresses that how a group session ends is crucial because that is the memory group members take with them. No matter how much time may have been spent reviewing past pregnancies or deceased babies, the group ends with everyone coming back to acknowledge the unborn babies who are here now. Reading an affirmation for each baby is a powerful way to close each meeting starting with the youngest fetus and ending with the one nearest birth. Each affirmation features some element of the baby's developmental stage (Kilvington & Brunies 1992). For example, an affirmation at week 10 is "The cartilage of your baby's pre-skeleton forms," and at week 18 is "Your baby is now sensitive to light that penetrates the uterine wall." Sometimes the affirmations can begin with the name of the deceased sibling; for example, "This affirmation is for Charlie's unborn sibling." The group becomes a safe place in which to talk about all the babies in all the families.

Summary of PAL group

Participating in a group and sharing feelings is good, not just for the person who is doing the sharing, but also for the other people taking part. Something happens in a group that is healing (Moyer 1993). In a way, it's a gift. This has been found in both face-to-face and online support groups (Gold et al. 2011). Nettle (1995) has suggested that obstetricians have lagged behind oncologists in the provision of support groups, primarily because of a lack of knowledge about what groups do and the benefits to be gained, and the relatively small number of patients obstetricians might identify as needing to attend one. Others suggest that helping parents understand their continued relationship to the deceased baby while embracing a new baby appears to decrease their risk of depression. There is also less chance of grief becoming complicated; for example, whereby it has not been processed at the expense of embracing the new baby (Attig 2001; Gaines 1997; O'Leary 2004; O'Leary & Thorwick 2006).

> I think saying things out loud is huge and you don't do that online. It's great to write, it's great to journal but when you say something out loud it's breaking a barrier. And sometimes you can't say things because you don't want to start crying. So the words actually can't come out because your crying stops it but I think it's really important to get past that and verbalize what's going on. Otherwise it gets hidden. It doesn't go away of course, it just doesn't get out. There's so much about honoring what you've been through and what you are going through now. Sometimes when you say something out loud it's not as big as it was before you said it.

To date there has been only one focused ethnographic study of a face-to-face PAL support group (Côté-Arsenault & Freije 2004). It found that parents learned how to cope with their pregnancy in a supportive environment where loss was the common thread, worry was normal, all babies were honored, new skills were gained for advocating for self and baby with providers, and personal growth was achieved. A home visiting program run by nurses, the aim of which was to normalize the pregnancy after loss experience, reduce anxiety and depression in pregnancy by teaching women skills to manage their anxiety, and facilitate prenatal attachment

(Côté-Arsenault et al. 2014) found that, compared to the control group, women felt an increased level of support and their anxiety was reduced; the differences, however, were not statistically significant.

BOX 12.2

Key points to observe in a PAL support group

- Parents attend as unique people and find a commonality.
- What is said in group stays in group.
- Group membership is open-ended; parents at varying gestational stages support each other within the context of the different phases of prenatal parenting.
- The facilitator should:
- Maintain a focus on the developmental stage of each baby in the group and the phases of prenatal parenting.
- Facilitate the parent relationship with their deceased baby alongside the baby in the current pregnancy.
- Listen empathetically.
- Probe gently for feelings.
- Not be afraid of silence and able to wait. There is always someone else in the group who is more uncomfortable than them.
- Use the group process to help parents problem solve, for example by asking "Does that sound familiar to any of you?"
- Facilitate group members helping each other rather than them being the "expert."
- Maintain balance in the group by being aware of who might be talking too much and those who aren't talking at all.
- Establish boundaries; the facilitator is not an educator or a nurse in this context.
- Avoid rescuing or fleeing; they do not "fix" they reflect back feelings.
- Be aware of their comfort level in relation to loss; they should not take on the pain of the parents.
- Close each session by coming back to the present and acknowledging the unborn babies in the room.

In an anonymous follow-up survey of 75 former PAL support group participants, all of the respondents said that their anxiety was reduced but, as other research has found, did not completely go away until the birth of their healthy babies (Côté-Arsenault & Dombeck 2001; Côté-Arsenault & O'Leary 2015). Most striking in the evaluations were parents reporting that the group helped them learn to advocate for themselves and their baby. This implies that the model of prenatal parenting, "the baby leading," helped them engage actively in their health care. Thus, given their obstetric history, it may be beneficial for physicians to routinely refer parents pregnant after loss to a support group just as they would refer a woman with gestational diabetes to a nutritionist. This would reframe behaviors which may be seen as pathological to normal in the light of their obstetric history.

Group support may also reduce the time physicians spend on psychosocial issues, thus permitting efficient but unhurried emphasis on medical issues (Nettles 1995). Parents gain increased knowledge about their problems and concerns, and potentially develop improved understanding about what can and cannot be done in their plan of care (Nettles 1995; O'Leary 2009). Other benefits may include fewer phone calls to the health care provider, increased patient satisfaction, and improved patient compliance (Nettles 1995).

Parents need a safe place in which to discuss their fears and anxieties in an open and caring environment (Côté-Arsenault & Freije 2004; Côté-Arsenault & O'Leary, 2015; O'Leary & Thorwick 2006). The group can provide parents with the opportunity to share and talk about their thoughts and feelings, which they may hide from their friends or extended family (Dyregrov et al. 2014a). The provision of psychosocial support to parents pregnant after loss has been described as at least as important as medical management of the pregnancy, and warranting the same degree of consideration (Aho et al. 2006; Condon 2006; O'Leary & Thorwick 2006; Turton et al. 2006).

The strongest argument favoring a PAL group is that parents offer and receive understanding, information, and support in ways that care providers, family, or friends are unable to. Only other bereaved parents truly understand their anxiety and fears when embarking on another pregnancy.

> In the support group you share life experiences. Maybe not the same but if you've suffered a loss you know what that feels like, you all have some commonality. With family, you may not have had somebody in your family that's had some kind of life experience or loss so all they see is your pain, they don't see your progression through it. They grieve for you, they grieve for the loss, they grieve for the grandchild, but they're also grieving for you as their child and all of your pain.

Parents attending such groups reported a greater understanding of their grief and attachment issues and, just as in an infant loss group (Cacciatore 2007), found comfort in their similarities with other parents (Côté-Arsenault & Freije 2004; McCreight 2004; O'Leary 2008).

> I've been able to get support from people so I know that the things I'm thinking and feeling are not unusual and that they're not out of the realm of being normal.
>
> That was an important part for me too, thinking of the babies as whole people before they were born and communicating with the babies [twins] about the loss and communicating that mommy's scared about this. I know that the babies know the chemical reactions when you're nervous or when you're grieving.

Summary

This chapter has addressed the difference between infant loss and PAL support groups and presented a model of intervention that combines the continued bond and attachment theories used in over 30 years of clinical practice. These parents know that pregnancy comes with no guarantees. They need professionals who understand that their fears and anxieties are *normal*. As with all infant mental health and educational intervention, following the lead of the parents will ultimately allow "the baby to lead," beginning in pregnancy.

Notes

1 Pregnancyafterlossupport.com and palsmagazine@gmail.com.
2 Adapted from *The Sacred Tree* (Bopp et al. 1989).

13

BEREAVED PARENTS RAISING CHILDREN

Regardless of how the loss occurred, this chapter explores the challenges parents face in rebuilding trust in the world as they move forward and raise their children. The chapter also explores ways in which the experience of loss can change parenting behaviors and how parents integrate their deceased child into their family.

Little research has addressed parenting after a perinatal loss. Historically what has been written has not necessarily been helpful. Often called the "replacement" (Grout & Romanoff 1999) or "vulnerable child," under the influence of a "Ghost" or "penumbra baby," the children may be seen as subject to increased risk of psychopathology, including attachment disorders (Cain & Cain 1964; Heller & Zeanah 1999; Kempson et al. 2008; Powell 1995; Poznanski 1972). Indeed, the long-term effects of the parents' heightened anxiety and fear during pregnancy have been found to affect the mental health needs of the subsequent child (O'Leary & Gaziano 2011). In a study assessing the mother–child attachment relationship with one-year-old children born after a loss, 45 percent of the infants had disorganized attachments compared with 15 percent in the "normal" non-bereaved population (Heller & Zeanah 1999). It is important to note that this study was undertaken with bereaved parents who were not necessarily offered supportive intervention at the time of loss or in the pregnancy that followed.

Protective parenting: rebuilding trust

When parents have lost a child through whatever cause, it is understandable that they exhibit overprotective behaviors raising subsequent children (Buckle & Fleming 2011; Lamb 2002; Pantke & Slade 2006; Rosenblatt 2000a). This is why parents continue to need support in dealing with the fear that this baby could also die (Armstrong et al. 2009; Côté-Arsenault & O'Leary 2015; O'Leary 2005). The fear, anxiety, and stress experienced during nine months of pregnancy take time to resolve. Parents also need time to truly believe they have a healthy baby. Anxiety levels can decrease but the symptoms of posttraumatic stress can remain in the moderate range at eight months (Armstrong et al. 2009) and even 16 months (Theut et al. 1992) after birth for some parents. Although no information was given on bereavement care for mothers who chose elective termination, one study found relational disharmony between the mother and subsequent child (Alexander et al. 2015) speculated to be the result of the mother's inability to resolve the grief associated with her decision, especially if the death occurred late in pregnancy. These parents have lost their sense of naivety and strive to do everything to avoid having to endure again the pain that results from the death of a child.

> *I was so very overprotective. I remember when he turned once and I was like, "Oh my God, I've been holding my breath waiting for him to die."*
>
> *I think we are maybe much more concerned about situations, a little bit more scared in the world than other people would be. Both of us make sure that all the safety rules are followed; you wear your helmet when you're doing this, be careful about that. I don't know if it stops us from doing stuff but it certainly colors the way we do those things; crossing the street, going sledding, whatever, so I think we're far more cautious.*

The reason for overprotectiveness is valid but the behavior is not. Overprotective parenting style and poor parent–child affectional bonds can impact children's later mental health (Armstrong & Hutti 1998; O'Leary & Gaziano 2011). Therefore bereaved parents must try harder than most to allow their children to be children. It can be helpful for parents to assess their overprotective behavior by comparing it to that of non-bereaved friends who they think are doing a good job in raising their children (O'Leary & Warland 2011).

> *There is something to be gained from having friends who have never experienced loss and are sort of skipping through the tulips, as I used to say. I can tone down to some degree the overprotectiveness. But I really think it's more of an emotional thing and it's our connecting with our kids.*

Overprotective behavior can understandably make it difficult for parents to leave their child in someone else's care. Leaving their child for the first time when they return to work can be a difficult and overwhelming experience for some parents because this situation evokes memories of leaving the hospital without their baby who died.

> *Actually the first time I left her she was nine months old and I just had a lot of panic attacks.*
>
> *Dropping him off the first day, saying goodbye at a new daycare place, I would feel really sad as I left, maybe also a little guilty.*

These parents need more reassurance that their child is safe, and thus often only ask a close family member to babysit.

> *They had their first babysitter when [my oldest daughter] was five, probably four and a half. We had [their grandmother]. I was comfortable with that so I could do that. But she was about the only person because she just lived really close and she was always there.*

Ten years after their loss these parents were still rarely away from their three subsequent children:

> *We never wanted to leave him [first subsequent child], which in hindsight was terrible for our [the parents'] relationship. Even now we rarely do. I think a lot of it is still, something could happen to them. We just need to do as much as we can because there is so much we can't control. That's why I stay home with the kids because … life is so short.*

As the above quotation illustrates, parents do need to regain their relationship as a couple. Care providers need to encourage parents not to wait until their children are older before they start doing things for themselves. This humorous account demonstrates why:

> *When I did get a babysitter and went out, the kids were just shocked that I looked good. They like, almost fell over. They were like* mom*! I was wearing a skirt and jacket and they said, "Are those your real legs?" Then I thought, maybe I need to go out more often.*

Teachers need to be aware that protective behavior on the part of previously bereaved parents can continue throughout their children's schooling:

> *I can't leave the boys with a neighborhood babysitter. I'm hiring a nanny for the summer and she has a Master's in child psych and is a middle school teacher, pretty high credentials. I've interviewed some other people; they might do a fine job but I just want them to have CPR, want to be of a more mature level and I need to know where they are. If I can't get a hold of them I just go crazy. I do let my mom take care of them and my nephew, who is in his twenties. That's about it. I feel safe with family. They go to private school now and I feel safe with them there.*

Just as they learned to advocate during their pregnancy (O'Leary & Warland 2012), these parents continue to need concrete, specific reassurance from those caring for their children. Parents should be encouraged to share their family story with those who look after their children because it explains why they are anxious and may stop them from being viewed as overprotective (ibid). Those looking after their children can ameliorate overprotective behavior by seeking more information from the parents and listening carefully to identify their needs:

The daycare providers helped to make it easier. They were really supportive and vali-dated what we needed to do. It was very personalized and it was a very good experience.

Similar to the reasoning behind parents' choice of health care provider for their pregnancy, this parent did not choose a particular day care provider because she was unclear of their expectations regarding children in the classroom:

They didn't provide us with much information. When we asked questions, they seemed to think we were questioning their ability to do their job instead of finding out just what's going on in the classroom. She was pretty upset with us for even asking the question. It wasn't very long after that that we pulled him out of that situation because we couldn't count on how things were being handled there. The kids in that class were probably three and four year olds and I think you need to know a whole lot about the behavior expectations at that age.

Parents may continue to worry about the physical health of their subsequent child or children (Theut et al. 1992). It is perfectly normal to worry about sickness in this way. Finding a pediatrician who will be sensitive to their history is important:

I've been very pro-active. I only see certain pediatricians now. I said, you should just put this on the front of my file, that this is my history and that you need to probably do a little more with me than you would an average parent. Dr. Smith has been our primary and he's just great. I've encountered a couple of other doctors who will say, "Lady, what's your problem?" and now I just won't see them. I say, put it on there so they read that so they know I'm just not your average parent waiting in here.

Loss changes the family landscape forever (Buckle & Fleming 2011), both for par-ents and the deceased baby's siblings. Worrying about sickness is not confined to the subsequent baby, nor bereaved parents. This family found that their older child who also experienced the loss of the baby lives with concerns too:

This fear is not confined to us, as our children also feel anxious when there is sickness. Recently when Sarah was quite sick with a high temperature, Gregory said, "She looks pale like Emma, is she going to die too?"

Some parents are aware they need help to not be overprotective and this should be noted by professionals:

I definitely would have benefited from more emotional support through parenting chil-dren after a loss. I kind of look back, I was so scared and I had so much anxiety that I think I realize it more now than when I was going through it. I was just so deter-mined to have a healthy child that maybe I didn't deal with some things in pursuit of parenthood.

Intentional parenting

Rather than describing parents' behavior as overprotective, it may be helpful to reframe it in a more positive light, as intentional parenting (O'Leary & Warland 2012). In this context, "intentional" means parents prefer a parenting style whereby spontaneity is avoided and deliberation, intent, and planning valued. Especially in regard to discipline, parents report that it is helpful when they are clear about rules:

> *I have rules but I always hear the children out. I don't do any physical disciplining whatsoever. I try and follow the love and logic type of parenting.*
>
> *I'm trying to find a balance which I realize is healthier for the boys, as I work on issues and let go a little bit. I have made a really conscious effort to keep myself in check about that. I really make a specific effort not to go overboard with them.*

Parents need to resume a healthy lifestyle too, trusting that their children will be safe even if they are not hovering over them:

> *I'm working really hard on trying to enjoy life and being a little bit more light-hearted about things, but it's definitely a challenge for me.*

A paradoxical parenting style

Realizing how lucky they are to be parents coupled with their understanding of the reality that children can die, leaves parents feeling vulnerable. One study reported that parents feel as though these children do not completely belong to them but are simply on loan (Green & Solnit 1964). These parents know things can happen that they have little or no control over. Similar to parents who have lost older children, the post-death approach to child-rearing of these parents can make them feel powerless to prevent harm (Buckle & Fleming 2011). Warland et al. (2011b) describe a "paradoxical" parenting style in parents raising children after a loss; that is, they are simultaneously *in control but out of control*, as this example demonstrates:

> *I remember not even turning the monitor on. My friends would ask why I wasn't afraid of SIDS [sudden infant death syndrome], and I think I didn't feel that way because I felt like if it was gonna happen, it was gonna happen. I am not going to be able to do anything about it. I am not going to like hear her last breath and know that it is her last breath. Do I want it to happen, NO, I try to do everything in my power to prevent it but beyond that if it is going to happen I am powerless to stop it. It is up to nature.*

Although this mother let her children experiment to help her let go of overprotective behavior, she also prepared herself for the worst:

> *I always did have pictures [in my mind] of them dying and being in a casket, and how I would plan the funeral. No one in the family did that. I was living the practical side, if they die, what will I do? Who will I call?*

Sharing the story of a deceased baby with the subsequent child

Parents may wonder when they should tell the subsequent child about the sibling before them. During a relationship-based parenting intervention in a subsequent pregnancy, parents naturally share the story of their deceased baby with the fetus. To avoid their children feeling that they were carrying a "burden" regarding being born after a loss, one family honored this as part of their story (O'Leary & Thorwick 2006):

> *Our subsequent children have known grief from conception onward, because losing Micah changed who we are and how we've parented our daughters. We actually think it is a gift—especially in a culture that is so afraid of grief. We feel like our daughters got a healthier start at a spiritual level, because Micah's life and death have always been a part of their being. It's a natural part of their being, not something they have to learn to cope with or manage or run away from.*

> *My subsequent child is now two and has seen pictures of her big brother. She's asked, "Who's that?" We told her that her brother died and is with the angels. She's been to the cemetery many times. She now talks about her brother on occasion. Out of the blue she'll say, "Ben died, Mommy." Or, "This is Ben's toy." She accepts the idea on her level of understanding, and I like that he's become a part of her idea of our family.*

Another mother saved the gifts that were given to her first child, who died, and gave one to each of his siblings as a gift from Bailey. *Madeline got a little blanket, Max got a couple little stuffed animals, and Isabelle got a little bunny. So they now have them in their room and that's their presents from their big brother.*

For other parents, sharing the information can take time and need guidance from a professional. Some children realize they may not have been born if their sibling had not died (Jonas-Simpson et al. 2014; Warland et al. 2011a). *We don't know if we would have been born, my brother and I.* One wise mother describes her response to her 12-year-old son's question:

> *"Mom, if she hadn't died, would I be here?" You could just see the profound meaning at that very moment in time. It just drained all energy from him. And I just put my arm around him and said, "You know, I don't know how all of this works but I really believe that you were meant to be a part of our family. I don't know if you would have been born a year later or if you would have been born at another time but I truly believe you were meant to be with us."*

Memory building: keeping the deceased baby in the family

How the family keeps the memory of their deceased baby alive is a personal choice, and an important goal for all family members (Fanos et al. 2009). Just as parents have a continued bond with and attachment to the deceased baby, so do children continue their sibling relationship to him (Erlandsson et al. 2010; Jonas-Simpson et al. 2015; Packman et al. 2006; Thompson et al. 2011).

Children often become the memory keepers for the missing sibling (Kempson & Murdock 2010; Jonas-Simpson et al. 2015; Limbo & Kobler 2009). In the preschool years children follow the lead of their parents. Art has been found to be a useful tool for helping children integrate a sibling into their lives and letting others know they have a missing brother or sister (Jonas-Simpson, et al. 2015). It is quite common for children from bereaved families to include their baby in pictures as a continued member of the family:

> When my daughter and her little friend draw pictures of their family, her little friend will say, "Remember to draw Connor." They'll have conversations about her brother Connor, that he's in heaven, how he died, and these little four- and five-year-old girls will have conversations about death and her brother in heaven.

Responses to grief are very individual for children as well as adults. It is important for professionals to be mindful that how parents respond to their children's requests for more information needs to be tailored to the language around death they already use (Limbo & Kolber 2009). Some bereaved siblings rely on their faith/belief system as a source of comfort (Thompson et al. 2011):

> I remember Darby drawing a picture of the family and she drew three. It wasn't elaborate, it was like sticks; it was mom and dad drawn and then there were three kids. Why are there three kids? You only have a brother. And she said, I have an angel.

> He will correct me if I say I have three children in front of other people. And I'm at least partially responsible for that because he had so many questions early on about Connor. The best way that I could describe it is to say, "He's your brother and he's an angel and he's looking out for you; he's your guardian angel. He's with us, he's with you all the time." So that must have impressed upon him that he's always got somebody behind him. He draws pictures of our family with Connor floating with wings above us. Often he will tell me things like, "If Connor were here he'd do this."

Keeping the memory of the deceased child within the family should not overtake family life:

> You can't ignore the fact that you had a child who passed away. But you can't make your house a memorial to that child either because then the other children suffer. You have to find a balance.

> I generally remind myself how blessed I am to have them, how fragile life is. You just forget sometimes. I think that's made a difference in how we try to treat them respectfully and not take them for granted too much. We try to make it known that Sydney is part of our family but not have it impact our everyday life too much.

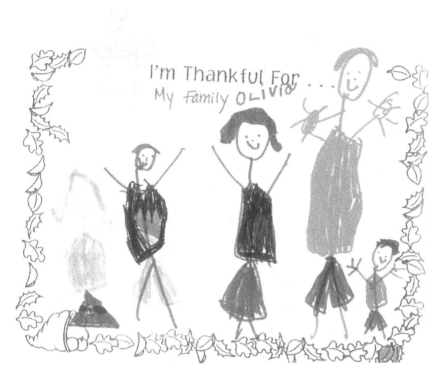

FIGURE 13.1

Losing Matthew still affects me every single day. There's really not a day that it doesn't cross my mind, some times in a positive way but it's not always fear based. I've thought a lot about, one of the coolest things about subsequent children is you just think they were in the same space, and I always wonder if they knew that somebody else was living in there. I think they do. That's why it's important for me to let them know that Matthew was there, that he's their brother, and to celebrate his birthday, that it is a significant day and we recognize it.

Children's view of their parents' parenting

Children can also link the way they were parented to the loss of their sibling, some understanding why their parents were overprotective, *Yeah probably a bit overprotective. I know it is for a reason*, and others feeling the opposite, *I found that they were very open to us having adventures and kind of being confident and independent.* Most adolescents in one study felt neither overprotected nor that they were a replacement (Warland et al. 2011a), and the researchers speculated that that was the case because their parents had undertaken professional counseling and/or peer support in the early years following their loss. This intervention may have assisted the parents to deal appropriately with their loss, thus enabling them to provide appropriate parenting to their subsequent child. Others whose parents did not have support described being held at a distance or feeling invisible (O'Leary et al. 2006c, 2011b).

Parents' altered view of self

Some parents recognize that their experience has had a positive effect on their parenting and their appreciation of the value of life (O'Leary et al. 2011):

> *This experience has fundamentally changed who I am. It's changed how I parent. It's changed everything—how I understand what life is about and how I live my life.*

Parents today are very aware of research demonstrating the effect of maternal stress on the unborn baby, and some may continue to worry that their continued anxiety about safety can be transferred to their children:

> *The kids definitely pick up on your anxiety and I realized it's important for me to work through this, to not hand this off to them too and that they respond. I have a lot of guilt about the anxiety I felt while they were in utero. I wonder how that affected them.*
>
> *They already were hearing so they knew what the anxiety was about. I do think as they get older I'm doing better, I'm more comfortable. I realize it's their job to separate from me more.*

It is important to focus on the positive gifts that can eventually result from the experience of losing a child:

> *I think I'm a better person, I think I'm much more sensitive, I think I have a lot more compassion. I think I'm more present in all my relationships with people, having that vulnerability. I know people would say, everything happens for a reason. At the time that's not real comforting but I do feel like this is my path, doing the Faith's Lodge[1] thing and that everybody that comes through gets a quilt. And the letters I've gotten from families talking about when they got home, being able to wrap themselves in something is a real comfort. It's a mission in my life to be able to provide comfort to families who walk through the same path. I think I'm instilling that in the boys.*

Twelve years after the loss of their first baby, this mother describes her continuing grief for her first son after birthing two healthy subsequent children: *[It's] maybe a journey of always moving towards learning to live with that grief in your life and to share it with the people who care about you and are concerned about you.* The continued bond with and attachment to a deceased child remains, as it should, part of the family story.

Summary

This chapter has addressed how parents move forward in raising children after a perinatal loss. They have experienced the worst possible outcome for parents, which subsequently changes their life view and how they parent other children. They understand that keeping the memory of their deceased baby alive is important for the family. They are naturally more protective of their surviving children but there is still little research on other aspects of parenting after a perinatal loss, especially the long-term impact on the mental health of all family members.

Note

1 http://faithslodge.org/.

14

WHAT ABOUT THE CHILDREN?

A child can live through anything, so long as he or she is told the truth and is allowed to share with loved ones the natural feelings people have when they are suffering.[1]

According to the Early Childhood Longitudinal Study, Birth Cohort (ECLS-B 2005), one in every four currently parenting women in the United States has experienced one or more reproductive losses during her lifetime (Price 2006). There are 26,000 stillbirths in the US each year, which is equal to the number of deaths caused by SIDS and prematurity combined (Hankins & Longo 2006), and an additional 19,000 newborn deaths in the first month of life. These statistics are echoed in other high-income countries across the globe (Flenady et al. 2011). Often these parents have other children who bear witness to (and will be impacted by) their grief. This chapter addresses the experiences of existing children at the time of loss and during the pregnancy that follows, and of the children born after loss, including those who are now teenagers and adults.

When birth goes wrong, parents' sense of self in relation to others changes, including their children (O'Leary & Thorwick 2008; Shainess 1963). Grieving parents display a variety of feelings: anxiety, insecurity, betrayal, abandonment, and vulnerability (Attig 2002), all of which can compromise their awareness of the emotions children may be encountering in their home. Rarely do parents know how to explain such a loss to their children or if they should even try; social norms and myths surrounding children and grief may confuse the issue (see the nearby box). They will often question if the older sibling is still a brother or sister. With little information, parents can feel powerless to alleviate their children's grief (Bartellas & Van Aerde 2003; Buckle & Fleming 2011; Schwab 2009), and may inadvertently neglect their needs, fail to respond to their overtures for care, or provide a secure base (Avelin et al. 2011; Davies 2006; Leon 1996).

BOX 14.1

- Myths about children and grief
- Adults should be able to teach their children about death and spirituality
- There is a stage like progression to children's experience of grief
- Adult grief does not impact children
- Parents, educators, and clergy are qualified and prepared to help
- Infants and toddlers are too young to grieve
- Adults should avoid topics that cause a child to cry
- An active playing child is not a grieving child
- Children are better off if they don't attend funerals.[2]

Whilst these myths about children and grief were written in 1983 many are still prevalent today. Children in families who experience a perinatal death suffer two losses: their anticipated sibling and the parents they knew before the loss (O'Leary & Gaziano 2011). An adult sibling explains, *When I was 16 my mom had a stillbirth, and I 'lost' my mom when that baby died. She became a different person.* Bereaved parents need guidance to help their children, both at the time of loss (Avelin et al. 2011; Cacciatore & Flint 2012; Limbo & Kobler 2009) and during the pregnancy that follows (O'Leary 2007; O'Leary & Gaziano 2011a). The first task is to help parents with their own grief and the second is to help them communicate with their children (Avelin et al. 2011; Davis & Limbo 2010). If the parents are okay, their children are much more likely to be okay too. Well-intended attempts to protect children from potential upset usually isolate them and impede their grieving process (O'Leary & Gaziano 2011).

The reactions of children and adolescents to grief are related to their developmental age (Sood et al. 2006). Even infants are aware of emotions and have a sensual awareness of a parent's grief, sadness, and depression (Lieberman et al. 2003; Limbo & Kobler 2009). Young children from infancy to 28 months sense emotions in the home and are likely to become more upset by the anxiety of their parents and their own fantasies than by exposure to death and dying (Erlandsson et al. 2010). The majority of children learn to recognize when something is dead at around three years of age. However, death, separation, and sleep can often be synonymous in the child's mind. Rosner et al. (2010) suggest that most kindergarten-aged children have a mature understanding of universality (all living things must die), but do not understand irreversibility (the physical body cannot ever be reanimated) or non-functionality (the dead body can no longer perform activities like a living body). Many children between the ages of three and seven in families who have experienced a perinatal loss do, however, understand that death is permanent (Dowden 1995; O'Leary & Gaziano 2011a). For example, after experiencing the loss of a full-term brother, on hearing that his friend's mother had gone to the hospital to have her baby one four-year-old child commented to his mother, *Yeah, but will she bring a baby home?*

One concern for children in bereaved families is that not only are they aware of their parents' grief but they also feel compelled to take it on (Jonas-Simpson 2014), as some adult subsequent children have reported (O'Leary & Gaziano 2011a). Parents need to reassure a young child that it is not her job to comfort them (Jonas-Simpson et al. 2015). Children also need to know that the family is a safe place within which to share feelings and that their parents will be there to listen to their fears, fantasies, and questions and validate their individual thoughts and feelings. An example is this mother reassuring her four year old when she cries:

> It was really hard for him to see me cry. I would tell him, I'm still okay when I'm cry-ing. Mommy's still okay. We had to work through that a lot. One time I went to the doctor and he wanted to come because he was going with me all the time when I was pregnant. I said, "No, I'm just going to go by myself with Grandma." He said, "Why can't I come?" and I responded, "Well it's going to be hard. I'm probably going to cry a lot." He jumped up and said, "But you said you would be okay! You can't go there and cry!" So we had to talk about how I'm going to cry there but I will come home and I will be okay.

Some children may perceive their parents' grief as too overwhelming and forgo their own expressions of grief or even fail to acknowledge their own feel-ings in order to avoid adding more pain within the family (Crenshaw 2002; Jonas-Simpson et al. 2015; O'Leary & Gaziano 2011a). One older adult sibling described herself as becoming "the perfect child" to make her parents happy again after the loss of her baby brother, a common means of coping expressed by many siblings (Buckle & Fleming 2011). *I was the perfect student. I don't know if it was ever conscious. I read all about the saints and suffering because I was suffering too.* This suggests the need to explore with those parents who speak of their child as being "so well behaved" the feelings that may lie beneath such behavior (O'Leary & Gaziano 2011a).

At the time of loss: meeting the baby

Siblings have the right to meet the dead baby to understand that she is really dead (Avelin et al. 2011). Yet there is a strong tendency for parents to not include young children, in the hope of sparing them from the same pain they are experiencing (Fanos et al. 2009; O'Leary 2007; Roose & Blanford 2011). Despite their desire to protect their child from pain it becomes painfully obvious that parents cannot hide the permanence of a baby missing from their family.

Whether or not a sibling has an opportunity to say farewell to a deceased baby can depend on the care parents receive in the hospital (Erlandsson et al. 2010). Most hospitals today offer parents the opportunity to spend time with their deceased baby, take photographs, and share the experience with extended family and friends

(Côté-Arsenault 2003; Warland 2000). There is strong agreement that these opportunities to bond with the deceased baby are helpful to the parents but less effort is made to include siblings or resources given to parents on helping their children when they go home. Parents report wanting support from hospital personnel, especially in relation to how a sibling might react on meeting the deceased baby (Avelin et al. 2011). Health care providers need to frame the loss in a way that is congruent with individual family values, beliefs and practices, and provide suggestions for involving children in creating keepsakes and rituals for meaning making (Limbo & Kobler 2009; Warland 2000).

Children can deal with the truth if they are prepared for it. Parents need to provide not only the facts but also information about how a child may be feeling, and what and what not to expect (Crenshaw 2002; Davis 2006; O'Leary 2007; O'Leary & Gaziano 2011a). A child who has been involved in a sibling's illness and death (for example, neonatally in a NICU) will have a better opportunity to grieve, express feelings, and gain information (Nolbris et al. 2014; Roose & Blanford 2011; Rosenberg et al. 2015).

Parents should be encouraged to discuss death in simple terms; for example, that it has a specific cause, involves cessation of bodily functions, and is irreversible. It is also universal (leaves die, plants die, animals die, and so do people). If the baby's death was early in pregnancy it sometimes helps to share pictures of fetal development, demonstrating visually that some babies are too small to live (O'Leary 2007; Ostler 2010).

Parents have also reported wanting to inform their child themselves so they can handle the reactions and questions before she meets the deceased baby (Avelin et al. 2011). The couple below told their daughter (who was almost three) rather than the people caring for her. Their child's behavior shows both magical thinking and her awareness of her parents' grief:

> We told her that her sister had died and she just immediately said, "Well that's okay mommy. I'm going to go to the nursery and find us a new baby." We said, "No, those babies belong to other people and they want them. Our baby is in heaven." She then responded, "Then I'm just going to fly up to heaven and get our baby for us." So she could see our pain and was very concretely trying to make it better.

Children may not understand the concept of death but need information on why their parents are sad and crying:

> Right from the moment that we knew about Emma's death, we were concerned about how we would tell the children; how we would involve them and what we would and would not offer them. As a midwife I had some idea of the kind of things which should be done for them and with them and what was best avoided; however, there were still times when we neglected them terribly, as we were immersed in our grief. As our grief continued, so our concern for them waxed and waned, depending on our ability to keep our own heads above water.

My feelings is, outwardly for my children, when they saw mommy's tummy getting big, even if my tummy wasn't getting big, if they knew there was a baby inside, something happened to that baby. They were young and their picture was a baby inside my tummy and it doesn't just go away. I really felt strongly that they needed to know what happened when the baby didn't come home and they saw us crying.

Involvement in the funeral

Whether to have children attend the funeral or memorial service is another decision parents need to consider. Children can be disenfranchised in their grief when their loss is not recognized, or they are not recognized as grieving (Corr 2008). Yet recognition and inclusion in family events and religious rituals has been assessed as an important part of supporting grieving siblings (Erlandsson et al. 2010; Kolber et al. 2007; Wilson 2001). Some parents feel this helps keep the baby in the family and also helps their children understand their parents' sadness (Avelin et al. 2011).

Children can be involved in memory creation at the time of loss (Carlson 2012; Erlandsson et al. 2010) through art—for example, drawing pictures to go with the baby in the coffin—making the invisible visible (Mitchell et al. 2011). This is especially helpful for children with limited language and higher cognitive understanding. One family brought their two children (age three and five) to the burial service for miscarried babies sponsored by a local hospital. The mother later found a picture her five-year-old son had drawn which demonstrated his awareness of her grief and the missing sibling. Selecting a toy to remain with their sibling can also be a helpful way to involved bereaved siblings (Warland 2000).

Siblings may be cared for by relatives to shield them from their parents' initial intense grief (Avelin et al. 2011). It is important to help grieving parents understand that sending a sibling away may be viewed as rejection at a time when the child is already confused about what is going on in the family (O'Leary & Gaziano 2011a). An alternative is to encourage parents to find someone the child knows and trusts to provide respite care during some hours of the day in their own home (Avelin 2011; O'Leary 2007). This person can temporarily share some of the parenting responsibilities such as reading stories to the child and alerting the parents to feelings the child may express about the loss.

The following case illustrates how one family helped their young child.

Dustin's story

Dustin was three when his newborn sister died hours after birth. His parents brought the siblings to the hospital before she died so they could see and hold her and took a picture of them together. Everyone said Dustin was too young to understand and that he probably wouldn't remember. His way of trying to make sense of what happened was visiting the cemetery. His mother related that, *He was the child in the family who once a week forced me to take him out to the grave the first year to year and a half.* When

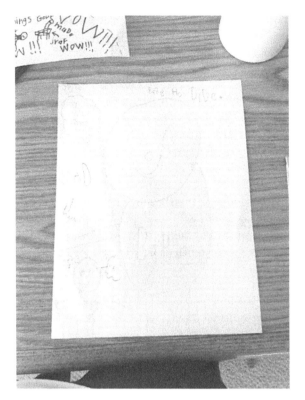

FIGURE 14.1

a baby brother was born a year later he was still processing magical thinking and the concept of what dead meant:

> *The first thing he asked on seeing that Larry was home was, "When do we get to bring Denise home, mom?" I said, "Dustin, do you remember where Denise went?"*
>
> *"Yeah, she went to visit God," he said. "Yes, that's right," I continued, "but what happens when you go to visit God?" He was quiet for a short time and then he looked at me and said, "You die. But can't she still visit us?" I told him, "Whenever you think about her she is visiting you and she will always be looking over us." He then laughed and said. "I've seen her make pictures in the clouds and with the stars so I know she loves me."*

The pregnancy that follows

> *When I became pregnant we had to consider how and when to tell them about the new baby.*

When parents enter a new pregnancy children have also lost their innocence; pregnancy does not mean a live baby will come home (O'Leary & Gaziano 2011a).

Children are intuitive, often noticing unsettling changes in their parents' behavior. They may feel their parents' anxieties and have similar fears (O'Leary 2007; O'Leary & Thorwick 2006; Warland & Warland 1996).

> When we first told her she was going to have another little brother or sister she said, "Is this one going to die like Jacob did?" We explained that we were going to do everything we [could] not to let that happen. We never promised her that it wasn't going to happen but we said we have good doctors and they're going to do what they can to keep it from happening. We're just basically telling her things that might happen. We're not looking into the future further than what we can control.

Just as during the loss, siblings need reassurance that they, their mother, and unborn sibling are all safe. They must be provided with information on how the pregnancy is progressing. Parents should be encouraged to cautiously share information so as not to take away their existing child's excited anticipation of being a big brother or sister again (O'Leary 2007):

> I just say to him [five year old], look we hope it will be alright but we don't, we just don't know. So I'm waiting to go in [to the doctor] and he says, "Will it be alright mommy?" Even yesterday, I'm not sure what—I think they were watching some video and someone was crying and Nicolas out of the blue said, "Ah mommy you were crying when you lost your baby." So obviously he's got a good memory and remembers.
>
> I can remember, they [three and five year olds] said, "Well this baby will live; this baby will live. And I told them, "I don't know. I absolutely don't know. I hope so but I really can't say. I can't tell you absolutely that this baby will live." Being honest with them and accepting that to myself was huge, and really hard.

Reassurance is especially important if there had been a crisis with the mother along with the loss of a baby. The sibling will most likely have been traumatized too. For example, one mother had been in intensive care herself when her baby died and shares how her four-year-old child responded to hearing she was pregnant again:

> He was excited that he was going to have a little brother but he was really worried. He asked if I was going to get really sick again, and he was very, very interested in what was going on; how the blood pressure was going to affect the baby and if the baby was going to die. So he was just a really nervous kid during that time. I told him that this is a different baby, this is a different time. Mommy is feeling better now, that it was going to be okay.

Her description makes apparent that the child is still traumatized by his experience of his mother losing a baby. Helping her through the pregnancy involved discussion in the support group on how her son was coping. She was encouraged to seek additional support with a child psychologist but the child's father would not agree to this (the mother and facilitator speculated that he was resistant because he was not ready to process his own experience of trauma). To help her child deal with his fear, the mother took him back to the hospital where the new baby would also be born:

> *I decided to take him to the hospital where I was going to deliver his brother, which happened to be the same place where his sister had died. We did a tour and he was very scared. He didn't want to sit on the bed, he didn't want to do anything. I just told him, this one will be different. I'll just be in a regular room. He was processing that the whole time. I think that was helpful but at the moment it was really hard for him. I knew I needed to do something like that because when I would go to my OB check-ups he would come along; it was the same OB and he would be scared.*

Supporting grieving children

The sibling relationship with a deceased baby is constructed through parental memories and expectations (Limbo & Kobler 2009). How children respond to and cope with the impact of their sibling's perinatal death may depend on the degree to which they were involved in or excluded from the experience and how their parents communicated with them about it (Avelin et al. 2014; Limbo & Kobler 2009). A school or daycare setting where children spend a good part of their time can be an important place in which to help bereaved children navigate their feelings and create space for acknowledging their grief (Jonas-Simpson et al. 2015). But teachers need education and supervision in order to know how to acknowledge a child's grief (Avelin et al. 2011). Studies exploring the role of teachers with grieving children in primary and secondary schools found that they perceive grief to be something that children do not easily forget and were aware of the importance of empathizing with them (Dyregrov et al. 2013). A further study by Dyregrov and colleagues (2014) found that teachers demonstrated limited knowledge about how child bereavement affects school performance, concentration, and learning. In turn, this restricted teachers' own efforts to arrange support for grieving children during the school day because of heavy workloads and lack of knowledge about grief, leaving them feeling guilty for not doing more. Classmates knowing the story can help children feel less isolated (Auman 2007; Holland 2008; Jonas-Simpson 2014) and provide on-going support for the sibling's grief and the sibling relationship. As one eight-year-old child said, *My best friend knows about him and some kids in my class know about him.*

Most children whose parents have been open about what happened in the family do want to share the loss of a sibling with their teacher or classmates (Jonas-Simpson 2014). This mother describes her subsequent child's experience:

> *The first thing he told the teacher at kindergarten readiness was that he had a brother who died and that he [the deceased brother] would be in kindergarten otherwise. When he started kindergarten he told me that whenever his class does anything to do with the family he always includes his brother. He asked the teacher if that was okay and she*

said that was fine. This meant so much to him (and to us!). He has included him in many ways in his school work both in kindergarten and first grade.

It is helpful for parents to ask what the child might want to share and then help them process what to say. For example, one mother purchased black wristbands[3] for her children (who were six and eight) to wear that represented the loss of a baby brother. She then helped them formulate words if classmates asked about the wristbands; what to say when they felt like sharing and also when they didn't.

When parents have difficulty in telling their children what happened, they need guidance on how to move forward. A teacher may see a child acting out the story in play or art work. This can open an opportunity to discuss the child's behavior and explore how she is managing at home, what parents have shared about the loss, and how the school can help. Teachers can ask, "Have you noticed any changes in your child's behavior?" They can encourage parents to share photographs and stories of the deceased sibling to help the child memorialize in a healthy way. Lots of books are available to help parents address their children's needs and children understand their feelings.[4]

Parents' ability to continue assessing how their children are coping can also help address potential worries such as children's belief that it was their fault the baby died (O'Leary & Gaziano 2011b), which they are often unable to express (Limbo & Kobler 2009). One sibling, aged four years when her eight-month-old brother died in his crib, did not reveal until she was an adult that she felt it was her fault because she had asked her mother to read *one more bedtime story* before she checked on the baby. Another adult sibling reflects on her feelings during her mother's repeated experience of miscarriage, which persisted until adulthood:

> *I remember lots of the miscarriages as a toddler/preschooler and my mom often feeling sad and alone. I was frightened and often overwhelmed. I still need to hear that what happened was not my fault and I couldn't fix it or make my mom feel better.*

The sibling relationship and sense of loss is neither short-lived nor forgotten (Sveen et al. 2014). Sibling grief can be as significant as that of a bereaved parent (DeVita-Raeburn 2004; Jonas-Simpson et al. 2015; Kempson & Murdock 2010) and continues beyond the physical death (Nolbris et al. 2014; Packman et al. 2006). *I will never recover but I do get used to her not being here.* Children will revisit and ask more questions as they mature to gain a new level of understanding regarding what happened at the time of the sibling's death. At approximately age seven or eight, children begin to understand the meaning of death and often miss the older sibling in a very different way, wanting more information:

> *In the last few months as her [seven-year-old] cognitive awareness has increased, so has her difficulty grasping what happened. We've been out to his grave a couple of times this summer and she has this deep, deep heart-wrenching sadness that overcomes her. She goes through phases too where she'll lay in bed crying, missing him, wanting to know him.*

Carol [age six] has started to ask more questions, just like her older brother did at that age, about the brother who died before they were born. It is definitely not as intense with her but interesting. She pretends he is in the room. She told me that she does not miss him because he is with her. She also has told me that she does not think it is fair that I got to see him and she did not!

In studies of bereaved teenagers who have experienced the death of a sibling as a result of SIDS, accident, cancer, or perinatal loss, all felt they had been emotionally affected by it and that the effects were long term (Johnson & Warland 2012; Rosenberg et al. 2015). As described by others at this age (Jonas-Simpson 2014), they had a more mature understanding of the parents' grief and seemed to be particularly sensitive to and understanding of their pain:

Dad doesn't talk about things as much as mum does and lets things go by. He thinks about things a lot, like lots of men do; thinks about it and thinks about it, which annoys mum because she likes to get things done. ... If I lost either of them I don't know what I would do. I don't know how they dealt with it and I don't understand how mom and dad have dealt with it. I have never been in that situation of losing someone. I just feel so sorry for them. (Teenage girl)

It's hard seeing mom suffering like this because we used to always go shopping and have fun and everything but now, she still likes going shopping but she hates seeing the pregnant people.

(Teenage girl)

As children mature they develop a greater understanding of how they and their missing sibling fits into their family (Johnson & Warland 2012; Jonas-Simpson et al. 2015; O'Leary et al. 2011). During the adolescent years some children move on from the pictures they drew when they were younger to wanting tattoos in memory of their missing sibling (Johnson & Warland 2012; Jonas-Simpson et al. 2015):

I guess I have always wanted to see what she would look like, that is something I have always wondered. I wanted to see if she would be like us, if I could see a bit of myself in her, or she could see a bit of herself in me. (Teenage boy)

It is kind of like losing a grandmother or grandfather. Mine died before I was born and [my relationship with] Emily feels like that.

(Teenage girl)

The impact of a loss continues into adulthood, as demonstrated in this quote from an adult:

I was born into a grieving family. Although I had always known I was loved, I had felt that, as a young child, I was held at arms' length. It also explained why my first memories of my parents' faces were of pain.

Some adults voice fear of having children themselves (O'Leary & Gaziano 2011). There's a lot of built up pain and anxiety about babies. I'm really worried that when *I want to have children this will happen to me*. Health care providers should gently probe more deeply with women and their partners who express a fear of labor and birth as one study found that fear of childbirth was a predisposing factor for postpartum depression (Räisänen et al. 2013). Although to our knowledge there have been no reported studies suggesting that women with infertility issues may also have been given messages inferring that pregnancy means disaster, when working with families seeking reproductive support family history regarding pregnancy should be explored for both parents as it may impact their ability to conceive (Quant et al. 2013).

How these adults came to terms with the ambiguous loss, their search for meaning and integration of this sibling relationship for many came later. Some helped elderly parents find where the baby was buried (O'Leary & Gaziano 2011b). One adult took her elderly mother and sisters to their sister's grave site and held a ceremony, something her mother had not been allowed to do at the time of her death (ibid). Still another found the grave of her deceased stillborn sister after her mother's death.

Children in bereaved families: who they become

The tragedy of loss actually results in gifts for many bereaved families, described as "post-traumatic growth" (Jonas-Simpson et al. 2015) or transformation (Davies & Limbo 2010). Children also benefit, many seeing subsequent knowledge and experience as gifts from their sibling. For example, both children alive at the time of the loss and children born after were found to share common foundational beliefs regarding being sensitive and nurturing to others, to feel a sense of sadness and curiosity about not knowing their sibling, and to feel comfortable around people who may be sad or grieving (O'Leary et al. 2011b). One mother suggested that her subsequent daughter's strong ethical stance stemmed from her *early experience of the worth of and danger inherent in life and belief in love that made her strive for justice in the world*. Children whose parents received supportive intervention during their pregnancy tend to report feeling loved and cherished by their parents (O'Leary et al. 2011a; Warland et al. 2011). This is in stark contrast to those whose parents did not get support, who described feeling invisible, held at a distance, and never "good enough" for their parents (O'Leary et al. 2006).

Regardless of how they were viewed by their parents, both adults and children who were subsequent children share a common gift of empathy for others (O'Leary & Gaziano 2011b; O'Leary et al. 2011b). Empathy involves both cognitive and affective components:

> Cognitive empathy involves a mental representation of another's internal state, while affective empathy involves the ability to recognize and vicariously experience another's emotions based on body language, facial expressions, and speech, and to identify one's own emotional state in response to another person.
>
> *(Cacciatore et al. 2015, p. 96)*

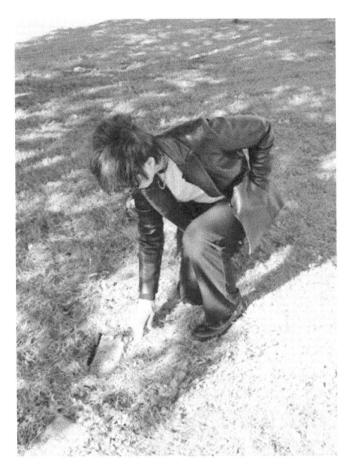

FIGURE 14.2

Quotes from a surviving twin, a mother about her adolescent and adult provide examples:

> *I feel protective [of other children]. I feel like I want to figure out why they are sad and stuff to help. Like, I just want them to be happy and get help if they need it.* (11-year-old surviving twin)

> *For his macho personality, he seems to be sensitive to other people's experiences. He has more girl buddies. He seems to be sensitive to what's going on with those girls. He'll mention things that are going on with them, things they're experiencing, if they're having a hard time.* (Mother with a 16-year-old child alive at the time of the loss)

> *A friend of mine lost a child to SIDS about eight and a half years ago. A lot of her friends didn't know what to say and avoided her at the grocery store. They were just scared or found it too painful to address her. And I just felt so pulled towards her. So I know I've been very sensitive. I really feel for people.*

> *(Adult subsequent child)*

Children who receive adequate support in relation to their grief seem to cope better (Sveen et al. 2013). Subsequent children as adolescents were found to be doing well (feeling loved, wanted, and special) while also remembering their sadness and even trauma when they first realized that they had another sibling (Warland et al. 2011). Children in bereaved families have also been described as mature beyond their years, having grown up faster than their peers, being sensitive, caring more deeply for others, being more tolerant of themselves and others, emotionally "strong" and having more of an adult understanding of life (Hogan 2006; Jonas–Simpson et al. 2015; O'Leary & Gaziano 2011a, 2011b; Steele et al. 2013).

> *He's more mature about other things because he's been exposed to death and he's thought so much about heaven and dying, so much more than other seven year olds.* (Mother talking about her subsequent child)
>
> *I've always been a lot more mature than kids my age. I didn't have time for immature high school kids. I went to class. I was more, concentrating on getting good grades. I'm here to work. I wasn't in to drinking.*
>
> *(21-year-old sibling)*

Their sensitivity and nurturing of others is reported by teachers too (O'Leary & Warland 2012):

> *Her teacher had said in school there was a little girl who has English as a second language. So Madeline, with the little bit of Spanish she learned, went over and in Spanish said, "Me llamo es Madeline." She noticed that she was feeling sad or a little bit of an outsider and included her by trying to find some common ground with her by using the little bit of Spanish that she knew. I see it in my family but seeing it in the out of the family situation too was kind of neat.*
>
> *(Mother talking about her six-year-old subsequent daughter)*

The impact of the loss of a sibling can also influence a remaining sibling's education and career goals (Rosenberg et al. 2015), some adults choosing to work in a caring profession, such as social work or chaplaincy, and aware that their career is directly related to being raised in a bereaved family (O'Leary et al. 2011a, 2011b). They universally voiced wanting parents to be aware of meeting the emotional needs of children (O'Leary & Gaziano 2011a, 2011b; O'Leary & Warland 2012; O'Leary et al. 2006; Warland et al. 2011a, 2011b). Boyraz et al. (2010) found that, on reflecting on who they are as a result of the loss, these adults found positive meanings, an important message for bereaved parents to understand—good things may emerge from their loss (Jonas–Simpson et al. 2015; O'Leary et al. 2011).

A possible explanation for these adults' and young children's sensitivity, ability to be with grieving people, and understanding of death can perhaps be found in the research on maternal emotions impacting the unborn baby. We speculate that being carried by grieving mothers can be seen as a gift in terms of understanding grief at a level that many adults don't otherwise experience until well into their adulthood, if ever:

> *She just has a heart for other people when they're sad, just what she can do to make them feel better. Even in the womb, I can count probably more than 20, 30 times when I was nervous, especially later in pregnancy, about her not being okay or not having felt her kick for a while, and she would kick.*
>
> *(Mother talking about her nine-year-old subsequent child)*

All children need age-appropriate information to help them understand the concept of death; open and honest communication is also vital (Hopkins 2002; Limbo & Kobler 2013). When children know the story of the deceased sibling's life, no matter how long that was, it is not a secret in the family. Communication skills within the family, including grandparents talking about their experiences of dealing with death and loss, are also important in terms of either helping or hindering children's involvement and in minimizing disenfranchised grief (Roose & Blanford 2011; Rosenberg et al. 2015).

Summary

This chapter has addressed ways to help children at the time of loss, in the pregnancy that follows and beyond. Most parents have no roadmap for themselves to prepare for perinatal loss, let alone their children. During this family crisis parents need professionals who can provide guidance on how to help their children. They must be encouraged to seek resources in their community to help them address their children's concerns (for example, parent educators, family life specialists, pediatric, or family nurse practitioners). Finally, this chapter has addressed the benefits children gain from being involved in rituals celebrating the life of the deceased baby and the gifts they may receive because of a missing baby in their family.

Notes

1 Eda LeShan: http://www.griefspeaks.com/id112.html.
2 Wolfelt, A. (1983). *Helping Chidlren Cope with Grief*. London, New York: Routledge.
3 Available from: www.missfoundation.org www.inmourningband.org.
4 See www.aplacetoremember.com; griefwatch.com.

15

FATHERS

It affects me too

Fathers are often neglected grievers. One reason for this is that, whilst perceptions are slowly changing, their role continues to be viewed as a source of support for the mother during pregnancy and birth, not necessarily a dyad within the plan of care. There is also a dearth of information regarding the experience of fathers during pregnancy, especially if it is not considered high risk. More information is available on fathers who have suffered a perinatal loss and their experience of the subsequent pregnancy. This chapter provides more in-depth information on fathers' experience of perinatal loss and suggests ways to meet their needs.

Father's role during pregnancy

The father's role during pregnancy is frequently marginalized; especially when their partner experiences a low-risk pregnancy, preterm birth, or perinatal loss (Condon 1985; Condon et al. 2004; McCreight 2004). Pregnancy is more than a significant phase in the genesis of the future father–infant attachment relationship. Fathers are essential to family health and well-being, the complement to the mother (May 1996). Their family background and relationship with the mother influence the infant's emotional development and future mental health (Barrows 2004; Condon 2006; Mauger 2004). Assessment of a father's psychological and emotional problems, especially in a low-risk pregnancy, is not common practice (Vreeswijk et al. 2013). However, they too have specific psychological, emotional, and physical needs, and desire options in terms of their role during the labor, birth, and postpartum experience (Bonnette & Broom 2011). Pregnancy offers a window of opportunity for recognizing and addressing men's attachment issues and mental health, as well as problems in a couple's relationship (Edvardsson et al. 2011).

The identity fathers ascribe to the unborn baby in a normal pregnancy has been found to be more strikingly similar to than different from that of mothers

(Condon 1985, 2006; Condon et al. 2013). While one study found that fathers focused more on the future baby (Seimyr et al. 2009), others found that the unborn baby was increasingly conceptualized by fathers as something separate from "her" pregnancy and "their" baby (Fletcher et al. 2014). Although fathers view themselves as "partner and parent," studies suggest that maternity care services view them as "not-patient and not-visitor" (Steen et al. 2012), with care centered on responding to the health needs of the mother–child dyad (Dubeau et al. 2011; deMontigny & Lacharité 2013). Lesbian partners have similarly described themselves as "like everyone else, but not quite," wanting to be recognized as equally invested in the pregnancy yet feeling invisible and drained of energy (Erlandsson et al. 2010). Bereaved lesbian mothers have reported experiencing a double-disenfranchisement, with social support often insufficient to meet their psychological needs (Cacciatore & Raffo 2011). Regardless of gender, partners are placed in an interstitial and undefined space, both emotionally and physically, which makes them feel disconnected from the pregnancy and on the periphery of events during labor; they struggle to find their role because of a lack of knowledge, believing that parenthood begins once the baby is born (Longworth & Kingdon 2011). In contrast, other studies have found that men attending an ultrasound scan come to occupy the same position as their partner in terms of "knowing" the baby and, for them, fatherhood begins during pregnancy (Bonnette & Broom 2011).

The meaning of fatherhood undergoes a dramatic transformation following a perinatal loss. Pregnancy and fatherhood are never the same again. As one father said, *Why did I have to lose a baby before I realized I was already a father?* (O'Leary & Thorwick 2006b, p. 1). Acknowledgment of parenthood is of central importance to bereaved fathers, regardless of the gestation of the deceased fetus (McCreight 2004; Murphy 1998); their needs, however, are often overlooked (Bonnette & Broom 2011). Bereaved fathers who have seen their baby during ultrasound screening tend to express a greater sense of loss than those who have not (Armstrong 2001; McCreight 2004). Bonnette and Broom (2011) found that fathers described the time spent with their stillborn baby as a coherent and valuable fathering experience. When asked about their prenatal relationship with their stillborn baby, the fathers in this study described an embodied and technological experience of fathering in utero and considered themselves to be fathers pre-perinatal and post-stillbirth, further supporting the notion that fatherhood emerges while a child is in the womb.

Fathers' grief

Men have been recognized as legitimate mourners from as long ago as biblical times (2 Samuel 12: 14–31). That childbirth is for fathers an emotionally demanding experience cannot be denied (Johansson et al. 2012), and it is greatly intensified when there is an unexpected outcome (Bonnette and Broom 2011; Harvey 2012;). Similar to bereaved fathers, fathers of babies born prematurely describe being unprepared, frustrated, helpless, anxious, and alone as the health care is focused on mother and baby (Harvey 2012). Armstrong (2001) found that the intensity of perinatal loss was greater than expected for men; their sense of lack of control over life events being the primary outcome of this experience. While first-time fathers in a low-risk pregnancy described the meaning they ascribed to childbirth as an interwoven process oscillating between euphoria and agony (Premberg et al. 2011), bereaved fathers merely felt agony. In the pregnancy that follows euphoria and agony co-exist.

Doka and Martin (2010) discuss two types of griever: intuitive and instrumental. While intuitive grievers experience grief through their feelings, instrumental grievers are reluctant to talk about feelings and cope using problem-solving, cognitive or behavioral patterns and directive activity (Penman et al. 2014). Men are more likely to avoid expressing emotions related to a loss and to be less willing to talk about the loss than women (DeFrain 1991; Schwab 1996); they are thus more likely to be instrumental grievers. *It's harder for me to open up my feelings. I don't come from a family where we open up our feelings a lot.* Doka and Martin's (2010) descriptions of instrumental grievers support those of an earlier study in which Staudacher (1991, p. 12) identified the following expectations of men: they must (a) be in control, (b) be confident, (c) be more concerned with thinking than feeling, (d) be rational and analytical, (e) be assertive, (f) be courageous, and (g) accomplish tasks and achieve goals. Men are not expected to: (a) lose control over a situation or themselves, (b) openly cry, (c) be afraid, (d) be dependent, (e) be insecure or anxious, (f) express the need for love or affection, or (g) express loneliness, sadness, or depression. In summary, studies show that men clearly do feel grief but are not expected to show it; as a result, their grief is often not recognized (Levang 1998; Stinson et al. 1992).

> *She can go online to support groups. But what can I do? Just hold it in and do nothing. And that's why I think it's tougher for a man. We just can't break down and start balling at the supper table. It's just not being a man.*

The psychological and spiritual adjustment that occurs during the transition to parenthood impacts the partner relationship (Figueiredo et al. 2008) and is more pronounced after perinatal loss. Some research suggests that women suffer more psychological distress than fathers and over a longer period of time following the loss of the expected child (Bohannon 1990–1991; Zeanah et al. 1995b). Yet their future hopes and dreams and disruption in the relationship with their partner can be as devastating for men as for women (McCreight 2004; Murphy 1998; Worth 1997).

The reality is that men grieve too (Frost & Condon 1996) and the intensity and quality of men's affective experience (closeness, tenderness, love, concern, etc.) during pregnancy may not differ from that of women (Condon 1985; O'Leary & Thorwick 2006; Zeanah et al. 1995). The full range of men's reactions to grief may not be tapped, as most measurements focus on emotional reactions, to which women are more responsive (Bonnette & Broom 2013; Cacciatore et al. 2012). Women may cope intuitively through expressive thoughts and emotions (Penman et al., 2014), while men are discouraged from expressing "feminine" emotions such as sadness and tenderness. As a result, men can experience significant psychological blocks in terms of expressing powerful feelings of grief that conflict with their sense of self and conception of the social world (Rosenberg 2009; Thompson 2001). Men's emotional reaction may be delayed due to external demands such as giving the news to family and friends, picking out the coffin alone, meeting with the person planning the memorial, or caring for other children at home (Cacciatore et al. 2012; Worth 1997). Men are also less likely to receive emotional support outside the marriage and thus rely on their spouse (O'Leary & Thorwick 2006; Thompson et al. 2011). They also tend to assume full responsibility for their bereaved state (McCreight 2004; O'Leary & Thorwick 2006; Staudacher 1991). This may provide one explanation for why studies have found that men's grief after a loss increases over time (Puddifoot & Johnson 1999; Stinson et al. 1992) and that their grief can even exceed that of their partners (Benfield et al. 1998; Zeanah et al. 1995).

An example of instrumental grieving is shown in this father's description of his behavior after the loss of his baby:

> I remember immediately after the funeral, when there were 50 people here in our house. And I'd be, "I just got to get out of here. I just have to go somewhere." On the side of our house we have a garden that I think I dug all by myself just so I could be out of the house. I think I tore it out with my hands rather than a shovel just because I wanted everyone just to leave me alone. I'm fine.

In his need to do something, another father coped by remodeling the basement:

> I went to the lumber yard and just started framing it. I'd come home at night and work on it, wired it, plumbed it, gathered the stone, did all the work on the fireplace, put all the cabinets in and the tiles down.

While one father went fishing, another used Tai Chi as a physical activity to help with his sense of anxiety:

> It's those quiet times you reflect back on yourself, start to think more about it and grieve for his loss. Other than that, I just don't let it out. I think the Tai Chi practice that I do in the morning has been more of a source of strength or substance for me than getting together with the guys.

These examples illustrate that men and women may grieve very differently.

Despair, the most severe response to loss, is thought to predict the most serious and long-lasting consequences in individuals, and men are just as likely as women to suffer (Stinson et al. 1992). The trauma for one father still lingers 17 years after the birth of two healthy children that followed three miscarriages and continued multiple early losses during their childbearing history. He believes both parents should be recognized as grieving:

> *With the mother you can see the bleeding. You can see the baby being physically expelled. I think the father's feelings have been downplayed, ignored. I wish I could bleed physically when she had a pregnancy loss to show people that I'm wounded too, that I hurt too. It's like depression. It's a disease but you can't see it. It's an intangible, a painful intangible that people need to recognize.*

Although men may not show their grief outwardly, the pressures created by grief are substantial and can be unrecognized, especially if they do not have the opportunity to openly grieve (Frost & Condon 1996; McCreight 2004; Staudacher 1991). This can cause their grief to be disenfranchised by those around them. One study reported that fathers felt their experience was misunderstood by others and they were not given adequate support as a grieving parent too (Wagner et al. 1997). An example of this phenomenon is shown in this father's description of returning to graduate study following the loss of his twins at 22 weeks gestation:

> *People can just be insensitive. I don't have the greatest memories of how my women professors handled it. I showed up, just totally finished, looked terrible. And people asked me, "What happened to you?" and I said, "Agnes lost the twins; we lost the twins." And I remember my hematology teacher said, "Oh I feel terrible for her. That's just awful for Agnes that she lost those twins." I replied, "Well I took it pretty hard too, you know." And she [professor] kind of stumbled at that point.*

Another father knew that he used work to "manage his grief":

> *I had to go back to work right away and I knew that. I think that's how I managed the grief. It's managing my grief as much as managing hers. Fifty percent is mine and 50 percent is hers. And I have to look at it where I have to manage it enough so I can continue to go back to work.*

In his wish to control how he returned to work after the loss of his son, this father invited co-workers to the memorial service:

> *Part of the reason for that was I didn't want to see them all for the first time weeks later. I wanted the initial encounter to be over with.*

In the subsequent pregnancy, he realized people thought he had moved on:

> *I got a lot of comments like, "Smile" or "Why are you upset?" It's people not thinking about knowledge that they already know. Nothing that directly affects them so they see business as usual and they want me to be happy like I used to be, just like everybody else.*

Similar to fathers who experience a preterm birth struggling to define their role (Harvey 2012), bereaved fathers commonly have neither guidelines nor adequate support to manage their grief (Armstrong 2001; O'Leary & Thorwick 2006; Worth 1997). Finding support can be hard for men because they often do not feel comfortable in a group setting (Carlson et al. 2013; O'Leary & Thorwick 2006b). Although agreeing to be interviewed during the subsequent pregnancy, one father said: *It's really tough letting someone in. Not only just into your door but letting someone have a peek at your life. I was taught you don't show feelings* (O'Leary & Thorwick 2006a). Support from male friends is also hard to find unless they encounter another man who has had a similar experience:

> *I realize guys are different than girls. My friends attended the funeral; they are supportive. They'll say, "How you doing? Oh it's too bad Derek's died." But you don't really get into in-depth conversations nor do I allow myself after a while. It's evident to me, early on when you talk to somebody that they really don't know where I'm coming from so I'm not going to sit here and open up all my feelings to somebody who really just can't relate anyway. Most of my talking out grief has really been with Susan.*

Regardless of the gestation of the deceased fetus, fathers are grateful when health care professionals validate their grief and fatherhood (Aho et al. 2011; Cacciatore et al. 2012; Davis et al. 2013). Fathers who are not viewed as equal partners at the time of loss typically have a more difficult time, as is the case for fathers in a low-risk pregnancy (Edwards et al. 2009). Fathers who receive intervention (a support package, contact with peer supporters or health care personnel) at the time of loss typically score lower on reaction to grief scales and demonstrate stronger personal growth six months post-loss (Aho et al. 2010, 2011). This support should continue in the pregnancy that follows.

Fathers and pregnancy after loss

There is a stark contrast in feelings towards the role of being a father and view of the unborn baby when pregnancy follows the death of baby. Armstrong (2001) identified that fathers demonstrate the following emotions and behaviors in a subsequent pregnancy: (1) anxiety about the outcome, (2) a heightened sense of risk, and (3) a need for increased vigilance. Four themes were further identified: recognition, preoccupation, stoicism and support (O'Leary & Thorwick 2006).

Recognition

Little is known or understood about how fathers cope because *nobody asks.* As found in the literature on fathers' experience of normal labor and birth (Harvey 2011; Johannsson et al. 2012; Longworth et al. 2011), during a perinatal loss and in the pregnancy that follows fathers often feel they are not recognized as bereaved parents too. Fathers can also experience an embodied grief at the time of loss that can follow into the subsequent pregnancy (Bonnette & Broom 2011; O'Leary et al. 2012). Lack of recognition can leave fathers feeling helpless (Harvey 2012; Weaver-Hightower 2102), which means they often carry indelible emotions from the previous loss into the next pregnancy.

> *You couldn't even feel like what you were feeling because you were seeing that [the memory of the previous loss]. Words, that's what I remember; what people said. You're helpless. You can't do anything, just sit there and listen to the nurses, the doctors. Okay we're going to do this. We're going to do that. Nothing you can do. That's the worst thing about it. You wish you could do something. They really don't say anything to me, just paid attention to her.*

Just as fathers in a normal pregnancy report wanting recognition during antenatal care (Erlandsson et al. 2010; Premberg et al. 2011; Steen et al. 2012), so do many bereaved fathers, some taking a more proactive role in the next pregnancy. Their sense of being recognized as an equal partner needing information is because, *It affects me too. Most men don't care about going to doctor visits, appointments and I haven't missed one yet.* Two fathers phoned various medical providers, one trying to get answers regarding why his wife was spotting and the other worried about his partner's energy level. They had no control over the last experience and found it frustrating that answers are still unavailable:

> *I called a couple of specialists and ended up at the perinatal clinic at the university. I wanted a definite answer [as to] why women spot and I was told sometimes there just is no reason. And that's just a hair pulling. It isn't right. It shouldn't be happening. Tell me why. And they can't.*
>
> *The first couple weeks of the second trimester she was still coming home, wanting to lie down, wanting to sleep. So I brought that up with the doctor. Basically the doctor's response was that the second trimester doesn't start for everybody on the fourteenth week and if you feel you're tired, get some sleep. But a couple weeks later I saw her full of energy again and I knew things were normal.*

Other fathers may assume a more active role, feeling they didn't do enough last time and had relied on the doctors rather than trusting their partner's intuition (O'Leary et al. 2011b; Warland et al. 2015). One mother was aware that her husband was still struggling with this:

> *He blamed himself I think a lot too because I kept saying she's not moving very much. We should go to the hospital. He's like, you're just being silly. It turns out she was slowly dying. So he's had a hard time with that.*

Fathers' prenatal attachment and their representations of the fetus were found to be interrelated; those reporting a higher quality of prenatal attachment were more likely to have balanced representations of their unborn baby, whereas those with a lower quality of attachment were more likely to show disengaged representations

(Vreeswik et al. 2014). This research is important to bear in mind with regard to fathers' prenatal attachment in pregnancies after loss.

Like mothers, fathers can also intuit that something is wrong. As his wife went past the due date in their second subsequent pregnancy, this father felt a strong sense that something bad was going to happen:

I remember walking with her and saying something is going to be wrong with the cord. Something bad is going to happen. We have to get this baby induced. I don't want anything to happen. I don't want anything to go wrong. As they were delivering Darby the cord was wrapped around her throat. And it immediately went from a nice calm thing to every doctor running in and lights flashing and I'm like, "Oh my God. I don't want this again. I've had this before. I don't want this." But everything turned out fine. It wasn't that it choked her off or anything like that. But if something had happened it would have been very bad.

Preoccupation

Lack of motivation or concentration at work can continue into the subsequent pregnancy (O'Leary & Thorwick 2006). Many people process their feelings while driving to work. One father said he thought about his two deceased babies at work so that he could be the stoic protector at home and not upset his wife in their subsequent pregnancy: *I start thinking about them and not what I am doing. I probably think about the kids at work more than I think about them at home.* Another father felt guilty that he was *moving on with the new baby.* He purposefully drove by the cemetery where his twins were buried every day on his way to work: *It's kind of nice just to go by and glance over there every day.*

Another father felt unmotivated at work following the loss of his daughter, behavior that continued into the subsequent pregnancy. This supports the findings of an earlier study, which found that bereaved fathers do not find work a retreat (Hughes & Page-Lieberman 1989). *I am just not interested in work anymore. It seems like—what's the point?* Regardless, barriers exist that make accepting and receiving help more difficult for fathers, which leaves them more at risk for developing complicated grief (Bonnette & Broom 2011; Rando 1986b). Similar to fathers in a low-risk pregnancy, support during paternal leave is inadequate, and even more so when there is no baby at home to care for. Bereaved people also might not receive medical help or legal compensation (Parks 2002).

One bereaved father (a police officer) felt conflicted in his need to keep in contact with his wife because he couldn't carry his cell phone at work in case it rang and the *bad guys [would] know where [he's] at*:

> *I work in a squad car so she can't get a hold of me like if I worked at a desk. I don't carry the cell phone with me. I leave it in the squad car. Every time I get back in the car, the first thing I do is check that cell phone. And I check the messages to make sure she doesn't call. Because you still have that 1 or 2 percent in the back of your mind that at any given time she could call and say there's a problem. How can we get down to the perinatal center and fast enough so they can save the baby?*

Stoicism

The societal norm of men being protectors, defenders, and problem-solvers makes it difficult for them to request and accept help (Rando 1986; Stinson et al. 1992). This has led to a stronger emphasis on the tendency of men to engage in supportive rather than expressive roles (Versalle & McDowell 2005), both at the time of loss and in the pregnancy that follows. Fathers' grief may be overlooked as they assume their role of caretaker for the mother (Cacciatore et al. 2012; O'Leary & Thorwick 2006a). Many see their role as protector of the family who needs to stay strong for the mother and hide their own fears and anxieties (Bonnette & Broom 2011; McCrieght 2004; McGreal et al. 2012); this sense can continue in the subsequent pregnancy (O'Leary & Thorwick 2006a). Fathers have described closing their door at work and crying or crying in their cars, never sharing these times with their partners: *I often think about the losses and fears when I'm driving.*

Some fathers believe it is their role to manage all the grief in the family, both at the time of loss and in their subsequent pregnancy because *the family has to keep going.* Fathers have also expressed similar feelings regarding their role in supporting other children at the time of loss (Miyoko 2012):

> *I've got to be that support for her then also be a father to our daughter and a husband. I'm the only one working, so it's juggling all these four things that I have to do.*

Stroebe and colleagues (2013) focused on a phenomenon called partner-oriented self-regulation (POSR): the avoidance of talking about loss and the need to remain strong in the partner's presence with the intention of protecting her. This behavior comes at a cost, not only for the man but also his partner; as this mother describes: *He's really nervous but he tries really hard not to act nervous because he thinks it agitates me more. But it agitates me more when he doesn't have any kind of a reaction.*

Support

In spite of acknowledging that fathers need support, when asked where they received it most stated from their partner (O'Leary & Thorwick 2006). Mothers often credit their partners with being stronger and helping them to stay positive; fathers, however, report feeling burdened by the role of the stable one (O'Leary 2002). They often stifle their own feelings of anxiety to protect the mother from these negative emotions, as described by these two fathers:

> *You don't know if everything's going to be okay. But you need to give some sort of reassurance. Otherwise what else would you say? Well, I don't think everything's okay. Maybe we should go into the doctor. Well, we were just there two days ago. You just can't keep going to the doctor every two days for confirmation that everything's okay. So the tremendous weight is just trying to be the, the solid wall and be strong for the whole family.*

I had to chuck my emotions out of the way—the sadness and loneliness—to fight through that. I had to go to a job and try to keep us together, take care of her however I could. She had enough emotions.

Keeping abreast of the father's process through the next pregnancy is crucial. He is the other grieving parent (Bonnette & Broom 2011). It is helpful to ask how the father is coping and to enquire of the mother if he doesn't attend prenatal visits. The father also needs reassurance regarding how this pregnancy will be treated differently and to be helped to understand the clinical data showing how and why the mother and baby are safe and that the pregnancy is proceeding normally. In our clinical practice we find that fathers tend to respond in one of two ways: by becoming more involved in the pregnancy or by distancing themselves out of a sense of self-preservation. Planning prenatal or home visits at times when the father is present demonstrates that his role is crucial and helps him gain an understanding of what is being done for the mother and baby.

The medical community needs to view fathers as part of the pregnant triad and should make an effort to both involve them in the pregnancy and support them (Harvey 2012; Iles et al. 2011). This is an important goal for all professionals working in the childbearing area. Bereaved fathers have described their immense gratitude for person-centered psychosocial care in the aftermath of stillbirth and in the pregnancy that follows, particularly when they feel validated as a grieving father and their child is acknowledged with reverence (Cacciatore et al. 2013; Davis et al. 2013; O'Leary & Thorwick 2006).

Summary

This chapter has described the father's role during pregnancy and shown how it changes following perinatal loss. We have stressed the need for fathers to be recognized and acknowledged as an important element of antenatal care. They can feel on the sidelines, in a low-risk pregnancy, at the time of loss, and in the pregnancy that follows, yet also strongly feel their role as a parent. Similar to bereaved fathers, a lesbian partner can also feel unacknowledged in her grief and during a subsequent pregnancy. Acknowledgment of their role as part of a triad in low-risk pregnancies can be a beginning. This may help professionals gain a better understanding of how to meet their needs at the time of loss and during the pregnancy that follows.

Postscript

At the time I was transcribing my interviews with fathers, I (JOL) was also supporting my sister Kate through her treatment for breast cancer which ultimately took her life. As I listened to one father after another describe his vigilance and fear regarding the wellbeing of his partner and unborn baby, I felt a familiarity in my experience with Kate. As the fathers described their need to repeatedly ask the mother how the baby was doing I realized that I, too, was having a similar experience. The first thing I did every morning was call to hear my sister's voice. I needed that reassurance she was still alive. My lack of control over her disease left me feeling helpless, much as expressed by the fathers during their interviews.

For many of the fathers, I was the first person to ask about their stories. They all agreed to the interview in order to help other fathers and were enormously surprised to have someone actually listen to their personal narratives. Some wept for the first time. They needed to release their feelings of helplessness. They had stayed strong through the pregnancy, fearing their concerns would add more stress to the mother. I remained quiet as they cried, offered to stop the interview when it seemed too painful, but always they wanted to continue. It was in transcribing their stories that I cried, realizing the depth of pain these men carried that was like mine, invisible to others in the health care setting we were trying to navigate. It resonated with me because I, too, held back my emotions to be strong for my sister, wanting to believe she would live. I could not let her see my fear and helplessness as I watched the cancer take her away from me and her beautiful family.

Like the fathers, I don't recall ever being asked by any care provider how I was doing. Kate was a Shiatsu therapist, an alternative healer, reluctant to access Western modalities, but, in trying to stay alive for her family, she eventually submitted. I desperately tried to do the right thing for my sister, believing that was my role as her advocate. I always questioned what they were doing and why they didn't offer alternative healing alongside the Western IV medication she hated. I was frustrated by the lack of coordination between hospital and clinic and having to repeat her history at each visit. In doing so I regret that I was challenging, sometimes rude, to her care providers. I share this personal account because bereaved fathers also often display emotions such as anger or frustration that may seem displaced—they are scared and advocating too. Any mother who is the focus of professional intervention at the time of loss and in the subsequent pregnancy is part of a whole family system, chosen or biological. All members are impacted and changed by the experience of perinatal loss and become part of the circle of caring for the baby that follows. All need to be heard.

16

HOLISTIC HEALTH CARE FOR BEREAVED PARENTS

Plato wrote that the greatest mistake in the treatment of disease is that there are physicians for the body and physicians for the soul, although the two cannot be separated.[1]

This chapter explores the use of complementary and alternative medicine (CAM) modalities—including mindfulness/relaxation, aromatherapy, guided imagery/ meditation, massage, physical activity and spirituality—with parents during their pregnancy following loss. While still in its infancy, research suggests that using mind–body therapies in conjunction with conventional prenatal care has health benefits for pregnant women (Beddoe & Lee 2008; Field et al. 2009; Hall & Jolly 2014; Hall et al. 2011; Huberty et al. 2014a, 2014b; Jallo et al. 2008, 2014; Urech et al. 2010; Thompson 2012). In light of research suggesting that parents pregnant after loss are at greater risk for anxiety and depression, the potential benefits result- ing from some types of CAM could be recommended during inter-conception care (Huberty et al. 2014a, 2014b). CAM may complement medical care and talk- ing therapy to restore a connection between body and mind (Hoffman et al. 2010; Huberty et al. 2014b; Thompson 2012). CAM can be used during pregnancy as a natural approach to health, such as in managing nausea (Frawley et al. 2014).

Impact of stress on the unborn baby

An important part of prenatal care is introducing mothers to resources to help them learn ways in which to cope with stress and anxiety (Fink et al. 2012). As stated earlier in this book, anxiety during pregnancy has been associated with shorter gestation and adverse implications for fetal neurodevelopment and childhood out- comes (Dunkel Schetter & Tanner 2012; Guardino & Dunkel Shetter 2014). Stress hormones may cause early contractions, onset of labor in some women (Christian 2012), and elevated blood pressure (Crosson 2012). There is also increasing evidence that stress and the maternal psycho-social environment have long-term implications for uterine artery blood flow and fetal/infant brain development (Davis et al. 2011; DiPietro 2010; DiPietro et al. 2006; Glover 2011; Glover et al. 2014; Hepper 2005; Teixeira et al. 2005). That said, linking developmental outcomes to prenatal and biological effects on the developing brain is challenging because reports on child temperament, development, and behavior are limited (DiPietro 2012). Psychological stress is difficult to measure, pregnancy itself is a state of hypercortisolism (ibid), and mild to moderate levels of psychological distress may enhance fetal maturation in healthy populations (DiPietro et al. 2006). Glover (2015) points out that the human hypothalamic–pituitary–adrenal (HPA) axis, which causes cortisol to function differently in animal and human pregnancy, with the maternal HPA axis becoming gradually less responsive to stress as pregnancy progresses. Therefore, an anxious woman can be reassured that there is only a weak, if any, association between her prenatal mood and her cortisol level. However, because maternal psychological distress can adversely affect early parenting (Davis & Sandman 2010) and prenatal maternal distress predicts postnatal maternal distress, pregnancy provides a key opportunity for maternal mental health intervention, particularly given the number of provider contacts occurring in prenatal care (DiPietro 2012; Leiferman et al. 2011).

Although aware that maternal stress has negative health implications for the unborn baby, it is important to reassure parents that the effects of prenatal maternal stress on child cognitive and emotional development postpartum have been found to be moderated when there is a secure attachment (Bergman et al. 2010). CAM may therefore be used to alleviate stress levels and provide health benefits for both parents and the unborn baby. There is currently little research evidence to suggest that mothers' anxiety in pregnancy, per se, impacts pregnancy outcome (DiPietro 2012; Glover 2015), as this mother attests:

> *I worried the subsequent baby would be affected by my anxiety. Perhaps she would be ruined for life or cry all night because of my anxious pregnancy. I worried needlessly. Sarah is as placid and well-adapted as the rest of our children. She is certainly not the emotional cripple that I imagined having.*

Physical wellness

Physical activity may be an opportune means of alleviating stress in a pregnancy after loss but health care providers rarely suggest it (Huberty et al. 2014b). Physical activity may also improve depressive symptoms in women with postpartum depression after stillbirth (Huberty et al. 2014a). Women who have experienced a loss may, however, experience barriers to physical activity such as avoiding walking in public (Huberty et al. 2014b), not wanting to see other pregnant women or babies, and not feeling motivated to be physically active. This behavior may continue in the subsequent pregnancy, as voiced by one mother who was pregnant three months after the loss of her stillborn son:

> *I hated walking around. If I saw other pregnant women walking around I would think in my head, "You just have no idea! You're running around here just being happy. What are you being so happy about? You have no idea what can happen to you!" I remember just feeling that way, standing in the store, people would be having a good time and I'm just thinking, "Don't you people know that the world ended a few months ago and I'm going through what I'm going through?"*

Sleep

It is well known that grief can disrupt sleep (Hardison et al. 2005), and for a prolonged period after pregnancy loss and during subsequent pregnancies (Patterson 2000). Mounting evidence indicates that disruption in normal sleep duration and quality is associated with a range of poor pregnancy outcomes, such as fetal growth restriction, high blood pressure, and diabetes (Palagini et al. 2014). These outcomes are in turn associated with increased risk of stillbirth (Helgadóttir et al. 2013).

Women pregnant after loss may be particularly receptive to CAM to manage sleep disruption, as this can be a concrete means of empowering and reassuring them they are doing all they can to protect the unborn baby. A range of CAM approaches can be used to improve the subjective quality of sleep; for example, *B. pinnatum* (moonwort) has been shown to decrease the sense of tiredness during the day, with no serious adverse reactions being detected (Lambrigger-Steiner et al. 2014).

Although little research has been conducted into their experiences with sleep, preoccupation may interfere with fathers' sleep patterns and so care providers should ask them about this issue. A number of fathers who were interviewed during their partners' subsequent pregnancy voiced difficulty around sleeping. When asked about worrying, one father stated:

> *I wake up in the middle of the night sometimes; 4 o'clock in the morning. I'll just start thinking about a funeral. What if we have to go through it again?*

This father describes worrying when he hears that his wife is up: *That whole night I was just tossing and turning, expecting to be woken up.* Another wasn't sleeping because he was worried about the baby's movements: *If the baby's not moving enough she won't sleep that night. She'll toss and turn and that keeps me up.*

Aromatherapy

Aromatherapy is a CAM resource that can be used to help reduce stress during pregnancy (Hall et al. 2011). Igarashi (2013) found a significant difference in women's tension and anger scores after using aromatherapy for longer than a five-minute period at different points during their pregnancy. Igarashi noted that an important step forward in both aromatherapy research and clinical practice is asking women to select a preferred fragrance.

Yoga

Grief is an embodied experience (Gudmundsdott 2009) that often manifests in physical ways. One father described grief as:

> [L]ike a semi was just put on your shoulder and they won't let it off. It's always an empty hole in your heart. It's just like someone grabbed your arm and stepped on it. You just feel empty.

There is little research that directly links yoga and grief counseling but the combination of mindfulness and yoga within a therapeutically supportive environment appears to be beneficial to a grieving person (Mitchell 2012). Yoga has three elements: breathe (pranayama), mind (mindfulness), and body (postures); it involves listening to the body and letting go of judgment and expectation (Balasubramaniam et al. 2013). Yoga has been found to be of benefit during pregnancy (Narendran et al. 2005) as well as improving depressive symptoms and quality of life (Saeed et al. 2010; Tsang et al. 2008). It may also help mothers to self-reflect, quiet their mind, and regain comfort in moving and using their bodies in a positive way (Remer 2012). This form of physical activity has been suggested for women who have experienced stillbirth (Huberty et al. 2014a) and may also benefit women who are pregnant after loss. For example, during a breathing and relaxation session in a PAL birth class, mothers were asked to begin deep breathing and to place their hands on their abdomens. One woman, 35 weeks into her pregnancy and with a history of multiple miscarriages, stated, I haven't touched that part of my body through this whole pregnancy. She had lost trust in her body to carry a baby to term and was extremely reluctant to touch any part of her body related to pregnancy or birth.

Another mother began yoga in her subsequent pregnancy as a means of doing some physical activity. Her description illustrates releasing embodied grief:

> Doing the stretches and the breathing; that's really helpful. The first couple of times I cried, being connected to my body or thinking about the [new] baby; that was something I had to push through. Now I'm more comfortable. I think that helped me to connect a little bit to her and talk to her. I saw it as a tool for getting through labor. I'm not carefree and I'm not naive. I feel like there's a little bit of joy missing but I've gotten very good at just letting my feelings be, instead of trying to fix them or change them or make them better, make me better. My new model now is, "It is what it is." I can't do anything else for her to make a certain outcome.

Touch/massage

Little research has been conducted into touch/massage for parents pregnant after loss. However, studies in other populations are showing the usefulness of these modalities. For example, one study with depressed mothers (Field et al. 2009) used a CAM model together with providing infant mental health training to home visitors. The experimental group received massages during their pregnancy and a special-ized home visitor trained in infant mental health while the control group had no massages and a home visitor with no special training. Those in the experimental group were 30 percent less likely to develop depression six months after childbirth compared to the control group. This study suggests that the use of CAM and a close relationship, with a consistent care giver were both important for mothers pregnant after loss (Côté-Arsenault et al.).

Many hospitals and clinics have integrated touch and massage into their practices. One study in a hospital in the US Midwest used healing touch combined with harp music to reduce pain and anxiety in post-operative patients (Lincoln et al. 2014).

Spirituality

A spiritual foundation in one's life can play an important role in ability to cope with fears and anxieties during a high-risk pregnancy (Breen et al. 2007; Price et al. 2007) and has been found to improve perception of perinatal loss in some faiths (Sutan & Miskam 2012). Spirituality is not necessarily bound to a religious denomination but described as the search for meaning, belief in a higher power, and/or the feeling of connectedness, all encompassing hope, love, peace, and comfort (Seth et al. 2011). Individuals who report higher levels of existential well-being and involvement in spiritual and or/religious activities may have fewer or less intense symptoms of depression (Brown et al. 2013; Wachholtz & Pargament 2005). Programs to train others in this area are becoming more prominent, the University of Minnesota being one of the first to integrate study of spirituality into its medical school. It defines spirituality not as religion but as helping people find purpose, meaning, and connection (www.csh.umn.edu)—all of which support the prenatal parenting model with parents pregnant after loss.

Praying with a sacred object has been found to be a rich experience that sup-ports finding a sense of meaning within the context of a significant life stressor (Miller et al. 2011). Parents may be encouraged to produce an "amulet" (Brett 2014) from a special object or symbol to represent their baby during pregnancy and birth. Some parents bring a picture of their deceased child when in labor with the subse-quent child to provide a spiritual presence.

The following examples illustrate ways in which parents have used spirituality in their subsequent pregnancies. This mother used prayer and a spiritual director:

> *For me, I do it with prayer. That's the way that I deal with the possibility of loss. "Let me be open and accept what is happening today." I have not trusted my body because*

it's betrayed me. Like it's something out there, that relates to the earlier miscarriages. I'm working with a spiritual director and we're just talking about doing some body forgiveness and integration of not feeling my body is going to betray me, words that I really don't want to apply to myself.

This father relied on prayer:

We're Catholic and looked at it first like a punishment. Why is God punishing me? Why? And nobody really has an answer. It's just what God meant, so why did God mean it. I don't know. We used to go to church once or twice a month. Now we go every week. We pray a lot more.

Whilst trying to decide with his wife whether to try for another baby, this father had a spiritual experience that revealed they were already pregnant. His story supports others who have written about a spiritual connection with a baby before birth (Chamberlain 2013):

I have very spiritual beliefs but I'm not a person who is a big believer in angels coming down and doing things. I believe there's a God that looks after us, so I believe that things can happen. I was going to sleep one night, it was kind of that half asleep and I was just sort of dreaming or just kind of laying there. And I heard a voice in my head that said, "It has happened." And then I sat up. And I just thought woo, what was that? And I thought, "She's pregnant right now! There's a baby in there and it's going to be okay." Ever since hearing that I've just felt like things are going to be fine.

Anger at God is a common feeling for some bereaved parents. In a five-year period one mother experienced the unexplained loss of two daughters at 32 weeks gestation, before and after the delivery of a full-term healthy daughter. Describing herself as a born-again Christian, she had been very angry at God:

It's like parenting. The kids can be angry at you, the kids can decide they aren't going to talk to you, it doesn't mean you stop loving them. I was at that point with God. I was so mad and so hurt and so angry. And I know God met me where I was at. I didn't have to worry. I finally said I was sorry. He knows my heart. It's like now, "Oh, what a surprise. She's pissed off." I'll be honest with you, if it weren't for my faith, and if it weren't for a belief that there's a better day I don't know how it would have been for me.

Mindfulness/relaxation

Mindfulness has its roots in the Pali word *sati*, meaning awareness, attention, remembering (Cacciatore & Flint 2012). Mindfulness-based stress reduction teaches people to direct their attention to the contents of experience (Thompson 2012), and has been found to be beneficial for people with a generalized anxiety disorder (Evans et al. 2008) and as a self-help treatment for anxiety and depression (Edenfield & Saeed 2012; Lee et al. 2007).

Mindfulness as a therapeutic approach to grief and loss is not necessarily about relaxation or achieving a particular state of mind but a skill allowing people to experience feelings of grief with less struggle and attempts at escape (Thompson 2012). Jallo and colleagues (2008, 2009) investigated the effects of mindfulness/relaxation guided imagery (R-GI) on perceived stress, anxiety, and corticotropin-releasing hormone (CRH) levels in pregnant African American women beginning in the second trimester. This prospective, longitudinal 12-week study of 59 women used a controlled randomized experimental design with two groups and asked participants in the intervention group to complete daily practice logs. They found state anxiety significantly decreased over time in the R-GI group and increased over time in the control group. There were no significant differences found in perceived stress or in CRH levels between groups.

Spiritually-based mantram repetition, defined as the practice of silently repeating a self-selected sacred word or phrase to redirect attention and calm oneself (Oman & Driskill 2003), was explored with a small group of military families to help them cope with childbirth-related fears (Humber et al. 2011). Humber and colleagues (2011) conducted an intervention in which women in late pregnancy received three two-hour sessions on mantram repetition. Although the intervention appeared to be ineffective in reducing cesarean section and other complications, mothers reported that using the mantram helped them cope with the confusing moments of uncertainty. These findings suggest that such interventions should be offered earlier and more frequently during the pregnancy to be most effective (Fink et al. 2012). Nevertheless, previous studies using mantram intervention found a significant reduction in perceived stress, anxiety, anger, and PTSD, and improvements in quality of life and spiritual well-being (Bormann et al. 2005, 2006, 2008).

A pilot study involving an eight-week mindfulness-based intervention to reduce stress and improve mood in pregnancy and early postpartum (Vieten & Austin 2008) found a greater decline in anxiety and negative affect in the experimental group, although at follow-up (three months postpartum) there was no significant difference. Progressive muscle relaxation combined with guided imagery during pregnancy was also effective in inducing self-reported relaxation and reduction of cardiovascular activity (Urech et al. 2010). DiPietro and colleagues (2008) measured fetal responses to maternal relaxation using guided imagery during the 32nd week of pregnancy and found significant alterations in fetal neurobehavior, including decreased heart rate, increased heart rate variability, suppression of motor activity, and normal increase in heart rate during movement. Others found that relaxation could improve the non-stress test results described in Chapter 5, reduce the basal fetal heart rate, and increase the number of fetal heart accelerations (Akbarzade et al. 2015). These studies support others (Fink et al. 2012) demonstrating that unborn babies are less stressed when the mother is relaxed. To date, there has been no research on using mindfulness guided imagery with parents pregnant after loss to help them cope with their anxiety and feelings towards the unborn baby. However, its use with low-risk mothers suggests that applying it with parents pregnant after loss would be beneficial.

Six months after the loss of triplets at 22 weeks gestation, and before becoming pregnant again, this mother took a 10-week mind–body class specific to people undergoing IVF. She learned body scanning, meditation, and centering. In her next round of IVF she became pregnant with triplets. To improve the babies' chance of survival, she made the decision to reduce to twins. When asked if she had communicated with the unborn babies while making this painful decision, replied that she had, using the skills she had learned in the mind–body class. *At the time there was no distinction between the three of them. One of you is dying and I don't know which one. I don't feel like I can give you a good explanation why.* She continued to use mindfulness, meditation, and centering, believing this helped her connect to the babies, and that her body was being as helpful as it could be: they were in this pregnancy together:

> *Ever since 17 weeks I can just sit in a chair and be completely still and relaxed. I'll listen to a meditation CD and the only thing that I feel is the twins. It's very clear that it's them. I sit in a chair with my hands on my belly, look out the window and focus on the way I'm breathing, trying to breathe more and more deeply.*

A mind–body class was offered to the mothers in JOL's PAL group, using guided imagery. From this experience a prenatal parenting CD was developed to help parents learn how the mother's body was protecting the unborn baby (O'Leary & Parker 1998). This progressive guided muscle relaxation intervention (Urech et al. 2010), similar to Vieten and Astin's (2008) Mindfulness Motherhood intervention,) also integrated connecting with the deceased baby as part of healing (Armstrong 2012) and recognized the unborn baby as a sibling.

Listening to the parenting CD was the only time during each day that this mother was able to focus on the baby in her subsequent pregnancy:

> *Every day I played the CD and that made me feel a lot better. I was just trying really hard to make it about this baby, not about what I had been through. I was really, really worried that she was going to suffer as a result of my stress and that I was going to put some burden on her. It was the only time of just being about her and me because I was still grieving for Davis.*

ATTEND (Attunement, Trust, Therapeutic touch, Egalitarianism, Nuance, and Death education; Cacciatore & Flint 2012) is another model of holistic care that involves mindful attunement to both self and other in the healing partnership. Attunement can be achieved through an emphasis on mindfulness, responsiveness, empathy, and self-awareness, and is recommended for traumatized people and bereaved parents as a means of helping them construct new meaning from their experience.

Evidence demonstrating the long-term effect on the child of maternal stress and anxiety during pregnancy sets the stage for the next era of psychiatric and collaborative interdisciplinary research. Its aim is to reduce the burden of maternal stress, depression, and anxiety in the perinatal period. It is critical to identify the signs, symptoms, and diagnostic thresholds that warrant prenatal intervention and to develop efficient, effective, and ecologically valid screening and intervention strategies (Dunkel Schetter & Tanner 2012).

It is important to remember that not only the first pregnancy following loss can be difficult but ones that follow too. The case study below uses a "problem formulation" (that is, reframing one's consciousness) approach to mindfulness guided imagery (Teasdale et al. 2000) to help one couple engage in their second subsequent pregnancy and separate the deceased son from the coming son.

CASE STUDY

Using guided imagery

In her first pregnancy, Julie felt very connected to her son, Eliot. At 18 weeks gestation she had a dream that he would not live but told no one, including her husband, Joe. At the 24-week ultrasound showing he was healthy, she wanted to take hope but couldn't forget the dream. At 27 weeks, a few days before Christmas, she knew he had stopped moving but avoided gaining positive proof until after the holidays. On January 3, her secret fear became a reality when Eliot was stillborn.

Pregnant again four months later, Julie joined the weekly support group. She took care of herself physically and read to her baby every night. She listened to the guided imagery relaxation CD, *Parenting Your Baby Before Birth* (O'Leary & Parker 1998) and told the group she always fell asleep before the section dealing with the baby. She shared that she could visualize a body but not a head. Remembering how connected she was to Eliot, the facilitator gently suggested she might be afraid to check in with the baby, fearful of the message he or she might convey, knowing that Eliot had communicated he could not stay. She cried as she acknowledged this was probably true. As her pregnancy progressed she continued to talk about her love for Eliot as she began attaching to the new baby. Emma was born at 40 weeks gestation, a healthy baby.

In the pregnancy that followed Emma's birth (third pregnancy), Julie learned she was having another boy. During a home visit, at 28 weeks pregnant, Julie admitted she had shut down. She said, *I know that I can bring girl babies into the world but I only know my body kills boys. I haven't wanted to think about this being a boy. I've struggled with letting him be an individual and I'm afraid.*

Her husband admitted that he had also been distant and somewhat removed from the pregnancy. Julie was less engaged compared to Emma's pregnancy, not talking about how much she loved being pregnant or reading information on fetal development. *I don't think about it because we don't really talk about it like we did with Emma.* He also confided his concern that his mother would acknowledge this boy as their first son because, when asked how many grandchildren she had, she never included Eliot.

Julie was open to a guided imagery experience to help her face her fear of preparing for the birth of this new son. With her husband, Joe, close by, Julie was asked to go to a place where she would feel safe and in control; a place where Joe could help her visualize when she was in labor. She went back to Eliot's pregnancy, choosing the family cabin where they had told Joe's parents they were pregnant, a place she had always loved. Unfortunately, rather than making her feel safe, the cabin brought back memories of Eliot's death. Realizing this place was no longer safe, she needed a different place to go when she was in labor with their second son. During the guided imagery she could visualize a body and a head but not the baby's facial features. It was also of interest to note that this little boy was positioned transversely, something we often see when parents are fearful. Part of the visualization involved getting Joe and Julie to encourage the baby to turn head down.

After the guided imagery, both Joe and Julie realized that neither of them had taken control in this pregnancy and were avoiding thinking about labor and birth. Fearing another loss, they could think about being pregnant but not about the baby inside. Once their feelings were verbalized they both felt ready to take control of what they could. This included talking with Joe's mother to help her understand that this was their third child, and second son, and that Eliot needed to be included as an important member of their family. Their son was born vaginally and healthy a few weeks later.

Summary

This chapter has explored CAM therapy as an overlooked but important component of care for bereaved parents, both at the time of loss and during the pregnancy that follows. In addition to referral to support groups or cognitive therapy, professionals need to discuss the benefits of CAM as a resource to relieve stress and help connect to the unborn baby. Offering a list of resources during inter-conception counseling and as part of care before entering the new pregnancy can be helpful. If parents initially refuse to engage in CAM therapy, it can be offered more than once throughout the course of the pregnancy.

Note

1 http://www.science20.com/scientist/blog/physician_quotes-64984

REFERENCES

ACOG. (2009). ACOG Practice Bulletin No. 107: Induction of labor. *Obstetric Gynecology*, 114(2 Pt 1): 386–397.

Adeyemi, A., Mosaku, K., Ajenifuja, O., Fatoye, F., Makinde, N., & Ola, B. (2008). Depressive symptoms in a sample of women following perinatal loss. *Journal of the National Medical Association*, 100(12): 1463–1468.

Adolfsson, A. (2010). Applying Heidegger's interpretive phenomenology to women's miscarriage experience. *Psychology Research and Behavior Management*, 3: 75–79.

Aho, A., Tarkka, M., Astedt-Kurki, & Kaunonen, M. (2006). Fathers' grief after the death of a child. *Mental Health Nursing*, 26(8): 647–663.

Akbarzade, M., Rafiee, B., Asadi, N., & Zare, N. (2015). The effect of maternal relaxation training on reactivity of non-stress test, basal fetal heart rate, and number of fetal heart accelerations: A randomized controlled trial. *International Journal of Community Based Nursing and Midwifery*, 3(1): 51–59.

Alderman, L.C., Chisholm, J., Denmark, F., & Salbod, S. (1998). Bereavement and stress of a miscarriage: As it affects the couple. *Omega*, 37(4): 317–327.

Alexander, M., Votino, C., De Noose, L., Cos Sanchez, T. et al. (2015). The impact of prior medical termination of pregnancy on the mother's early relationship with a subsequent infant. *Journal of Maternal-Fetal & Neonatal Medicine*, Early Online: 1–6. DOI: 10.3109/14767058.2015.1043260.

Alhusen, J. (2008). A literature update on maternal–fetal attachment. *Journal of Obstetric, Gynecological and Neonatal Nursing*, 37(3): 315–328.

Almog, B., Levin, I., Wagman, I., Kapustiansky, R., Lessing, J.B., Amit, A., & Azem, F. (2010). Adverse obstetric outcome for the vanishing twin syndrome. *Reproductive Biomedicine Online*, 20(2): 256–260. DOI: 10.1016/j.rbmo.2009.11.015.

Ainsworth, M., Blehar, M., Waters, E., & Wall, S. (1978). *Patterns of attachment: A psychological study of the Strange Situation*. Hillsdale, NJ: Lawrence Erlbaum.

Amarapurkar, R. (Producer/Director). (2010). *Jananee* [*The Mother*]. English subtitles. India, Samvedana Film Foundation.

American Psychiatric Association (APA). (2013). *Diagnostic and statistical manual of mental disorders* (5th ed.). Washington, DC: American Psychiatric Association.

American Society for Reproductive Medicine. (2012). Evaluation and treatment of recurrent pregnancy loss: A committee opinion. *Fertility and Sterility*, 98(5): 1103–1111. http://www.asrm.org/Guidelines/.

Angelfire. (2004). *Multifetal pregnancy reduction* (Islamic View). http://www.angelfire.com/la/IslamicView/Reduction.html.

Archer, J. (1999). *The nature of grief: The evolution and psychology of reactions to loss*. New York: Routledge.

Armstrong, C. (2012). Envisioning connection through guided imagery. In R.A. Neimeyer (Ed.) *Techniques of grief therapy: Creative practices for counseling the bereaved*. New York: Routledge, pp. 256–262.

Armstrong, D. (2001). Exploring fathers' experiences of pregnancy after a prior perinatal loss. *Maternal Child Nursing*, 26(3): 147–153.

Armstrong, D. & Hutti, M. (1998). Pregnancy after perinatal loss: The relationship between anxiety and prenatal attachment. *Journal of Obstetric, Gynecologic, and Neonatal Nursing*, 27(2): 183–189.

Armstrong, D. & Shakespeare-Finch, J. (2011). Relationship to the bereaved and perceptions of severity of trauma differentiate elements of posttraumatic growth. *Omega*, 63(2): 125–140.

Armstrong, D., Hutti, M., & Myer, J. (2009). The influence of prior perinatal loss on parents' psychological distress after the birth of a subsequent healthy infant. *Journal of Obstetric, Gynecologic, and Neonatal Nursing*, 38: 654–666. DOI: 10.1111/j.1552-6909.2009.01069.x.

Artlett, C., Smith, B., & Jimenez, S. (1998). Identification of fetal DNA and cells in skin lesions from women with systemic sclerosis. *New England Journal of Medicine*, 338(17): 1186–1191.

ASRM. (2006). http://www.asrm.org/.

Attig, T. (2001). Relearning the world: Making and finding meanings. In R.A. Neimeyer (Ed.) *Meaning reconstruction and the experience of loss*. Washington, DC: American Psychological Association, pp. 33–53.

Attig, T. (2013). *Holiday sorrows and precious gifts*. http://www.griefsheart.com/holidaysorrows.php.

August, E.M., Salihu, H.M., Wedleselasse, H., Biroscak, B.J. et al. (2011). Infant mortality and subsequent risk of stillbirth: A retrospective cohort study. *BJOG: An International Journal of Obstetrics and Gynaecology*, 118(13): 1636–1645.

Auman, M.J. (2007). Bereavement support for children. *Journal of School Nursing*, 23(1): 34–39.

Austin, M. & Priest, S.R. (2005). Clinical issues in perinatal mental health: New developments in the detection and treatment of perinatal mood and anxiety disorders. *Acta Psychiatrica Scandinavica*, 112: 97–104.

Avelin, P., Erlandsson, K., Hildingsson, I., & Rådestad, I. (2011). Swedish parents' experiences of parenthood and the need for support to siblings when a baby is stillborn. *Birth*, 38(2): 150–158.

Avelin, P., Gyllenswärd, G., Erlandsson, K. & Rådestad, I. (2014). Adolescents' experiences of having a stillborn half-sibling. *Death Studies*, 38(9): 557–562.

Back, A.L., Arnold, R.M., & Quill, T.E. (2003). Hope for the best, and prepare for the worst. *Annals of Internal Medicine*, 138(5): 439–443.

Badenhorst, W. & Hughes, P. (2007). Psychological aspects of perinatal loss. *Best Practices Research & Clinical Obstetric Gynaecology*, 21(2): 249–259.

Balasubramaniam, M., Telles, S., & Doraiswamy, P.M. (2013). Yoga on our minds: A systematic review of yoga for neuropsychiatric disorders. *Front Psychiatry*, 25(3): 117.

Balk, D. (2011). Does coping with bereavement occur in states? In K. Doka & A. Tucci (Eds) *Beyond Kubler-Ross: New perspectives on death, dying, and grief*. Washington, DC: Hospice Foundation of America, pp. 45–60.

Barnett, B. (2005). Early intervention, prevention, and perinatal psychiatry. *The Signal*, 13(1): 1–7.

Barone, L., Lionetti, F., & Dellagiulia, A. (2014). Maternal–fetal attachment and its correlates in a sample of Italian women: A study using the Prenatal Attachment Inventory. *Journal of Reproductive and Infant Psychology*, 32(3). http:///www.tandfonline.comloi/cjri20.

Barret, J.F., Hannah, M.E., Hutton, E.K., Willan, A.R., et al.—Twin Birth Study Collaborative Group (2013). A randomized trial of planned cesarean or vaginal delivery for twin pregnancy. *New England Journal of Medicine*, 369(14): 1295–1305.

Barr, P. (2006). Relation between grief and subsequent pregnancy status 13 months after perinatal bereavement. *Journal of Perinatal Medicine*, 34(3): 207–211.

Bartellas, E. & Van Aerde, J. (2003). Bereavement support for women and their families after stillbirth. *Journal of Obstetrics & Gynaecology Canada*, 25(2): 131–138.

Bassam, A., Khunda, S., & Hussan, E. (2011). Obstetric outcome of subsequent pregnancy following intrauterine death. *Journal of the Faculty of Medicine, Baghdad*, 53(3), 265–268.

Beddoe, A. & Lee, K. (2008) Mind–body interventions during pregnancy. *Journal of Obstetrics, Gynecology, and Neonatal Nursing*, 37(2): 165–175.

Bell, D. (2012). Next steps in attachment theory. *Journal of Family Theory & Review*, 4: 275–281.

Bennett, S.M., Litz, B.T, Lee, B.S., & Maguen, S. (2005). The scope and impact of perinatal loss: Current status and future directions. *Professional Psychology: Research and Practice*, 36: 180–187.

Benute, G., Nomura, R., Liao, A., deLourdes Brizot, M., de Lucia, M., & Zugaib, M. (2012). Feelings of women regarding end-of-life decision making after ultrasound diagnosis of a lethal fetal malformation. *Midwifery*, 289: 472–475.

Benute, G., Nozzella, D., Prohaska, C., Liao, A., Lucia, M., & Zugaib, M. (2012b). Twin pregnancies: Evaluation of major depression, stress, and social support. *Twin Research and Human Genetics*, 16(2): 629–633.

Bergman, K., Sarkar, P., Glover, V., & O'Connor, T. (2010). Maternal prenatal cortisol and infant cognitive development: Moderation by infant–mother attachment. *Biological Psychiatry*, 67(11): 1026–1032.

Bergner, A., Beyer, R., Klapp, B.F., & Rauchfuss, M. (2009). Mourning, coping and subjective attribution after early miscarriage. *Psychotherapie, Psychosomatik, Medizinische Psychologie*, 59(2): 57–67.

Bhattacharay, S., Prescott, G.J., Black, M., & Shetty, A. (2010). Recurrence of stillbirth in a second pregnancy. *BJOG*, 117: 1243–1247.

Bianchi, D.W. (2000). Fetal cells in the mother: From genetic diagnosis to diseases associated with fetal cell microchimerism. *European Journal of Obstetrics & Gynecology and Reproductive Biology*, 92(1): 103–108.

Bianchi, D.W., Farina, A., Genova, M., Weber, W., Williams, J.M., & Klinger. K.W. (1998). PCR quantitation of fetal cells in maternal blood after voluntary interruption of pregnancy: Implications for diseases associated with microchimerism. *American Journal of Human Genetics*, 63: A6.

Bicking, K.C., Baptiste-Roberts, K., Zhu, J., & Kjerulff, K. (2014). Effect of miscarriage history on maternal–infant bonding during the first year postpartum in the First Baby Study: A longitudinal cohort study. *BMC Women's Health*, 14: 83. http://www.biomedcentral.com/1472–6874/14/83.

Black, B. & Wright, P. (2012). Posttraumatic growth and transformation as an outcome of perinatal loss. *Illness, Crisis & Loss*, 20(3): 225–237.

Black, M., Shetty, A., & Bhattacharay, S. (2008). Obstetric outcomes subsequent to intrauterine death in the first pregnancy. *BJOG: An International Journal of Obstetrics and Gynaecology*, 115: 269–274.

Blair, M.M., Glynn, L.M., Sandman, C.A., & Davis, E.P. (2011). Prenatal maternal anxiety and early childhood temperament. *Stress*, 14(6): 644–651.

Blickstein, I. & Perlman, S. (2013). Single fetal death in twin gestations. *Journal of Perinatology & Medicine*, 41(1): 65–69.

Boelen, P.A, Van Den Hout, M.A., & Van Den Bout, J.V. (2006). A cognitive-behavioral conceptualization of complicated grief. *Clinical Psychology: Science and Practice*, 13(2): 109–128Bolton, S.C. (2005). Women's work, dirty work: The gynaecology nurse as 'other'. *Gender, Work & Organization*, 12(2): 169–186.

Bonnette, S. & Broom, A. (2011).On grief, fathering and the male role in men's accounts of stillbirth. *Journal of Sociology*, 48(3): 248–265.

Bopp, J., Bopp, M., Brown, L., & Lane, P. (1989). *The sacred tree: Reflections on Native American spirituality* (3rd ed). Twin Lakes, WI: Lotus Light.

Bormann, J., Becker, S., Gershwin, M., Kelly, A., Pada, L. et al. (2006). Relationship of frequent mantram repetition to emotional and spiritual well-being in healthcare workers. *Journal of Continuing Education in Nursing*, 37(5): 218–224.

Bormann, J., Gifford, A., Shiverly, M., Smith, T., Redwine, L. et al. (2006). Effects of spiritual mantram repetition on HIV outcomes: A randomized controlled trial. *Journal of Behavioral Medicine*, 29(4): 359–376.

Boss, P. (2006). *Loss, trauma, and resilience: Therapeutic work with ambiguous loss.* New York: W.W. Norton & Co.

Bouchard, G. (2011). The role of psychosocial variables in prenatal attachment: An examination of moderational effects. *Journal of Reproductive & Infant Psychology*, 29(3): 197–207.

Bourne, S. & Lewis, E. (1984). Pregnancy after stillbirth or neonatal death: Psychological risks and management. *Lancet*, 2(8393): 31–33.

Bourquiqnon, A., Briscoe, B., & Nemzer, L. (1999). Genetic abortion: Considerations for patient care. *Journal of Perinatal & Neonatal Nursing*, 13(2): 47–58.

Bowlby, J. (1969). *Attachment, separation and loss.* New York: Basic Books.

Bowman, T. (1995). Beginning an ending with effective closure. Reflections from a group leader's notebook. In *Family Information Services Professional Resource Materials.* Minneapolis, MN: Family Information Services, pp. 60–61.

Boyraz, G., Horne, S., & Sayget, T. (2010). Finding positive meaning after loss: The mediating role of reflection for bereaved individuals. *Journal of Loss and Trauma*, 15(3): 242–258.

Brady, G., Brown, G., Letherby, G., Bayley, J., & Wallace, L. (2008). Young women's experience of termination and miscarriage: A qualitative study. *Human Fertility*, 11(3): 186–190.

Breen, G., Price, S., & Lake, M. (2007). Spirituality and high-risk pregnancy: Another aspect of patient care. *AWHONN Lifelines*, 10(6): 466–473.

Brett, M. (2014). *The Amulet.* Cork, Ireland: Anamnesis City Print Limited.

Brewin, C.R., Dalgleish, T., & Joseph, S. (1996). A dual representation theory of posttraumatic stress disorder. *Psychological Review*, 103(4): 670–686.

Brier, N. (2008). Grief following miscarriage: A comprehensive review of the literature. *Journal of Women's Health*, 17: 415–464.

Brigham, S.A., Conlon, C., & Farquharson, R.G. (1999). A longitudinal study of pregnancy outcome following idiopathic recurrent miscarriage. *Human Reproduction*, 4: 2868–2867.

Britt, D.W. & Evans, M.I. (2007). Sometimes doing the right thing sucks: Frame combinations and multi-fetal pregnancy reduction decision difficulty. *Social Science & Medicine*, 65: 2342–2356. DOI: 10.1016/j.socscimed.2007.06.026.

Brown, D., Carney, J., Parrish, M., & Klem, J. (2013). Assessing spirituality: The relationship between spirituality and mental health. *Journal of Spirituality in Mental Health*, 15: 107–122.

Buckle, J. & Fleming, S. (2011). *Parenting after the death of a child: A practitioner's guide.* New York: Routledge.

Cacciatore, J. (2007). Effects of support groups on post-traumatic stress responses in women experiencing stillbirth. *Omega: Journal of Death and Dying*, 55(1): 71–90.

Cacciatore, J. (2010). The unique experiences of women and their families after the death of a baby. *Social Work in Health Care*, 49: 134–148.

Cacciatore, J. (2012). Selah: A mindfulness guide through grief. In R.A. Neimeyer (Ed.) *Techniques of grief therapy: Creative practices for counselling the bereaved*. London: Routledge, pp. 16–19.

Cacciatore, J. & Flint, M. (2012). ATTEND: Toward a mindfulness-based bereavement care model. *Death Studies*, 36(1): 61–82.

Cacciatore, J., Ra°destad, I., & J. Frøen. (2008). Effects of contact with stillborn babies on maternal anxiety and depression. *Birth*, 35(4): 313–320.

Cacciatore, J. & Raffo, Z. (2011). An exploration of lesbian maternal bereavement. *Social Work*, 65(2): 169–177.

Cacciatore, J., Frøen, J., & Killian, M. (2013). Condemning self, condemning other: Blame and mental health in women suffering stillbirth. *Omega*, 35(4): 342–359.

Cacciatore, J., LaCasse, J., Lietz, C., & McPherson, J. (2014). A parent's tears: Primary results from the Traumatic Experiences and Resiliency Study. *Omega*, 69(3): 183–205.

Cacciatore, J., Thieleman, K., Killian, M., & Tavasolli, K. (2014). Braving human suffering: Death education and its relationship to empathy and mindfulness. *Social Work Education*, 34(1): 91–109. DOI: 10.1080/02615479.2014.940890.

Cain, A. & Cain, B. (1964). On replacing a child. *Journal of the American Academy of Child Psychiatry*, 3(3): 443–445.

Calhoun, L. & Tedeshi, R. (2001). Posttraumatic growth: The positive lessons of loss. In R.A. Neimeyer (Ed.) *Meaning reconstruction and the experience of loss*. Washington, DC: American Psychological Association, pp. 157–172.

Campbell, S.S. (1998). *Called to heal: Traditional healing meets modern medicine in Southern Africa today*. Cape Town, South Africa: Zebra Press.

Campbell-Jackson, L., Bezance, J., & Horsch, A. (2014). "A renewed sense of purpose": Mothers' and fathers' experience of having a child following a recent stillbirth. *BMC Pregnancy and Childbirth*, 14: 423. DOI: 10.1186/s12884-014-0423-x.

Carlson, R. (2012). Helping families create keepsakes. *International Journal of Childbirth Education*, 27(2): 86–91.

Carlson, R., Lammert, C., & O'Leary, J.M. (2012). The evolution of group and online support for families who have experienced perinatal or neonatal loss. *Illness, Crisis and Loss*, 20(3): 275–293.

Casper, M.J. (1998). *The making of the unborn patient: A social anatomy of fetal surgery*. New Brunswick, NJ: Rutgers University Press.

Caughey, A., Cahill, A., Guise, J.M., & Rouse, D. (2014). Safe prevention of the primary cesarean delivery. *Obstetric Care Consensus*, 1: 1–19.

Center for Reproductive Rights. (n.d.). The world's abortion laws 2012. http://world abortionslaws.com.

Chamberlain, D. (1997). Early and very early parenting: New territories. *Journal of Prenatal and Perinatal Psychology and Health*, 12(2): 51–59.

Chamberlain, D. (1998). *Babies Remember Birth*. Los Angeles, CA: Jeremy P. Tarcher, Inc.

Chamberlain, D. (2003). Communicating with the mind of a prenate: Guidelines for parents and birth professionals. *Journal of Prenatal and Perinatal Psychology and Health*, 18(2): 95–108.

Chamberlain, D. (2013). *Windows to the womb: Revealing the conscious baby from conception to birth*. Berkely, CA: North Atlanta Books.

Chapman, K. & Chapman, R. (1990). Premonition of foetal death. *Stress Medicine*, 6(1): 43–45.

Cheek, D. (1996). Use of the telephone and hypnosis in reversing true preterm labor at 26 weeks: The value of ideomotor questioning in a crisis. *Pre- and Peri-natal Psychology Journal*, 10(4): 273–287.

Cheng, C., Volk, A., & Marini, Z. (2011). Supporting fathering through infant massage. *Journal of Perinatal Education*, 20(4): 200–209. DOI: 10.1891/1058-1243.20.4.200.

Chez, R. (1995). After hours. *Obstetrics & Gynecology*, 85(6): 1959–1061.

Choi, H., Van Riper, M., & Thoyre, S. (2012). Decision making following a prenatal diagnosis of Down syndrome: An integrative review. *Journal of Midwifery and Women's Health*, 57(2): 156–164.

Choi, H., Van Riper, M., & Thoyre, S. (2012). Decision making following a prenatal diagnosis of Down's syndrome: An integrative review. *Journal of Midwifery & Women's Health*, 57(2): 156–164.

Christian, L. (2012). Psychoneuroimmunology in pregnancy: Immune pathways linking stress with maternal health, adverse birth outcomes, and fetal development. *Neuroscience and Biobehavioral Review*, 36(1): 350–351.

Cleirigh, C. & Safren, S. (2008). Optimizing the effects of stress management interventions in HIV. *Health Psychology*, 27(3): 297–301.

Clifford, K., Rai, R., & Regan, L. (1997). Future pregnancy outcome in unexplained recurrent first trimester miscarriage. *Human Reproduction*, 12: 387–389.

Collopy, K.S. (2004). "I couldn't think that far": Infertile women's decision making about multi-fetal reduction. *Research in Nursing and Health*, 27: 75–86.

Comparetti, A.M. (1981). The neurophysiologic and clinical implications of studies on fetal motor behavior. *Seminars in Perinatology*, 5: 183–189.

Condon, J. (1985). The parental–fetal relationship: A comparison of male and female expectant parents. *Journal of Psychosomatic Obstetrics and Gynaecology*, 4(4): 271–284.

Condon, J. (1987). Prevention of emotional disability following stillbirth: The role of the obstetric team. *Australian and New Zealand Journal of Obstetrics & Gynecology*, 27: 323.

Condon, J. (2006). What about dad? Psychosocial and mental health issues for new fathers. *Australian Family Physicians*, 35(9): 690–692.

Condon, J. & Corkindale, C. (1997). The correlates of antenatal attachment in pregnant women. *British Journal of Medical Psychology*, 66(2): 167–183.

Condon, J., Boyce, P., & Corkindale, C. (2004). The first-time fathers' study: A prospective study of the mental health and well-being of men during the transition to parenthood. *Australia and New Zealand Journal of Psychiatry*, 38: 56–64.

Condon, J., Corkindale, C., Boyce, P., & Gamble, E. (2013). A longitudinal study of father-to-infant attachment: Antecedents and correlates. *Journal of Reproductive and Infant Psychology*, 31(1): 15–30.

Connolly, K.J., Edelmann, R.J., Bartlett, H., Cooke, I.D., Lenton, E., & Pike, S. (1993) Counselling: An evaluation of counselling for couples undergoing treatment for in-vitro fertilization. *Human Reproduction*, 8: 1332–1338.

Corr, C. (2008). Children's emerging awareness of death. In K. Doka & A. Tucci (Eds) *Living with grief: Children, adolescents and loss*. Washington, DC: Hospice Foundation of America.

Corr, C. (2011). Anticipatory grief and mourning. In K. Doka & A. Tucci (Eds) *Beyond Kubler-Ross: New perspectives on death, dying and grief*. Washington, DC: Hospice Foundation of America, pp. 17–30.

Costa Segui, M. (1995). The prenatal period as the origin of character structures. *International Journal of Prenatal and Perinatal Psychology and Medicine*, 7(3): 309–322.

Côté-Arsenault, D. (2003). Weaving babies lost in pregnancy into the fabric of the family. *Journal of Family Nursing*, 9(1): 23–37.

Côté-Arsenault, D. & Denney-Koelsch, E. (2011). "My baby is a person": parents' experiences with life-threatening fetal diagnosis. *Journal of Palliative Medicine*, 14(12): 1302–1308. DOI: 10.1089/jpm.2011.0165.

Côté-Arsenault, D. & Dombeck, M.T. (2001). Maternal assignment of fetal personhood to a previous pregnancy loss: Relationship to anxiety in the current pregnancy. *Health Care for Women International*, 22(7): 649–665.

Côté-Arsenault, D. & Donato, K. (2011). Emotional cushioning in pregnancy after perinatal loss. *Journal of Reproductive and Infant Psychology*, 29(1): 81–92.

Côté-Arsenault, D. & Freije, M.M. (2004). Support groups helping women through pregnancies after loss. *Western Journal of Nursing Research*, 26(6): 650–670.

Côté-Arsenault, D. & Mahlangu, N. (1998). Impact of perinatal loss on the subsequent pregnancy and self: Women's experiences. *Journal of Psychosomatics in Obstetric and Gynecologic & Neonatal Nursing*, 28(3): 274–282.

Côté-Arsenault, D. & Marshall, R. (2000). One foot in–one foot out: Weathering the storm of pregnancy after perinatal loss. *Research in Nursing and Health*, 23: 473–485.

Côté-Arsenault, D. & Moore, S. (2014). Exploring women's experiences of pregnancy after loss through diary entries. Unpublished manuscript.

Côté-Arsenault, D. & Morrison, D. (2001). Women's voices reflecting changed expectations for pregnancy after perinatal loss. *Journal of Nursing Scholarship*, 33(3): 239–244.

Côté-Arsenault, D. & O'Leary, J.M. (2015). Understanding the experience of pregnancy subsequent to perinatal loss. In P. Wright et al. (Eds) *Perinatal and pediatric bereavement*. New York: Springer, pp. 169–181.

Côté-Arsenault, D., Bidlack, D., & Humm, A. (2001). Women's emotions and concerns during pregnancy following perinatal loss. *American Journal of Maternal/Child Nursing,* 26(3), 128–134.

Côté-Arsenault, D., Donato, K., & Earl, S.S. (2006). Watching and worrying: Early pregnancy after loss experiences. *MCN: American Journal of Maternal/Child Nursing*, 31: 356–363.

Côté-Arsenault, D., Krowchuk, H., Hall, W.J., & Denney-Koelsch, E. (2015). We want what's best for our baby: Prenatal parenting of babies with lethal conditions. *Journal of Prenatal and Perinatal Psychology and Health*, 29(3): 157–176.

Côté-Arsenault, D., Schwartz, B.S., Krochuk, H., & McCoy, T. (2007). Evidence-based intervention with women pregnant after perinatal loss. *MCN: American Journal of Maternal/Child Nursing*, 39(3): 177–186.

Couto, E.R., Couto, E., Vian, B., Gregorio, Z., Nomura, M.L., Zaccaria, R., & Junior, R.P. (2009). Quality of life, depression and anxiety among pregnant women with previous adverse pregnancy outcomes. *Sao Paulo Medical Journal*, 127(4): 185–189.

Cowchock, F.S., Meador, K.G., Floyd, S.E., & Swamy, G.K. (2011). Spiritual needs of couples facing pregnancy termination because of fetal anomalies. *Journal of Pastoral Care and Counseling*, 65(1–2): 4–10.

Creedy, D.K., Shochet, I.M., & Horsfall, J. (2000). Childbirth and the development of acute trauma symptoms: Incidence and contributing factors. *Birth*, 27(2): 104–111.

Crenshaw, D. (2002). The disenfranchised grief of children. In K.J. Doka (Ed.) *Disenfranchised grief: New directions, challenges, and strategies for practice*. Champaign, IL: Research Press, pp. 293–306.

Crosson, J. (2012). Psychoneuroimmunology, stress and pregnancy. *International Journal of Childbirth Education*, 27(2): 76–79.

Crowther, M. (1995). Perinatal death: Worse obstetric and neonatal outcome in a subsequent pregnancy. *Journal of the Royal Army Medical Corps*, 141(2): 92–97.

Cuisinier, M., Kuijper, J., Hoodgduin, C., de Graauw, C., & Janssen, H. (1996). Miscarriage and stillbirth: Time since the loss, grief intensity and satisfaction with care. *European Journal of Obstetrics & Gynecology*, 52(2): 163–168.

Culling, V. (2013). *Holding on and letting go: Facing an unexpected diagnosis in pregnancy.* Wellington, New Zealand:Vicki Culling Associates.

Cumming, K., Bolsover, L. et al. (2007). The emotional burden of miscarriage for women and their partners: Trajectories of anxiety and depression over 13 months. *BJOG: An International Journal of Obstetrics & Gynaecology,* 114(9): 1138–1145.

Currier, J.M., Neimeyer, R.A., & Berman, J.S. (2008). The effectiveness of psychotherapeutic interventions for the bereaved: A comprehensive quantitative review. *Psychological Bulletin,* 134: 648–661.

Davies, B. (2006). Sibling grief throughout childhood. *The Forum,* Jan/Feb, p. 4.

Davies, B. & Limbo, R.K. (2010). The grief of siblings. In N.B.Webb (Ed.) *Helping bereaved children: A handbook for practitioners* (3rd ed). New York: Guilford Press, pp. 69–90.

Davies, B., Baird, J., & Gudmundsdottir, M. (2013). Moving family-centered care forward: Bereaved father's perspective. *Journal of Hospice & Palliative Nursing,* 15(3): 163–170.

Davis, C., Lehman, D., Silver, R., Wortman, C., & Ellard, J. (1996). Self-blame following a traumatic event: The role of perceived avoidability. *Personality and Social Psychology Bulletin,* 22: 557–567.

Davis, D.L. (2016). *Empty cradle, broken heart: Surviving the death of your baby* (3rd ed). Golden, CO: Fulcrum.

Davis, D.L., Stewart, M., & Harmon, R.J. (1989). Postponing pregnancy after perinatal death: Perspectives on doctor advice. *Journal of the American Academy of Child and Adolescent Psychiatry,* 28(4): 481–487.

Davies, E.P. & Sandman, C.A. (2011). The timing of prenatal exposure to maternal cortisol and psychosocial stress is associated with human infant cognitive development. *Child Development,* 81(1): 131–148.

Davies, E.P., Glynn, L., Waffarn, F., & Sandman, C. (2011). Prenatal maternal stress programs infant stress regulation. *Journal of Child Psychology & Psychiatry,* 52(2): 119–129.

DeBackere, K.J., Hill, P.D., & Kavanaugh, K.L. (2008). The parental experience of pregnancy after perinatal loss. *Journal of Obstetric, Gynecologic, & Neonatal Nursing,* 37(5): 525–537.

deMontigny, F., Girard, M.E., Lacharite, C., Dubeau, D., & Devault, A. (2013). Psychosocial factors associated with paternal postnatal depression. *Journal of Affective Disorders,* 150(1): 44–49.

De Pascalis, L., Monti, F., Agostini, F., Fagandini, P. Giovanni, B., La Sala, G., & Blickstein, I. (2007). Psychological vulnerability of singleton children after the "vanishing" of a co-twin following assisted reproduction. *Twin Research and Human Genetics,* 11(1): 93–98.

deVries, J.,Visser, G., & Prechtl, H. (1982). The emergence of fetal behavior: I. Qualitative aspects. *Early Human Development,* 7: 301–322.

Diniz, D. (2007). Selective abortion in Brazil: The anencephaly case. *Developing World Bioethics,* 7: 64–67.

DiPietro, J. (2004). The role of prenatal maternal stress in child development. *Current Directions in Psychological Science,* 13(2): 271–274.

DiPietro, J. (2005). Neurobehavioral assessment before birth. *Mental Retardation and Developmental Disabilities Research,* 11: 21–24.

DiPietro, J. (2010). Psychological and psychophysiological considerations regarding the maternal–fetal relationship. *Infant and Child Development,* 19(1): 27–38. DOI: 10.1002/icd.651.

DiPietro, J. (2012). Does maternal psychological stress harm the developing fetus? Lecture PowerPoint slides. www.researchconnections.org/…/pdf/DiPietro_Janet_StressMtg2012.pdf.

DiPietro, J., Hodgson, D., Costigan, K., Hilton, S. & Johnson, T. (1996). Fetal Neurobehavioral Development. *Child Development,* 67: 2553–2567 DiPietro, J.A., Costigan, K., Nelson, P.,

Gurewitsch, E., & Laudenslager, L. (2008). Fetal response to induced maternal relaxation during pregnancy. *Biological Psychology*, 77(1): 11–19.

DiPietro, J.A., Novak, M.F., Costigan, K.A., Atella, L.D., & Resuing, S.P. (2006). Maternal psychological distress during pregnancy in relation to child development at age two. *Child Development*, 77(3): 573–587.

Dirix, C., Nijhuis, J., Jongsma, H., & Hornsta, G. (2009). Aspects of fetal learning and memory. *Child Development*, 80(4): 1251–1258. DOI: 10.1111/j.1467-8624.2009.01329.x.

Doan, H. & Zimerman, A. (2003). Conceptualizing prenatal attachment: Toward a multidimensional view. *Journal of Prenatal and Perinatal Psychology and Health*, 18: 11–148.

Doan, H. & Zimerman, A. (2008). Prenatal attachment: A developmental model. *International Journal of Prenatal and Perinatal Psychology and Medicine*, 20(1/2): 20–28.

Doka, K.J. (1989). *Disenfranchised grief: Recognizing hidden sorrow.* Lexington, MA: Lexington.

Doka, K.J. (2002). *Disenfranchised grief: New directions, challenges, and strategies for practice.* Champaign, IL: Research Press.

Dowden, S. (1995). Young children's experience of sibling death. *Journal of Pediatric Nursing*, 10(1): 72–79. DOI:10.1016/S0882-5963(05)80109-5

Duncan, C. & Cacciatore, J. (2015). A systematic review of the peer-reviewed literature on self-blame, guilt, and shame. DOI: 10.1177/0030222815572604.

Dunkel, C., Schetter, C., & Tanner, L. (2012). Anxiety, depression and stress in pregnancy: Implications for mothers, children, research, and practice. *Current Opinion in Psychiatry*, 25(2): 141–148.

Dyregrov, A. (2001). Telling the truth or hiding the facts: An evaluation of current strategies for assisting children following adverse events. *Association for Child Psychology and Psychiatry Occasional Papers*, 17: 25–38.

Dyregrov, A. & Dyregrov, K. (1999). Long-term impact of sudden infant death: A 12–15-year follow-up. *Death Studies*, 23(7): 635–661.

Dyregrov, A. & Regel, S. (2012). Early intervention following exposure to traumatic events: Implications for practice from recent research. *Journal of Loss and Trauma*, 17: 271–291.

Dyregrov, A., Dyregrov, K., & Idsoe, T. (2013a). Teachers' perceptions of their role facing children in grief. *Emotional & Behavioral Difficulties*, 18(2): 125–134.

Dyregrov, K., Dryregrov, A., & Johnsen, I. (2013b). Participants' recommendations for the ideal grief group: A qualitative study. *Omega*, 67(4): 363–377.

Dyregrov, K., Dryregrov, A., & Johnsen, I. (2014a). Positive and negative experiences from grief group participation: A qualitative study. *Omega*, 68(1): 45–62.

Dyregrov, K., Endsjo, M., Idsoe, T., & Dyregrov, A. (2014b). Suggestions for the ideal follow-up for bereaved students as seen by school personnel. *Emotional & Behavioral Difficulties*, 20(3): 289–301.

Earle, S., Foley, P., Komaromy, C., & Lloyd, C.E. (2008). Conceptualizing reproductive loss: A social sciences perspective. *Human Fertility*, 11(4): 259–262.

Eastward, E. (2001). *The natram handbook* (4th ed). Tomales, CA: Nilgiri Press.

Edenfield, T. & Saeed, S. (2012). An update on mindfulness meditation as a self-help treatment for anxiety and depression. *Psychological Research and Behavioral Management*, 5: 131–141.

Ehring, T., Ehlers, A., & Glucksman, E. (2008). Do cognitive models help in predicting the severity of posttraumatic stress disorder, phobia and depression after motor vehicle accidents? A prospective longitudinal study. *Journal of Consulting and Clinical Psychology*, 76: 219–230.

Eichhorn, N. (2012). Maternal fetal attachment: Can acceptance of fetal sentience impact the maternal–fetal attachment relationship? *Journal of Prenatal and Perinatal Psychology and Health*, 27(1): 47–55.

Eisenberg, D. (2004). Abortion in Jewish law. *Jewish World Society Today*. http://www.aish.com/societyWork/sciencenature?Abortion_in_Jewish_Law.asp.

Emerson, W. (1998). The vulnerable infant. *International Journal of Prenatal and Perinatal Psychology and Medicine*, 10(1): 5–17.

Engelkemeyer, S. & Marwit, S. (2009). Posttraumatic growth in bereaved parents. *Journal of Traumatic Stress*, 21(3): 344–346.

Erlandsson, K., Avelin, P., Säflund, K., Wredling, R., & Rådestad, I. (2010). Siblings' farewell to a stillborn sister or brother and parents' support to their older children: A questionnaire study from the parents' perspective. *Journal of Child Health Care*, 14(2): 151–160.

Evans, M.I. & Britt, D.W. (2008). Fetal reduction. *Current Opinion in Obstetrics and Gynecology*, 20(4): 386–393.

Evans, M.I., Ciorica, D., Britt, D.W., & Fletcher, J.C. (2005). Update on selection reduction. *Prenatal Diagnosis*, 25: 807–813.

Evans, P. (1999). Long term fetal microchenerism in peripheral blood mononuclear cell subsets in healthy women and women with scleroderma. *Blood*, 93(6): 2033–2037.

Evans, S., Ferrando, S., Findler, M., Stowell, C., Smart, C., & Haglin, D. (2008). Mindfulness-based cognitive therapy for generalized anxiety disorder. *Journal of Anxiety Diorders*, 22(4): 716–721.

Evans, W.G., Tulsky, J.A., Back, A.L., & Arnold, R.M. (2006). Communication at times of transitions: How to help patients cope with loss and re-define hope. *Cancer Journal*, 12(5): 417–424.

Fanos, J.H., Little, G.A., & Edwards, W.H. (2009). Candles in the snow: Ritual and memory for siblings of infants who died in the intensive care nursery. *Journal of Pediatrics*, 154: 849–853. DOI: 10.1016/j.peds.2008.11.053.

Fedor-Freybergh, P.G. (2008). Psychosomatic characteristics of prenatal and perinatal period as the environment of infant. *International Journal of Prenatal & Perinatal Psychology & Medicine*, 23(3): 3–28.

Fedor-Freybergh, P.G. (1992). The unborn baby. Presentation at the International Prenatal and Perinatal Psychology and Medicine, Krakow, Poland.

Fedor-Freybergh, P.G. & Maas, L. (2011). Continuity and indivisibility of integrated psychological, spiritual and somatic life processes. *International Journal of Prenatal & Perinatal Psychology & Medicine*, 23 (Suppl 1): 135–142.

Fernandez, R., Harris, D., & Leschied, A. (2011). Understanding grief following pregnancy loss: A retrospective analysis regarding women's coping responses. *Illness, Crisis & Loss*, 19(20): 143–163.

Fertl, K.I., Bergner, A., Beyer, R., Klapp, B.F., & Rauchfuss, M. (2009). Levels and effects of different forms of anxiety during pregnancy after a prior miscarriage. *European Journal of Obstetrics, Gynecology, & Reproductive Biology*, 142(1): 23–29.

Field, N. (2006). Unresolved grief and continuing bonds: An attachment perspective. *Death Studies*, 30: 739–756.

Field, N., Packman, W., Ronen, R., Pries, A., Davis, B., & Kramer, R. (2013). Type of continued bonds expression and its comforting versus distressing nature: Implications for adjustment among bereaved mothers. *Death Studies*, 37(10): 889–912.

Field, T. (2010). Touch for social emotional and physical well-being. *Developmental Review*, 30(4): 367–383.

Field, T., Diego, M., Hernandez-Reif, M., Deeds, O., & Figueiredo, B. (2009). Pregnancy massage reduces prematurity low birthweight and postpartum depression. *Infant Behavior and Development*, 32(4): 454–460.

Findeisen, B. (1992). The long term psychological impact of pre- and perinatal experiences. *International Journal of Prenatal and Perinatal Studies*, 4(1): 14.

Finer, L. & Fine, J. (2013). Abortion law around the world: Progress and pushback. *American Journal of Public Health*, 103(4): 585–589.

Fink, N., Urech, C., Cavelti, M., & Alder, J. (2012). Relaxation during pregnancy: What are the benefits for mother, fetus and the newborn? A systematic review of the literature. *Journal of Perinatal & Neonatal Nursing*, 26(4): 296–306.

Flenady, V., Middleton, P., Smith, G.C., Duke, W., Erwich, J.J. et al. (2011). Stillbirths: The way forward in high-income countries. *Lancet*, 377(9778): 1703–1717.

Fletcher, R., May, C., & George, J. (2014). Fathers' prenatal relationship with "their" baby and "her" pregnancy—implications for antenatal education. *International Journal of Birth and Parent Education*, 1(3): 23–27.

Fonagy, P. (1998). Prevention, the appropriate target of infant psychotherapy. *Infant Mental Health Journal*, 19(2): 124–150.

Fonagy, P. (2000). The development of psychopathology from infancy to adulthood: The mysterious unfolding of disturbance in time. Presentation at the World Association of Infant Mental Health Conference, Montreal, Canada.

Fox, N., Rebarber, A., Silverstein, M., Roman, A., Klauser, C., & Saltzman, D. (2013). The effectiveness of antepartum surveillance in reducing the risk of stillbirth in patients with advanced maternal age. *European Journal of Obstetrics and Gynecology and Reproductive Biology*, 170 (2): 387–390.

Fraiberg, S. & Fraiberg, L. (1987). *Selected writings of Selma Fraiberg*. Ohio: Ohio State University Press.

Fraiberg, S., Adelson, E., & Cherniss, D. (1980a). Treatment modalities. In S. Fraiberg (Ed.) *Clinical studies in infant mental health: The first year of life*. New York: Basic Books.

Fraiberg, S., Adelson, E., & Shapiero, V. (1980b). Ghost in the nursery: A psychoanalytic approach to the problems of impaired infant–mother relationships. In S. Fraiberg (Ed.) *Clinical studies in infant mental health: The first year of life*. New York: Basic Books, pp. 164–166.

Fraiberg, S., Shapiro, V., Bennett, V., & Pawl, J. (1980c). Brief crisis intervention: Two cases. In S. Fraiberg (Ed.) *Clinical studies in infant mental health: The first year of life*. New York: Basic Books, pp. 78–102.

France, E., Hunt, K., Ziebland, S., & Wyke, S. (2013). What parents say about disclosing the end of their pregnancy due to fetal abnormality. *Midwifery*, 29(1): 24–32.

Frawley, J., Adams, J., Broom, A., Steel, A., Gallois, C., & Sibbritt, D. (2014). Majority of women are influenced by nonprofessional information sources when deciding to consult a CAM practitioner during pregnancy. *Journal of Complimentary and Alternative Medicine*, 20(7): 571–577.

Frias, A., Luikennaar, R., Sullivan, A., Lee, R., Porter, T., Branch, W., & Sliver, R. (2004). Poor obstetric outcome in subsequent pregnancies in women with prior fetal death. *Obstetrics and Gynecology*, 104: 521–526.

Frøen, N.P., Cacciatore, J., McClure, E., Kuti, O., Jokhio, H., Islam, A., & Shiffman, J. (2011). Stillbirths: Why they matter. *Lancet*, 377: 1353–1366.

Gains, R. (1997). Detachment and continuity: The two tasks of mourning. *Contemporary Psychoanalysis*, 33(4): 549–571.

Galinsky, M. & Schopler, J. (1994). Negative experiences in suport groups. *Social Work in Health Care*, 20: 77–95.

Gamble, J., Creedy, D., Webser, J., & Moyle, W. (2002). A review of the literature on debriefing or non-directive counseling to prevent postpartum emotional distress. *Midwifery*, 18(1): 72–79.

Gaudet, C. (2010). Pregnancy after perinatal loss: Association of grief, anxiety and attachment. *Journal of Reproductive and Infant Psychology*, 28(3): 240–251.

Gaudette, H. & Jankowski, K. (2013). Spiritual coping and anxiety in palliative care patients: A pilot study. *Journal of Health Care Chaplaincy*, 19: 131–139.

Gawron, L., Cameron, K., Phisuthikul, A., & Simon, M. (2013). An exploration of women's reasons for termination timing in the setting of fetal abnormalities. *Contraception*, 88: 109–115.

Geerinck-Vercammen, C.R. & Kanhai, H.H.H. (2003). Coping with termination of pregnancy for fetal abnormality in a supportive environment. *Prenatal Diagnosis*, 23(7): 543–548.

Gerber-Epstein, P., Leichtentritt, R., & Benyamini, Y. (2009). The experience of miscarriage in first pregnancy: The women's voices. *Death Studies*, 33: 1–29.

Gesell, A. (1940). *The first five years of life: A guide to the study of the preschool child*. New York: Harper & Row.

Gilbert, K. (2002). Taking a narrative approach to grief research: Finding meaning in stories. *Death Studies*, 26(3): 223–239.

Glenn, M. & Cappon, R. (2013). Essential clinical principles for prenatal and perinatal psychology practitioners. *Journal of the Association for Prenatal and Perinatal Psychology and Health*, 28(1): 20–42.

Glover, V. (1997). Maternal stress or anxiety in pregnancy and emotional development of the child. *British Journal of Psychiatry*, 171:105–106.

Glover, V. (2011a). Annual research review: Prenatal stress and the origins of psychopathology: An evolutionary perspective. *Journal of Child Psychology and Psychiatry*, 52(4): 356–367.

Glover, V. (2011b). The effects of prenatal stress on child behavioural and cognitive outcomes start at the beginning. In R.E. Tremblay, R.E. Bivin, & R. DeV Peters (Eds) *Encyclopedia of early childhood development* [online]. Montreal, Quebec: Centre of Excellence for Early Childhood Development, pp.1–5.

Glover, V. (2012). Effects of prenatal anxiety, depression and stress on fetal and child development: Mechanisms and questions. Presentation at the Marce International Conference, Paris, France.

Glover, V. (2015). Prenatal stress and its effects on the fetus and child: Possible underlying biological mechanisms. In M. Antonelli (Ed.) *Perinatal programming of neurodevelopment: Advances in neurobiology*. New York: Springer, pp. 269–283. DOI: 10.1007/978-1-4939-1372-5_13.

Glover, V., O'Connor, T., O'Connell, K., & Capron, L. (2014). How prenatal depression, anxiety, and stress may affect child outcome. *Zero to Three*, 34 (4): 22–28.

Gold, K.J., Boggs, M., & Mugisha, E. (2011). After pregnancy loss: Internet forums help women understand they are not alone. *Women's Health Issues*, 22(1): e67–e72. DOI: 10.1016/j.whi.2011.07.006.

Gold, K.J., Leon, I., & Chames, M.C. (2010). National survey of obstetrician attitudes about timing the subsequent pregnancy after perinatal death. *American Journal of Obstetric Gynecology*, 202: 357.

Gold, K.J., Leon, I., & Chames, M.C. (2010). National survey of obstetrician attitudes about timing the subsequent pregnancy after perinatal death. *American Journal of Obstetric Gynecology*, 202: 357–356.

Gomes-Pedro, J., Nugent, J.K., Young, J.G., & Brazelton, T. (2013). *The infant and family in the 21st century*. New York: Routledge.

Gordon, L., Thornton, A., Lewis, S., Wake, S., & Sahhar, M. (2007). An evaluation of shared experience group for women and their support persons following prenatal diagnosis and termination for a fetal abnormality. *Prenatal Diagnosis*, 27: 835–839.

Grady, J. & O'Leary, J.M. (Eds) (1993). *Heartbreak pregnancies: Unfulfilled promises*. Minneapolis, MN: Abbott Northwestern Hospital (out of print).

Graham, M.A., Thompson, S.C., Estrada M., & Yonekura, M. (1987). Factors affecting psychological adjustment to a fetal death. *American Journal of Obstetrics and Gynecology*, 157: 254–257.

Green, M. & Solnit, A. (1964). Reactions to the threatened loss of a child: A vulnerable child syndrome. *Pediatrics*, 34(1): 58–66.

Grout, L. & Romanoff, B. (1999). The myth of the replacement child: Parents' stories and practices after perinatal death. *Death Studies*, 24(2): 93–113.

Guardion, C. & Dunkel Schetter, C. (2014). Understanding pregnancy anxiety. *Zero to Three*, 34(4): 12–21.

Gudmundsdottir, M. (2009). Embodied grief: Bereaved parents' narratives of their suffering body. *Omega*, 59(3): 253–269.

Gudmundsdottir, M. & Chesla, C.A. (2006). Building a new world: Habits and practices of healing following the death of a child. *Journal of Family Nursing*, 12(2): 143–164.

Hagman, G. (2001). Beyond decathexis: Toward a new psychoanalytic understanding and treatment of mourning. In R. Neimeyer (Ed.) *Meaning reconstruction and the experience of loss*. Washington, DC: American Psychological Association, pp. 13–31.

Hall, H. & Jolly, K. (2014). Women's use of complementary and alternative medicines during pregnancy: A cross-sectional study. *Midwifery*, 30(5): 499–505.

Hall, H., Griffiths, D., & McKenna, L. (2011). The use of complementary and alternative medicine by pregnant women: A literature review. *Midwifery*, 27(6): 817–824.

Hammerschlag, C. (1993). *The theft of spirit: A journey to spiritual healing with Native Americans*. Toronto: Simon & Schuster.

Hankins, G. & Longo, M. (2006). The role of stillbirth prevention and late preterm (near-term) births. *Seminars in Perinatology*, 3(1): 20–23. DOI: org/10.1053/j.semperi.2006.01.011.

Hardison, H.G., Neimeyer, R.A., & Lichstein, K.L. (2005). Insomnia and complicated grief symptoms in bereaved college students. *Behavioral Sleep Medicine*, 3(2): 99–111.

Hauck, F.R., Thompson, J.M.D., Tanabe, K.O. et al. (2011). Breastfeeding and reduced risk of sudden infant death syndrome: A meta-analysis. *Pediatrics*, 128(1): 103–110.

Hawkins, A., Stenzel, A., Taylor, J., Chock, V., & Hudgins, L. 2013). Variables influencing pregnancy termination following prenatal diagnosis of fetal chromosome abnormalities. *Journal of Genetic Counseling*, 22: 238–248. DOI: 10.1007/s10897-012-9539-1.

Hayton, A. (2007). *Untwinned: Perspectives on the death of a twin before birth*. Wren Publications (online).

Hayton, A. (2008). *A silent cry: Wombtwin survivors tell their stories*. Wren Publications (online).

Hayton, A. (2011*). Womb twin survivors: The lost twin in the dream of the womb*. Wren Publications (online).

Hayton, A. (2014). *Ripples from the womb: How therapist can help the sole survivor when a twin dies before birth*. Wren Publications (online).

Heazell, A.E. & Frøen, J.F. (2008). Methods of fetal movement counting and the detection of fetal compromise. *Journal of Obstetric Gynaecology*, 28(2): 147–154.

Heazell, A., Barrett, J., Ladhani, N., et al. (2015). International Consensus Statement meeting on care of the family pregnant subsequent to stillbirth. Satellite meeting following the International Stillbirth Alliance Conference, 4 October, Vancouver, British Columbia, Canada.

Helgadóttir, L.B.I., Turowski, G., Skjeldestad, F.E., Jacobsen, A.F., Sandset, P.M., Roald, B., & Jacobsen, E.M. (2013). Classification of stillbirths and risk factors by cause of death—a case-control study. *Acta Obstetrica et Gynecologic Scandinavica*, 92(3): 325–333.

Heller, S. & Zeanah, C. (1999). Attachment disturbances in infants born subsequent to perinatal loss: A pilot study. *Infant Mental Health Journal*, 20(2): 188–199.

Henshaw, S.K. (1998). Unintended pregnancy in the US. *Family Planning Perspective*, 30(24): 9–46.

Hepper, P. (1996). Fetal memory: Does it exist? What does it do? *Acta Pediatrica*, 416: 16–20.

Hepper, P. (2005). Unraveling our beginnings. *The Psychologist*, 18: 474–477.

Hepper, P. & Shaidullah, S. (1994). The beginnings of mind: Evidence from the behavior of the fetus. *Journal of Reproductive and Infant Psychology*, 12(3): 143–154.

Hilder, L., Zhichao, Z., Parker, M., Jahan, S., & Chambers, G.M. (2014). Australia's mothers and babies 2012. Perinatal Statistics Series No. 30. Cat. no. PER 69. Canberra: AIHW.

Hillman, S.C., Morris, R.K., & Kilby, M.D. (2010). Single twin demise: Consequence for survivors. *Seminars in Fetal and Neonatal Medicine*, 15(6): 319–326.

Hoffman, S., Sawyer, A., Witt, A., & Oh, D. (2010). The effect of mindfulness-based cognitive therapy on anxiety and depression: A meta-analytic review. *Journal of Consulting and Clinical Psychology*, 78(2): 169–183.

Hogan, N. (2006). Understanding adolescent sibling bereavement. *The Forum*, Jan/Feb/March: 5–6.

Holland, J.M. (2008). How schools can support children who experience loss and death. *British Journal of Guidance & Counselling*, 36(4): 411–424.

Holland, J.M., Currier, J.M., & Neimeyer, R.A. (2014). Validation of the Integration of Stressful Life Experiences Scale–Short Form in a bereaved sample. *Death Studies*, 38(4): 234–238.

Hopkins, A. (2002) Children and grief: The role of the early childhood educator. *Young Children*, 57: 40–47.

Horsch, A., Graz, M., Cevery-Macherel, M., Pierrenhumbert, B., du Chene, L., & Tolsa, J. (2014). Expressive writing intervention for mothers following the birth of their premature baby. Poster presentation at the World Association of Infant Mental Health conference, Edinburgh, ScotlandHouwen, van der K., Schut, H., van den Bout, J., Stroebe, M., & Stroebe, W. (2010). The efficacy of a brief internet-based self-help intervention for the bereaved. *Behavior Research and Therapy*, 48(5): 359–367. DOI: 10.1016/j.brat.2009.12.009.

Hruby, R. & Fedor-Freybergh, P. (2013). Prenatal and perinatal medicine and psychology towards integration neurosciences: General remarks and future. *International Journal of Prenatal and Perinatal Psychological Medicine*, 25(1–2): 121–138.

Huberty, J.L., Coleman, J., Rolfsmeyer, K., & Wu, S. (2014a). A qualitative study exploring women's beliefs about physical activity after stillbirth. *BMC Pregnancy and Childbirth*, 14: 26.

Huberty, J.L., Leiferman, J.A., Gold, K.J., Rowedder, L., Cacciatore, J., & Bonds, D. (2014b). Physical activity and depressive symptoms after stillbirth: Informing future interventions. *BMC Pregnancy and Childbirth*, 14: 391.

Hughes, P., Turton, P., & Evans, C. (1999). Stillbirth as risk for depression and anxiety in the subsequent pregnancy. *British Medical Journal*, 318(7200): 1721–1724.

Hughes, P., Turton, P. Hopper, E., & Evans, C. (2002). Assessment of guidelines for good practice in psychosocial care of mothers after stillbirth: A cohort study. *Lancet*, 360: 114–118.

Hughes, P., Turton, P., Hopper, E., McGauley, G.A., & Fonagy, P. (2001). Disorganized attachment behavior among infants born subsequent to stillbirth. *Journal of Child Psychology and Psychiatry*, 42(6): 791–801.

Hunt, K., France, E., Ziebland, S., Field, K., & Wyke, S. (2009). My brain couldn't move from planning a birth to planning a funeral: A qualitative study of parents' experiences of decisions after ending a pregnancy for fetal abnormality. *International Journal of Nursing Studies*, 46: 111–1121.

Hunter, L. Borman, J. Bedlding, W., Sobo, E. Axman, L. et al. (2011). Satisfaction and use of a spiritually based mantram intervention for childbirth-related fears in couples. *Applied Nursing Research*, 24(3): 138–148.

Hutti, M., Armstrong, D., & Myers, J. (2011). Health care utilization in the pregnancy following perinatal loss. *Maternal Child Nursing*, 36(2): 104–111.

Hutti, M., Armstrong, D., Myers, J., & Hall, L. (2015). Grief intensity, psychological well-being, and the intimate partner relationship in the subsequent pregnancy after a perinatal loss. *Journal of Obstetric, Gynecologic & Neonatal Nursing*, 44: 42–50. DOI: 10.1111/1552–8909.12539.

Igarashi, T. (2013). Physical and psychologic effects of aromatherapy inhalation on pregnant women: A randomized controlled trial. *Journal of Complimentary and Alternative Medicine*, 19(10): 805–810.

Imber-Black, E. (2004). Rituals and healing process. In F. Walsh & M. McGoldrick (Eds) *Living beyond loss: Death in the family* (2nd ed). New York: Norton & Co., pp. 340–357.

Jallo, N., Bourguignon, C.A.G., Taylor, A.G., J., Ruiz, J., & Goehler, L. (2009). The bio-behavioral effects of relaxation guided imagery on maternal stress. *Advances in Mind–Body Medicine*, 24(4): 12–22.

Jallo, N., Bourguignon, C., Taylor, A., & Utz, S. (2008). Stress management during pregnancy: Designing and evaluating a mind–body intervention. *Family Community Health*, 31(3): 190–203.

Jallo, N., Ruiz, R.J., Elswick, R.K., & French, E. (2014). Guided imagery for stress and symptom management in pregnant African American women. *Evidenced Based Complimentary and Alternative Medicine*, http://dx.doi.org/10.1155/2014/840923, PMID:24719646.

Janssen, H., Curisinier, M., Hoogduin, K., & de Graauw, K. (1996). Controlled prospective study on the mental health of women following pregnancy loss. *American Journal of Psychiatry*, 153(2): 226–230.

Jauniaux, E., Ben-Ami, I., & Maymon, R. (2013). Do assisted-reproduction twin pregnancies require additional antenatal care? *Reproductive Biomed Online*, 26(2): 107–119. DOI: 10.1016/j.rbmo.2012.11.008.

Johansson, M., Rubertsson, C., Rådestad, I., & Hildingsson, I. (2012). Childbirth—an emotionally demanding experience for fathers. *Sexual & Reproductive Health*, 3(1): 11–20. DOI: 10.1016/j.srhc.2011.12.003.

Jonas-Simpson, C. & McMahon, E. (2005). The language of loss when a baby dies prior to birth: Co-creating human experience. *Nursing Science Quarterly*, 18(2): 14–130. DOI: 10.1177/0894318405275861.

Johnson, S. & Warland, J. (2012). Our baby died: Adolescents' recollections of being raised in a family after the loss of a baby. Paper to ISPID/ISA International Conference on Stillbirth. Baltimore, MD.

Jonas-Simpson, C. (Prod.) (2014). *Always with Me: The Impact of Parental Grief on Children and Adolescent Grief*.

Jonas-Simpson, C., Steele, R., Granek, L., Davies, B., & O'Leary, J.M. (2015). Always with me: Understanding experiences of bereaved children whose baby sibling died. *Death Studies*, 39(4): 242–251.

Kaplan, L.A., Evans, L., & Monk, C. (2007). Effects of mothers' prenatal psychiatric status and postnatal caregiving on infant biobehavioral regulation: Can prenatal programming be modified? *Early Human Development*, 84(4): 249–256.

Katz-Rotham, B. (1993). *The tentative pregnancy: How amniocentesis changes the experience of motherhood*. New York: W.W. Norton & Co.

Kauffman, J. (2002). The psychology of disenfranchised grief: Liberation, shame and self-disenfranchisement. In K.J. Doka (Ed.) *Disenfranchised grief: New directions, challenges, and strategies for practice*. Champaign, IL: Research Press, pp. 61–77.

Kauffman, J. (2012). The empathic spirit in grief therapy. In R. Neimeyer (Ed.) *Techniques of grief therapy: Creative practices for counseling the bereaved*. New York: Routledge, pp. 12–15.

Keen, E. (1975). *A primer in phenomenological psychology*. New York: Holt, Reinhart & Winston.

Keesee, N., Currier, J., & Neimeyer, R. (2008). Predictors of grief following the death of one's child: The contribution of finding meaning. *Journal of Clinical Psychology*, 64(10): 1145–1163.

Kempson, D. & Murdock, V. (2010). Memory keepers: A narrative study on siblings never known. *Death Studies*, 34: 738–756.

Kempson, D., Murdock, V., & Conley, V. (2008). Transgenerational grief: The "ghost" of the sibling never known. *Journal of Illness, Crisis and Loss*, 16(4): 271–284.

Kersting, A. & Wagner, B. (2012). Complicated grief after perinatal loss. *Journal of the American Academy of Psychoanalysis and Dynamic Psychiatry*, 39(3): 187–194.

Kersting, A., Dolemeyer, R., Steinig, J., Walter, F., Kroker, K., Bauist, K., & Wagner, B. (2013). Brief internet-based intervention reduces posttraumatic stress and prolonged grief in parents after the loss of a child during pregnancy: A randomized controlled trial. *Psychotherapy and Psychosomatics*, 82: 372–381.

Kersting, A., Kroker, K., Schlicht, S., Baust, K., & Wagner, B. (2011). Efficacy of cognitive behavioral internet-based therapy in parents after the loss of a child during pregnancy: Pilot data from a randomized controlled trail. *Archives of Women's Mental Health*, 14: 465–477.

Kesternbaum, C.J. (2011). Secure attachment and traumatic life events. *Journal of the American Academy of Psychoanalysis and Dynamic Psychiatry*, 39: 409–419.

Khosrotehrani, K., Kirby, L., Johnson, K., Lau, J., Dupuy, A., Cha, D., & Bianchi, D. (2003). The influence of fetal loss on the presence of fetal cell microchimerism: A systematic review. *Arthritis & Rheumatism*, 48(11): 3237–3241.

Kilvington, C. & Brunies, R. (1992). *Affirmations for your healthy pregnancy. Daily affirmations with fetal developmental stages.* St. Paul, MN: Affirmation Press.

Kim, H. (2012). Drowning in plain sight. *Journal of the American Medical Association*, 307(18): 1923–1924.

Klass, D. (1993). Solace and immortality: Bereaved parents' continued bond with their children. *Death Studies*, 17: 343–368.

Klass, D. (2001). The inner representation of the dead child in the psychic and social narratives of bereaved parents. In R. Neimeyer (Ed.) *Meaning reconstruction and the experience of loss*. Washington, DC: American Psychological Association, pp. 77–94.

Klass, D. & Goss, R. (1999). Spiritual bonds to the dead in cross-cultural and historical perspective: Comparative religion and modern grief. *Death Studies*, 23(6): 547–567.

Klass, D., Silverman, P., & Nickman, S. (Eds) (1996). *Continuing bonds: New understandings of grief*. Washington, DC: Taylor & Francis.

Klein, S., Bolsover, D., Lee, A., Alexander, D., Maclean, M., & Jurgens, J. (2007). The emotional burden of miscarriage for women and their partners: Trajectories of anxiety and depression over 13 months. *BJOG: An International Journal of Obstetrics and Gynaecology*, 114: 1138–1145.

Kolber, K., Limbo, R., & Kavanaugh, K. (2007). Meaningful moments: The use of ritual in perinatal and pediatric death. *MCN: The American Journal of Maternal Child Nursing*, 32(5): 288–297.

Kolk, van der B.A. (1994). The body keeps the score: Memory and the evolving psychobiology of posttraumatic stress. *Harvard Review of Psychiatry*, 1(5): 253–265.

Koloroutis, M. & Trout, M. (2012). *See me as a person: Creating therapeutic relationships with patients and their families.* Minneapolis, MN: Creative Health Care Management.

Korenromp, M., Godelieve, C.M.L., Page-Christiaens, C.M.L., van den Bout, J., Mulder, E.J.H. et al. (2005). Psychological consequences of termination of pregnancy for fetal anomaly: Similarities and differences between partners. *Prenatal Diagnosis,* 25(13): 1226–1233.

Korenromp, M., Page-Christiaens, C.M.L., van den Bout, J., Mulder, E.J.H., Hunfeld, J.A.M. et al. (2007). A prospective study on parental coping 4 months after termination of pregnancy for fetal anomalies. *Prenatal Diagnosis,* 27(8): 709–716.

Kozhimannil, K., Attanasio, L., Jou, J., Joarnt, L., Johnson, P., & Gjerdingen, D. (2014). Potential benefits of increased access to doula support during childbirth. *American Journal of Managed Care,* 20(6): e340–e352.

Kozhimannil, K., Hardeman, R., Attanasio, L., Blauer-Peterson, C., & O'Brien, M. (2013). Doula care, birth outcomes, and costs among Medicaid beneficiaries. *American Journal of Public Health,* 103(4): e113–e121.

Krueger, C., Holditch-Davis, D., Quint, S., & DeCasper, A. (2004). Recurring auditory experience in the 28-to 34-week-old fetus. *Infant Behavior & Development,* 27: 537–543.

Kuebelbeck, A. (2003) *Waiting with Gabriel: A story of cherishing a baby's brief life.* Chicago, IL: Loyola Press.

Kuebelbeck, A. & Davis, D. (2011). *A gift of time: Continuing your pregnancy when your baby's life is expected to be brief.* Baltimore, MD: Johns Hopkins University Press.

Lally, R. (2014). *For Our Babies Campaign.* Forourbabies.org.

Lamb, E.H. (2002). The impact of previous perinatal loss on subsequent pregnancy and parenting. *Journal of Perinatal Education,* 11: 33–40.

Lambrigger-Steiner, C., Simões-Wüst, A.P., Kuck, A., Fürer, K., Hamburger, M., & von Mandach, U. (2014). Sleep quality in pregnancy during treatment with Bryophyllum pinnatum: An observational study. *Phytomedicine,* 21(5): 753–757.

Lamont, K., Scott, N.W., Jones, G.T., & Bhattacharya, S. (2015) Risk of recurrent stillbirth: Systematic review and meta-analysis. *British Medical Journal,* 350: 3080. DOI: http://dx.doi.org/10.1136/bmj.h3080.

Lander, D. & Graham-Pole, J. (2008–2009). Love letters to the dead: Resurrecting an epistolary art. *Omega,* 58(4): 313–333.

Lang, A., Fleiszer, A.R., Duhamel, F., Sword, W., et al. (2011). Perinatal loss and parental grief: The challenge of ambiguity and disenfranchised grief. *Omega,* 63(2): 183–196.

Lao, M.R., Calhoun, B.C., Bracero, L.A., Wang, Y., Seybold, D.J. et al. (2009). The ability of the quadruple test to predict adverse perinatal outcomes in a high-risk obstetric population. *Journal of Medical Screening,* 16(2): 55–59.

Lawrence, R.A. & Lawrence, R.M. (2011). *Breastfeeding a guide for the medical profession* (7th ed). Maryland Heights, MO: Mosby/Elsevier.

Lazare, A. (1979). Unresolved grief. In A. Lazare (Ed.) *Outpatient psychiatry: Diagnosis and treatment.* Baltimore, MD: Williams & Wilkins.

Lee, L., McKenzie-McHarg, K., & Hosch, A. (2013). Women's decision making and experience of subsequent pregnancy following stillbirth. *Journal of Midwifery & Women's Health,* 28(4): 431–439.

Lee, S.H., Ahn, S.C., Lee, Y.J., Yook, K.H., & Suh, S.Y. (2007). Effectiveness of a meditation-based stress management program as an adjunct to pharmacotherapy in patients with anxiety disorder. *Journal of Psychosomatic Research,* 62(2): 189–195.

Lee, Y.M., Cleary-Goldman, J., & D'Alton, M.E. (2006). Multiple gestations and late preterm (near-term) deliveries. *Seminars in Perinatology,* 30(2): 103–112.

Liefer, M. (1977). Psychological changes accompanying pregnancy and motherhood. *Genetic Psychology Monographs,* 95: 55–96.

Leifer, M. (1980). *Psychological effects of motherhood.* New York: Praeger.

Leiferman, J., Swibas, T., Koiness, K., Marshall, J.A., & Dunn, A.L. (2011). My baby, my move: Examination of perceived barriers and motivating factors related to antenatal physical activity. *Journal of Midwifery and Women's Health,* 56: 33–40.

Leon, I.G. (1986). The invisible loss: The impact of perinatal loss on siblings. *Journal of Psychosomatic Obstetrics & Gynecology,* 5: 1–14.

Leon, I.G. (1990). *When a baby dies: Psychotherapy for pregnancy and newborn loss.* New Haven, CT: Yale University Press.

Leonard, L. & Denton, J. (2006). Preparation for parenting multiple birth children. *Early Human Development,* 82(6): 371–378.

Lepore, S., Cohen, R., Wortman, C., & Wayment, H. (1996). Social constraints, intrusive thoughts, and depressive symptoms among bereaved mothers. *Journal of Personality and Social Psychology,* 77: 1041–1060.

Leviton, R. (2002). Unraveling the biography in your biology: Medical intuition training with Caroline Myss and C. Norman Shealy. *Intuition: A Magazine for the Higher Potential of the Mind,* 1(4): 26–31.

Leroy, F., Olaleye-Oruene, T., Schomerus, G., & Bryan, E. (2002). Yoruba customs and beliefs pertaining to twins. *Twin Research,* 5(2): 132–136.

Lewis, E. (1979). Inhibition of mourning by pregnancy: Psychopathology and management. *British Journal of Medicine,* 11(27): 27–28.

Lewis, I. (1987). Coping with the loss of a twin. *Tavistock Clinic,* 23(4), 158–160.

Li, J., Laursen, T., Precht, D., Olsen, J., & Mortensen, P. (2005). Hospitalization for mental illness among parents after the death of a child. *New England Journal of Medicine,* 352: 1190–1196.

Li, J., Precht, D., Mortensen, P., & Olsen, J. (2003). Mortality in parents after the death of a child in Denmark: A nationwide follow-up study. *Lancet,* 361: 363–367.

Lichtenthal, W. & Cruss, D. (2010). Effects of directed written disclosure on grief and distress symptoms among bereaved individuals. *Death Studies,* 34(6): 475–499.

Lichtenthal, W. & Neimeyer, R. (2012). Directed journaling to facilitate meaning-making. In R. Neimeyer (Ed.) *Techniques of grief therapy: Creative practices for counseling the bereaved.* New York, Routledge, pp. 1165–1168.

Lieberman, A.F., Compton, N.C., Van Horn, P., & Ghosh Ippen, C. (2003.) *Losing a parent to death in the early years.* Washington, DC: Zero to Three Press.

Limbo, R. & Kobler, K. (2009). "Will our baby be alive again?" Supporting parents of young children when a baby dies. *Nursing for Women's Health,* 13(4): 303–311.

Limbo, R. & Kobler, K. (2013). *Meaningful moments: Ritual and reflection when a child dies.* La Crosse, WI: Gundersen Health System.

Lincoln, V., Nowak, E., Schommer, B., Briggs, T., Fehrer, A., Wax, G. (2014). A retrospective analysis. *Holist Nursing Practice,* 28(3): 164–170.

Lipton, B. (2005). *The Biology of Belief.* Santa Rosa, CA: Elite Books, Energy Psychology Press.

Lisonkova, S., Sabr, Y., Butler, B., & Joseph, K. (2012). International comparisons of preterm birth: Higher rates of late preterm birth are associated with lower rates of stillbirth and neonatal death. *BJOG: An International Journal of Obstetrics and Gynaecology,* 119: 1630–1639.

Lisonkova, S., Hutcheon, J., & Joseph, K. (2012). Sudden infant death syndrome: A re-examination of temporal trends. *BMC Pregnancy and Childbirth,* 12(1): 59. DOI: 10.1186/1471-2393-12-59.

Little, C. (2010). Nursing considerations in the case of multi-fetal pregnancy reduction. *Maternal Child Nursing,* 35(3): 166–171.

Littman, L., Zarcadoolas, C., & Jacobs, A. (2009). Introducing abortion patients to a culture of support: A pilot study. *Archives of Women's Mental Health,* 12: 419–431.

Lund, M., Kamper-Jørgensen, M., Nielsen, H.S., Lidegaard, Ø., & Andersen, A.M. (2012). Prognosis for live birth in women with recurrent miscarriage: What is the best measure of success? *Obstetric Gynecology*, 119: 37–43.

MacKinnon, C., Smith, N., Henry, M., Berish, M. et al. (2014). Meaning-based group counseling for bereavement: Bridging theory with emerging trends in intervention research. *Death Studies*, 0: 1–8. DOI: 10.1080/07481187.2012.738768.

Mahande, M., Daltveit, A., Obure, J., Mmbaga, B., et al. (2013). Recurrence of preterm birth and perinatal mortality in northern Tanzania: Registry-based cohort study. *Tropical Medicine and International Health*, 18(8): 962–967. DOI: 10.1111/tmi.12111.

Mahler, S., Pine, M.M., & Bergman, A. (1973). *The psychological birth of the human infant*. New York: Basic Books.

Maifeld, M., Hahn, S., Titler, M.G., & Mullen, M. (2003). Decision making regarding multifetal pregnancy reduction. *Journal of Obstetric, Gynecologic and Neonatal Nursing*, 32(3): 357–369.

Malkinson, R. (2012). Rational Emotive Body Imagery (REBI). In R. Neimeyer (Ed.) *Techniques of grief therapy: Creative practices for counseling the bereaved*. New York: Routledge, pp. 136–138.

Malm, M., Lindgren, H., & Radestad, I. (2010). Losing contact with one's unborn baby: Mothers' experiences prior to receiving news that their baby has died in utero. *Journal of Death and Dying*, 62(4): 353–367.

Malone, F., Craigo, S., Chelmow, D., & D'Alton, M. (1996). Outcome of twin gestations complicated by a single. *Obstetrics & Gynecology*, 88(1): 1–5.

Main, M., Kaplan, N., & Cassidy, J. (1985). Security in infancy, childhood, and adulthood: A move to the level of representation. In I. Bretherton & E. Waters (Eds) *Growing points of attachment theory and research. Monographs of the Society for Research in Child Development*, 50(1–2): 66–107.

Mansour, R., Gamal, St., Aboulghar, M., Kamal, O., & Hesham, A. (2010). The impact of vanishing fetuses on the outcome of ICSI pregnancies. *Fertility and Sterility*, 94(6): 2430–2432.

Marshall, S.L., Gould, D., & Roberts, J. (1994). Nurses' attitudes towards termination of pregnancy. *Journal of Advanced Nursing*, 20: 567–576.

Martin, J.A., Hamilton, B., Sutton, P., Ventura, S. et al (2010). Births: Final data for 2006. *National Vital Statistics Reports*, 57(7): 1–101.

Mayers, P., Parkes, B., Green, B., & Turner, J. (2005). Experiences of registered midwives assisting with termination of pregnancies at a tertiary level hospital. *Health SA Gesondheid*, 10(1): 15–25. DOI: 10.4102/hsag.v10i1.185.

McCarty, W. (2000). *Being with babies: What babies are teaching us* (Rev ed). *Vol. 2: Supporting Babies' Innate Wisdom*. Santa Barbara, CA: Wondrous Beginnings.

McCarty, W. (2004). *Welcoming consciousness: Supporting babies' wholeness from the beginning of life—An integrated model of early development*. Santa Barbara, CA: Wondrous Beginnings.

McClowery, S.G., Davies, E.B., May, K.A., Kulenkamp, E.J., & Martinson, I.M. (1987). The empty space phenomenon: The process of grief in the bereaved family. *Death Studies*, 11(5): 361–374.

McCoyd, J. (2007). Pregnancy interrupted: Loss of a desired pregnancy after diagnosis of fetal anomaly. *Journal of Psychosomatic Obstetrics & Gynecology*, 28(1), 37–48.

McCoyd, J. (2009). Discrepant feeling rules and unscripted emotion work: Women coping with termination for fetal anomaly. *American Journal of Orthopsychiatry*, 79(4): 441–451.

McCoyd, J. (2010). Authoritative knowledge, the technological imperative and women's responses to prenatal diagnostic technologies. *Cultural Medical Psychiatry*, 34: 560–614.

McCoyd, J. (2013). Preparation for prenatal decision-making: A baseline of knowledge and reflection in women participating in prenatal screening. *Journal of Psychosomatic Obstetrics and Gynecology*, 34(1): 3–8.

McCreight, B.S. (2004). A grief ignored: Narratives of pregnancy loss from a male perspective. *Sociology of Health and Illness*, 26(3): 326–350.

McEwen, A. (2013). A genetic counselor's perspective on facing an unexpected diagnosis: Loving Michael and letting go. In V. Culling (Ed.) *Holding on and letting go: Facing an unexpected diagnosis in pregnancy.* Wellington, New Zealand: Vicki Culling Associates, pp. 5–8.

McIlwraith, C. (2013). When letting go can be the most difficult parenting decision of all. In V. Culling (Ed.) *Holding on and letting go: Facing an unexpected diagnosis in pregnancy.* (Wellington, New Zealand: Vicki Culling Associates, pp. 9–11.

McKane, P., Larder, C., & Derman, Q. (2013). Preconception/interconception health in Michigan: Using data to inform programs. *Pulse: Monthly newsletter from the Association of Maternal and Child Health Programs.* http://www.amchp.org/AboutAMCHP/Newsletters/Pulse/Documents/Pulse_SeptOct13.pdf

McKeon Pesek, E. (2002). The role of support groups in disenfranchised grief. In K.J. Doka (Ed.) *Disenfranchised grief: New directions, challenges, and strategies for practice.* Champaign, IL: Research Press, pp. 127–133.

McLean, P. (2013). Hope springs eternal. In V. Culling (Ed.) *Holding on and letting go: Facing an unexpected diagnosis in pregnancy.* Wellington, New Zealand: Vicki Culling Associates, pp. 996–104.

Mehran, P., Simbar, M., Shams, J., Ramezani-Tehrani, F., & Nasiri, N. (2013). History of perinatal loss and maternal–fetal attachment behaviors. *Women's Birth*, 26(3): 185–189.

Mendelson, T., DiPietro, J.A., Costigan, K.A., Chen, P., & Henderson, J.L. (2011). Association of maternal psychological factors with umbilical and uterine blood flow. *Journal of Psychosometric Obstetric Gynaecology*, 32(1): 3–9.

Michael, S.T. & Snyder, C.R. (2005). Getting unstuck: The roles of hope, finding meaning, and rumination in the adjustment to bereavement among college students. *Death Studies*, 29: 435–458.

Miesnik, S., Cole, J., & Jones, T. (2015). Integration of a mental health professional in a multidisciplinary team caring for the pregnant woman after diagnosis of fetal anomaly. *Journal of Obstetric, Gynecologic, & Neonatal Nursing, Special Issue: Convention Proceedings*, 44(s1): S18–S19.

Mills, T.A., Ricklesford, C., Cooke, A., Heazell, A.E.P., Whitworth, M., & Lavender, T. (2014). Parents' experiences and expectations of care in pregnancy after stillbirth or neonatal death: A metasynthesis. *BJOG: An International Journal of Obstetrics and Gynaecology*, 121(8): 915–919.

Mitchell, D. (2012). Moving and breathing through grief. In R. Neimeyer (Ed.) *Techniques of grief therapy.* New York: Routledge, pp. 67–69.

Mitchell, G., Dupuis, S., & Jonas-Simpson, C. (2011). Countering stigma with understanding: The role of theatre in social change and transformation. *Canadian Theatre Review*, 146: 22–27. DOI: 10.1353/ctr.2011.0029.

Moore, T., Parrish, H., & Perry Black, B. (2010). Interconception care for couples after perinatal loss: A comprehensive review of the literature. *Journal of Perinatal and Neonatal Nursing*, 25(3): 44–51.

Morin, L. & Lim, K. (2011). Ultrasound in twin pregnancies. *Journal of Obstetric Gynecology Canada*, 33(6): 643–656.

Mosquera, C., Miller, R.S., & Simpson, L.L. (2012). Twin–twin transfusion syndrome. *Seminars in Perinatology*, 36(3): 182–189. DOI: 10.1053/j.semperi.2012.02.006.

Moulder, C. (1994). Towards a preliminary framework for understanding pregnancy loss. *Journal of Reproductive and Infant Psychology*, 12(1): 65–67.

Moyer, B. (1993). *Healing and the mind*. New York: Doubleday.

Murphy, F. (1998). The experience of early miscarriage from a male perspective. *Journal of Clinical Nursing*, 7(4): 325–332.

Nadeau, J. (2001). Family construction of meaning. In R. Neimeyer (Ed.) *Meaning reconstruction and the experience of loss*. Washington, DC: American Psychological Association, pp. 95–111.

Narendran, S., Nagarathna, R., Narendran, V., Gunasheela, S., & Nagendra, H.R. (2005). Efficacy of yoga on pregnancy outcome. *Journal of Alternative Complementary Medicine*, 11: 237–243.

National Center for Education Statistics (2006). *Early Childhood Longitudinal Study, Birth Cohort*. Washington, DC: NECS.

Neilsen-Gatti, S., Watson, C., & Siegel, C. (2011). Step back and consider: Learning from reflective practice in infant mental health. *Young Exceptional Children*, 14(2): 32–45.

Neimeyer, R.A. (1996). Bereavement and the quest for meaning: Rewriting stories of loss and grief. *Hellenic Journal of Psychology*, 3: 181–188.

Neimeyer, R.A. (1998). Can there be a psychology of loss? In J.H. Harvey (Ed.) *Perspectives on loss: A source book*. Philadelphia, PA: Taylor & Francis.

Neimeyer, R.A. (2000). Searching for the meaning of meaning: Grief therapy and the process of reconstruction. *Death Studies*, 24(6): 541–558.

Neimeyer, R.A. (2002). Traumatic loss and the reconstruction of meaning. *Journal of Palliative Medicine*, 5(6): 935–942.

Neimeyer, R.A. (2014). The changing face of grief: Contemporary directions in theory, research and practice. *Progress in Palliative Care*, 22: 125–130.

Neimeyer, R.A. & Currier, J.M. (2009). Grief therapy: Evidence of efficacy and emerging directions. *Current Directions in Psychological Science*, 18: 352–356.

Neimeyer, R.A. & Jordan, J. (2002). Disenfranchisement as empathic failure: Grief therapy and the co-construction of meaning. In K.I. Doka (Ed.) *Disenfranchised grief: New directions, challenges, and strategies for practice*. Champaign, IL: Research Press, pp. 95–118.

Neimeyer, R.A. & Thompson, B.E. (2014). Meaning making and the art of grief therapy. In B.E. Thompson and R.A. Neimeyer (Eds.) *Grief and the expressive arts: Practices for creating meaning*. New York: Routledge, pp. 3–13.

Neimeyer, R.A., Klass, D., & Dennis, M. (2014). A social constructionist account of grief: Loss and the narrative of meaning. *Death Studies*, 38(8): 485–498.

Neimeyer, R.A., Prigerson, H., & Davis, B. (2002). Mourning and meaning. *American Behavioral Scientist*, 46: 235–251.

Nettles, J.B. (1995). Support groups: A neglected resource in obstetrics and gynecology. *Obstetrical & Gynecological Survey*, 50(7): 495–496.

Newman, R.B. & Luke, B. (2000). *Multifetal pregnancy: A handbook for care of the pregnant patient*. Philadelphia, PA: Lippincott William & Wilkins.

Nicholson, J., Slade, P., & Gletcher, J. (2010). Termination of pregnancy services: Experiences of gynaecological nurses. *Journal of Advanced Nursing*, 66(10): 2245–2256.

Nicolson, S. (2015). Let's meet your baby as a person: From research to preventive prenatal practice and back again with the newborn behavioral observation. *Zero to Three*, 36(1): 29–38.

Nijkamp, J.W., Korteweg, F.J., Holm, J.P., Timmer, A., Erwich, J.J., & van Pampus, M.G. (2013). Subsequent pregnancy outcome after previous foetal death. *European Journal of Obstetrics & Gynecology and Reproductive Biology*, 166: 37–42.

Nikcević, A.V., Kuczmierczyk, A.R., & Nicolaides, K.H. (2007). The influence of medical and psychological interventions on women's distress after miscarriage. *Journal of Psychosomatic Research*, 63(3): 283–290.

Nolbris, M.J., Karin Enskär, K., & Hellström, A.L.(2014). Grief related to the experience of being the sibling of a child with cancer. *Cancer Nursing*, 37(5): E1–E7.

Norwitz, E.R., Edusa, V., & Park, J.S. (2005). Maternal physiology and complications of multiple pregnancy. *Seminals Perinatology*, 29(5): 338–348.

Nugent, K. (2015). The newborn behavioral observation (NBO) system as a form of intervention and support for new parents. *Zero to Three*, 36(1): 2–10.

O'Leary, J.M. (2004). Grief and its impact on prenatal attachment in the subsequent pregnancy. *Archives of Women's Mental Health*, 7(1): 7–18.

O'Leary, J.M. (2005). The baby who follows the loss of a sibling: Special considerations in the postpartum period. *International Journal of Childbirth Education*, 20(4): 28–30.

O'Leary, J.M. (2007). Pregnancy and infant loss: Supporting parents and their children. *Zero to Three*, 27(6): 42–49.

O'Leary, J.M. (2009). Never a simple journey: Pregnancy following perinatal loss. *Bereavement Care*, 28(2): 12–17.

O'Leary, J.M. (2012). The impact infant loss can have on children. *Inside Out: The Journal for the Irish Association for Humanistic & Integrative Psychotherapy*, 67(2): 24–30.

O'Leary, J.M. & Gaziano, C. (2011). The experience of adult siblings born after loss. *Attachment: New Directions in Psychotherapy and Relational Psychoanalysis*, 5(3): 246–272.

O'Leary, J.M. & Parker, L. (1998). *Parenting your baby before birth: A relaxation experience for parents during pregnancy*. www.aplacetoremember.com.

O'Leary, J.M. & Thorwick, C. (1993). Parenting during pregnancy: The infant as the vehicle for intervention in high risk pregnancy. *International Journal of Prenatal & Perinatal Psychology & Medicine*, 5(3): 303–310.

O'Leary, J.M. & Thorwick, C. (1997). Impact of pregnancy loss on subsequent pregnancy. In J.R. Woods, Jr. & J.L. Esposito Woods (Eds) *Loss during pregnancy or in the newborn period*. Pitman, NJ: Janetti Publications, pp. 431–445.

O'Leary, J.M. & Thorwick, C. (2006a). *When pregnancy follows a loss: Preparing for the birth of a new baby*. www.aplacetoremember.com.

O'Leary, J.M. & Thorwick, C. (2006b). Fathering perspective during pregnancy post perinatal loss. *Journal of Obstetrics, Gynecologic, and Neonatal Nursing*, 35(1): 78–86.

O'Leary, J., Gaziano, C., & Thorwick, C. (2006b). Born after loss: The invisible child in adulthood. *Journal of Prenatal and Perinatal Psychology and Health*, 21(1): 3–23.

O'Leary, J.M. & Thorwick, C. (2008). Attachment to the unborn child and parental mental representations of pregnancy following perinatal loss. *Attachment: New Directions in Psychotherapy and Relational Psychoanalysis*, 2(2): 292–320.

O'Leary, J.M. & Warland, J.M. (2012) Intentional parenting of children born after a perinatal loss. *Journal of Loss and Trauma*, 17(2): 137–157.

O'Leary, J.M. & Warland, J.M. (2013). Untold stories of infant loss: The importance of contact with the baby for bereaved parents. *Journal of Family Nursing*, 19(3): 324–347.

O'Leary, J.M., Thorwick, C., & Parker, L. (2012a). *The baby leads the way: Supporting the emotional needs of families' pregnant following perinatal loss*. Minneapolis, MN: www.aplacetoremember.com.

O'Leary, J.M., Warland, J., & Parker, L. (2011a). Prenatal parenthood. *Journal of Prenatal Educators*, 20(4): 218–220.

O'Leary, J.M., Warland, J., & Parker, L. (2011b). Bereaved parents' perception of the grandparents' reactions after perinatal loss and in the pregnancy that follows. *Journal of Family Nursing*, 17(3): 330–356.

O'Leary, J.M., Warland, J. & Parker, L. (2012b). Childbirth preparation for families pregnant after loss. *International Journal of Childbirth Educations*, 27(2): 44–50.

Oman, D. & Driskill, J. (2003). Holy name repetition as a spiritual exercise and therapeutic technique. *Journal of Psychology and Christianity*, 22(1): 5–19.

Ostler, T. (2010). Grief and coping in early childhood. *Zero to Three*, 31(1): 29–35.

Ouyang, F., Zhang, J., Betrán, A., Zujing Yang, Z., Souza, J., & Merialdi, M. (2013). Recurrence of adverse perinatal outcomes in developing countries. *Bulletin of the World Health Organization*, 91: 357–367.

Packman, W., Horsley, H., Davies, B., & Kramer, R. (2006). Sibling bereavement and continuing bonds. *Death Studies*, 30(9): 817–841.

Palagini, L., Gemignani, A., Banti, S., Manconi, M., Mauri, M., & Riemann, D. (2014). Chronic sleep loss during pregnancy as a determinant of stress: Impact on pregnancy outcome. *Sleep Medicine*, 15: 853–859.

Pantke, R. & Slade, P. (2006). Remembered parenting style and psychological well-being in young adults whose parents had experienced early child loss. *Psychology and Psychotherapy: Theory, Research and Practice*, 79: 69–81.

Parker, L. & O'Leary, J.M. (1989). Impact of prior prenatal loss upon subsequent pregnancy: The function of the childbirth class. *International Journal of Childbirth Education*, 4(3): 7–9.

Parkes, C. (2002). Grief: Lessons from the past, visions for the future. *Death Studies*, 26(5): 367–385.

Parish, S.L. & Cloud, J.M. (2006). Financial well-being of young children with disabilities and their families. *Social Work*, 51: 223–232.

Parish, S.L., Rose, R.A., Dababnah, S., Yoo, J., & Cassiman, S.A. (2012). State-level income inequality and family burden of US families raising children with special health care needs. *Social Science & Medicine*, 74: 399–407.

Pawl, J. (1995). The therapeutic relationship as human connectedness: Being held in another's mind. *Zero to Three*, 15(4): 1–5.

Pearson, J. (2009). *Parent–infant pathways: An educator's guide to providing information and support to new parents.* Minneapolis, MN: Aardvark Press.

Pearson, J. (2016). *Pathways to positive parenting: Helping parents nurture healthy development in the earliest months.* Washington, DC: Zero to Three.

Peat, A.M., Stacey, T., Cronin, R., & McCowan, L.M. (2012). Maternal knowledge of fetal movements in late pregnancy. *Australia and New Zealand Journal of Obstetrics and Gynaecology*, 52(5): 445–449.

Pennebaker, J.W. (1997). *Opening up: The healing power of expressing emotion.* New York: Guilford Press.

Pennebaker, J.W. & Beall, S. (1986). Confronting a traumatic event: Toward an understanding of inhibition and disease. *Journal of Abnormal Psychology*, 95: 274–281.

Pennebaker, J.W., Mayner, T.J., & Francis, M.E. (1997). Linguistic predictors of adaptive bereavement. *Journal of Personality and Social Psychology*, 72(4): 863–871.

Peppers, L. & Knapp, R. (1980). *Motherhood and mourning: Perinatal death.* New York: Praeger.

Perry, B. & Szalavitz, M. (2006). *The boy who was raised as a dog.* New York: Basic Books.

Peterson, S.E., Nelson, J.L., Gadi, V.K., Aydelotte, T.M., Oyer, D.J. et al. (2012). Prospective assessment of fetal–maternal cell transfer in miscarriage and pregnancy termination. *Human Reproduction*, 27(9): 2607–2612.

Peterson, S.E., Nelson, J.L., Gadi., V.K., & Gammill, H.S. (2013). Fetal cellular microchimerism in miscarriage and pregnancy termination. *Chimerism*, 4(4): 136–138. DOI: 10.4161/chim.24915.

Phillips, R. (2013). The sacred hour: Uninterrupted skin-to-skin contact immediately after birth. *Newborn and Infant Nursing Reviews*, 13(2): 67–72.

Pies, C., Strouse, C., & Hussey, W. (2013). Best Babies Zone: A collaborative initiative to improve birth outcomes and transform communities. *Pulse: Association of Maternal and Child Health*, September/October. http://www.amchp.org/AboutAMCHP/Newsletters/Pulse/Documents/Pulse.

Pinborg, A., Lidegaard, O., la Cour Freiesleben, N., & Andersen, A.N. (2005). Consequences of vanishing twins in IVF/ICSI pregnancies. *Human Reproduction*, 20: 2821–2829.

Pitts, R. (2000). Title unknown. Unpublished Master's thesis. University of St. Thomas, St. Paul, MN.

Porreco, R., Harmon, R., Murrow, N., Schultz, L., & Hendricx, M.L. (1995). Parental choices in grand multiple gestation: Psychological considerations. *Journal of Maternal–Fetal & Neonatal Medicine*, 4(3): 111–114.

Powell, M. (1995). Sudden infant death syndrome: The subsequent child. *British Journal Social Work*, 25(2): 227–240.

Poznanski, E. (1972). The replacement child: A saga of unresolved grief. *Behavioral Pediatrics*, 81(9): 1190–1193.

Prati, G. & Pietrantoni, L. (2009). Optimism, social support, and coping strategies as factors contributing to posttraumatic growth: A meta-analysis. *Journal of Loss and Trauma*, 14(5): 364–388.

Price, S. (2006). Prevalence and correlates of pregnancy loss history in a national sample of children and families. *Maternal Child Health Journal*, 10: 489–500.

Price, S. (2008). Stepping back to gain perspective: Pregnancy loss history, depression and parenting capacity in the Early Childhood Longitudinal Study, Birth Cohort (ECLS-B). *Death Studies*, 32(2): 97–122.

Price, S., Lake, M., Breen, G., Carson, G., Quinn, C., & O'Connor, T. (2007). The spiritual experience of high-risk pregnancy. *Journal of Obstetrics, Gynecology, and Neonatal Nursing*, 36(2): 63–70.

Priegerson, H., Horowitz, M., Jacobs, S., Parkes, C., Alsan, M. et al. (2009). Prolonged grief disorder: Psychometric validation of criteria proposed for DSM-V and ICD-11. *PLOS Medicine*, 6(8): 1–12.

Quant, H.S., Zapantis, A.L., Nihsen, M., Bevilacqua, K., Jindal, S., & Pal, L. (2013). Reproductive implications of psychological distress for couples undergoing IVF. *BMJ Open*, 30: 1451–1458.

Radestad, I., Hutti, M., Saflund, K., Onelov, E. & Wredling, R. (2010). Advice given by health-care professionals to mothers concerning subsequent pregnancy after stillbirth. *Acta Obstetrica et Gynecologica Scandinavica*, 89(8): 1084–1086.

Räisänen, S., Lehto, S.M., Nielsen, S.H., Gissler, M., Kramer, M., & Heinonen, S. (2013). Fear of childbirth predicts postpartum depression: A population-based analysis of 511 422 singleton births in Finland. *British Medical Journal Open*, 3: e004047.

Rando, T.A. (1986). *Parental loss of a child*. Champaign, IL: Research Press Co.

Rando, T.A. (2000a). On the experience of traumatic stess in anticipatory and postdeath mourning. In T.A. Rando (Ed.) *Clinical dimensions of anticipatory mourning: Theory and practice in working with dying, their loved ones, and their caregivers.* (pp. 155–221), Champaign, Il: Research Press.

Rando, T. (2000b). *Clinical dimensions of anticipatory mourning.* Champaign, IL: Research Press, pp. 155–221.

Range, L., Kovac, S., & Marion, M. (2000). Does writing about the bereavement lessen grief following sudden, unintentional death. *Death Studies*, 24(2): 115–134.

Raphael-Leff, J. (2004). Transitions to parenthood in societies in transition: Mental Health priorities in perinatal disturbances. *The Signal*, 12(3/4): 6–13.

Riches, G. & Dawson, P. (1998). Lost children, living memories: The role of photographs in processes of grief and adjustment among bereaved parent. *Death Studies*, 22(2): 121–140.

Rillstone, P. & Hutchinson, S. (2001). Managing the re-emergence of anguish: Pregnancy after a loss due to anomalies. *Journal of Obstetric, Gynecologic, & Neonatal Nursing*, 30(3): 291–298.

Robertson Blackmore, E., Côté-Arsenault, D., Tang, W., Glover, V., Evans, J. et al. (2011). Previous prenatal loss as a predictor of perinatal depression and anxiety. *British Journal of Psychiatry: The Journal of Mental Science*, 198(5): 373–378.

Robinson, M., Baker, L., & Nackerud, L. (1999). The relationship of attachment theory and perinatal loss. *Death Studies*, 32(3): 257–270.

Robson, S.J., Leader, L.R., Dear, KB., & Bennett, M.J. (2009). Women's expectations of management in their next pregnancy after an unexplained stillbirth: An internet-based empirical study. *Australian & New Zealand Journal of Obstetrics & Gynaecology*, 49(6): 642–646.

Roca, de Bes, M., Guitierrez Maldonado, J., & Gris Martinez, J.M. (2008). Psychosocial risks associated with multiple births resulting from assisted reproduction: A Spanish sample. *Fertility and Sterility*, 92(3): 1059–1066.

Rochman, D. (2013). Death-related versus fond memories of a deceased attachment figure: Examining emotional arousal. *Death Studies*, 37(8): 704–724.

Romanoff, B. (2001). Research as therapy: The power of narrative to effect change. In R Neimeyer (Ed.) *Meaning reconstruction and the experience of loss*. Washington, DC: American Psychological Association, pp. 245–257.

Romanoff, B. & Terenzio, M. (1998). Rituals and the grieving process. *Death Studies*, 22(8): 697–711.

Ronen, R., Packman, W., Field, N., Davis, B., Kramer, R., & Long, J. (2009–2010). The relationship between grief and adjustment and continued bonds for parents who have lost a child. *Omega*, 60(1): 1–31.

Roos, S. (2012). Making meaning of flashbacks. In R. Neimeyer (Ed.) *Techniques of grief therapy: Creative practices for counseling the bereaved*. New York: Routledge, pp. 99–101.

Roose, R.E. & Blanford, C.R. (2011). Perinatal grief and support spans the generations: Parents' and grandparents' evaluations of an intergenerational perinatal bereavement program. *Journal of Perinatal & Neonatal Nursing*, 25: 77–85.

Roscignol, C., Savage, T., Kavanaugh, K., Moro, T., Kilpatrick, S. et al. (2012). Divergent views of hope influencing communications between parents and hospital providers. *Quality Health Research*, 22(9): 1232–1246. DOI: 10.1177/1049732312449210.

Rosenberg, A., Postier, A., Osenga, K., Kreicbergs, U., Neville, B. et al. (2015). Long-term psychosocial outcomes among bereaved siblings of children with cancer. *Journal of Pain & Symptom Management*, 49(1): 55–65.

Rosenblatt, P. (1996). Grief that does not end. In D. Klass, P. Silverman, & S. Nickman (Eds) *Continuing bonds: New understandings of grief*. Washington, DC: Taylor & Francis, pp. 245–257.

Rosenblatt, P. (1983). *Bitter, bitter tears: Nineteenth-century diarists and twentieth-century grief theories*. Minneapolis, MN: University of Minneapolis Press.

Rosenblatt, P. (2000a). Parents talking in the present tense about their dead child. *Bereavement Care*, 19(3): 35–38.

Rosenblatt, P. (2000b). Protective parenting after the death of a child. *Journal of Personal and Interpersonal Loss*, 5(4): 343–360.

Rosner, R., Kruse, J., & Hagl, M. (2010). A meta-analysis of interventions for bereaved children and adolescents. *Death Studies*, 34: 99–136.

Rubin, R. (1975). Maternal tasks in pregnancy. *Maternal Child Nursing*, 4(3): 143–153.

Rubio, C., Simon, C., Vidal, F., Rodrigo, L., Pehlivan, T. et al. (2003). Chromosomal abnormalities and embryo development in recurrent miscarriage couples. *Human Reproduction*, 18(1): 182–188.

Saeed, S.A., Antonacci, D.J., & Bloch, R.M. (2010). Exercise, yoga, and meditation for depressive and anxiety disorders. *American Family Physician*, 81: 981–986.

Salihu, H., August, E., de la Cruz, C., Mgos, M., Wedleselasse, H., & Alio, A. (2013). Infant mortality and the risk of small size for gestational age in the subsequent pregnancy: A retrospective cohort study. *Maternal Child Health*, 17: 1044–1051.

Samuelsson, M., Radestad, I., & Segesten, K. (2001). A waste of life: Fathers' experience of losing a child before birth. *Birth*, 28(2): 124–130.

Sandelowski, M. & Barroso, J. (2005). The treavesty of choosing after positive prenatal diagnosis. *Journal of Obstetric, Gynecologic, & Neonatal Nursing*, 34(3): 307–318.

Sandman, C.A., Davis, E.P., Buss, C., & Gynn, L.M. (2011). Exposure to prenatal psychobiological stress exerts programming influences on the mother and fetus. *Neuroendocrinology*, 95(1): 7–21.

Sandman, C., Davis, E., & Glynn, L. (2012). Prescient human fetuses thrive. *Psychological Science*, 23(1): 93–100.

Segal, D. (2001). Toward an interpersonal neurobiology of the developing mind: Attachment relationships, "mindsight," and neural integration. *Infant Mental Health Journal*, 22(1–2): 67–94.

Seimyr, L., Sjogren, B., Wells-Nystrom, B., & Nissen, E. (2009). Antenatal maternal depressive mood and parental–foetal attachment at the end of pregnancy. *Archives of Women's Mental Health*, 12: 269–279.

Sell-Smith, J. & Lax, W. (2013). A journey of pregnancy loss: From positivism to autoethnography. *The Qualitative Report*, 18(92): 1–17.

Seth, S., Goka, T., Harbiso, A., Hollier, L., Peterson, S. et al. (2011). Exploring the role of religiosity and spirituality in amniocentesis decision-making among Latinos. *Journal of Genetic Counseling*, 20(6): 660–673.

Schwab, R. (1996). Gender differences in parental grief. *Death Studies*, 20: 103–113.

Seoud, M.A., Toner, J.P., Kruithoff, C., & Muasher, S.J. (1992). Outcome of twin, triplet, and quadruplet in vitro fertilization pregnancies: The Norfolk experience. *Fertility & Sterility*, 57(4): 825–834.

Seth, S., Goka, T., Harbiso, A., Hollier, L., Peterson, S. et al. (2010). Exploring the role of Religiosity and Spirituality in Amniocentesis decision-making among Latinos. *Journal of Genetic Counseling*, 20(6), 660–673.

Schwab, R. (2009). *Child's death: Encyclopedia of death and dying*. Flossmoor, IL: Advameg, Inc. http://www.deathreference.com/Gi-Ho/Grief.html.

Shainess, N. (1963). The structure of the mothering encounter. *Journal of Nervous and Mental Disease*, 136: 146–161.

Shear, K. (2012a). Get straight about grief. *Depression and Anxiety*, 29(6): 461–464.

Shears, K. (2012b). Grief and mourning gone awry: Pathway and course of complicated grief. *Dialogues in Clinical Neuroscience*, 14: 119–128.

Shek, N.W., Hillman, S.C., & Kilby, M.D. (2014). Single-twin demise: Pregnancy outcome. *Best Practice & Research Clinical Obstetrics & Gynaecology*, 28(2): 249–63. DOI: 10.1016/j.bpobgyn.2013.11.003.

Shonkoff, J.P., Boyce, W.T., & McEwen, B.S. (2009). Neuroscience, molecular biology and the childhood roots of health disparities. *Journal of the American Medical Association*, 301(21): 2252–2259.

Shore, A. (1994). *Affect regulation and the origin of the self: The neurobiology of emotional development*. Englewood Cliffs, NJ: Lawrence Erlbaum.

Sigel, D. (1998). The developing mind: Toward a neurobiology of interpersonal experience. *The Signal*, 6(3–4): 1–10.

Silver, R. (2007). Fetal death. *Clinical Expert Series*, 109(1): 153–167.

Simmons, R.K., Singh, G., Maconochie, N., Doyle, P., & Green, J. (2006). Experience of miscarriage in the UK: Qualitative findings from the National Women's Health Study. *Social Science & Medicine*, 63(7): 1934–1946.

Simmons, H.A. & Goldberg, L.S. (2011). High-risk pregnancy after perinatal loss: Understanding the label. *Midwifery*, 27(4): 452–457.

Simpson, J. & Elias, S. (2006). Fetal cells in maternal blood: Overview and historical perspective. *Annals of the New York Academy of Sciences*, 731: 1–8.

Slade, A. (2000). The development and organization of attachment: Implications for psychoanalysis. *Journal of the American Psychoanalytic Association*, 48: 1147–1174.

Slade, A. (2002). Keeping the baby in mind: A critical factor in perinatal mental health. *Zero to Three*, 22(6): 10–16.

Smart, L.S. (1993–1994). Parental bereavement in Anglo-American history. *Omega*, 28(1): 49–61.

Smyth, J. & Pennebaker, J. (2008). Exploring the boundary conditions of expressive writing: In search of the right recipe. *British Journal of Health Psychology*, 13: 1–7.

Soliday, E. & Tremblay, K. (2013). Provider trust: A useful concept in maternal care. *Journal of Prenatal and Perinatal Psychology and Health*, 27(3): 193–205.

Song, J., Floyd, F., Seltzer, M., Greenberg, J., & Hong, J. (2010). Long-term effects of child death on parents' health-related quality of life: A dyadic analysis. *Family Relations*, 59(3): 122–134.

Sood, A.B., Razdan, A., Weller, E.B., & Weller, R.A. (2006). Children's reactions to parental and sibling death. *Current Psychiatry Reports*, 8(2): 115–120.

Sowden, M., Sage, N., & Cockburn, J. (2007). Coping and adjustment in pregnancy: Giving babies a better start. In J. Cockburn & M.E. Pawson (Eds) *Psychological challenges in obstetrics and gynecology: The clinical management*. London: Springer, pp. 91–106.

Sroufe, L.A. (2005). Attachment and development: A prospective, longitudinal study from birth to adulthood. *Attachment and Human Development*, 7(4): 349–367.

Stacey, T., Thompson, J.M., Mitchell, E.A., Ekeroma, A., Zuccollo, J., & McCowan, LM. (2011). Maternal perception of fetal activity and late stillbirth risk: findings from the Auckland Stillbirth Study. *Birth*, 38(4): 311–316.

St. John, A., Cooke, M., & Goopy, S. (2006). Shrouds of silence: Three women's stories of prenatal loss. *Australian Journal of Advanced Nursing*, 23(3): 8–12.

Statham, H. (2002). Prenatal diagnosis of fetal abnormality: The decision to terminate the pregnancy and the psychological consequences. *Fetal and Maternal Medicine Review*, 13: 213–247.

Stephansson, O., Dickman, P., & Cnattingius, S. (2003). The influence of interpregnancy interval on the subsequent risk of stillbirth and early neonatal death. *Obstetrics and Gynecology*, 102(1): 101–108.

Stray-Pedersen, B. and Stray-Pedersen, S. (1984). Etiologic factors and subsequent reproductive performance in 195 couples with a prior history of habitual abortion. *American Journal of Obstetric Gynecology*, 148: 140–146.

Stray-Pedersen, B. & Stray-Pedersen, S. (1988). Recurrent abortion: The role of psycho-therapy. In R.W. Beard & F. Ship (Ed.) *Early pregnancy loss: Mechanisms and treatment*. New York: Springer-Verlag, pp. 433–440.

Steele, A., Kaal, J., Thompson, A., Barrera, M., Compast, B. et al. (2013). Bereaved parents and siblings offer advice to health care providers and researchers. *Journal of Pediatric Hematology & Oncology*, 35(4): 253–259.

Stepp-Gilbert, E. (2007). *Manual of high risk pregnancy and delivery* (5th ed). St. Louis: Mosby.

Strean, W. (2009) Laughter prescription. *Canadian Family Physician*, 55: 965–967.

Stroebe, M., Hansson, R.O., Stroebe, W., & Schut, H. (2001). Introduction: Concepts and issues in contemporary research on bereavement. In M.S. Stroebe, R.O. Hansson, W. Stroebe, & H. Schut (Eds.) *Handbook of bereavement research: Consequences, coping and care*. Washington, DC: American Psychological Association Press, pp. 3–22.

Stroebe, M., Schut, H., & Boerner, K. (2010). Continuing bonds in adaptation to bereavement: Toward a theoretical integration. *Clinical Psychology Review*, 30: 259–268. DOI: 10.1016/j.cpr.2009.11.007.

Stroebe, M., Schut, H., & Stroebe, W. (2006). Who benefits from disclosure? Exploration of attachment style differences in the effects of expressing emotions. *Clinical Psychology Review*, 26(1), 66–85.

Stroebe, M., Schut, H., & Stroebe, W. (2007). Health outcome of bereavement, *Lancet*, 370 (9603),1960–73.

Stroebe, M., Stroebe, W., van de Schoot, R., Schut, H., Abakoumkin, G., & Li, J. (2014). Guilt in bereavement: The role of self-blame and regret in coping with loss. *PLoS, ONE*, 9(5): e06606. DOI: 10.1371/journal.pone.0096606.

Stormer, N. (2003). Seeing the fetus: The role of technology and image in the maternal–fetal relationship. *Journal of the American Medical Association*, 289(13): 1700–1701.

Sullivan, A., Kean, L., & Cryer, A. (2006). *A midwife's guide to antenatal investigations*. London: Churchill Livingston.

Sun, H.L., Sinclari, M., Kernohan, G.W., Chang, H., & Paterson, H. (2011). Sailing against the tide: Taiwanese women's journey from pregnancy loss to motherhood. *American Journal of Maternal Child Nursing*, 36(2): 127–133.

Sutan, R. & Mikam, H. (2012). Psychosocial impact of perinatal loss among Muslim women. *BMC Women's Health*, 12(15). DOI: 10.1186/1472-6874-12-15.

Sutcliffe, A. & Derom, C. (2006). Follow-up of twins: Health, behaviour, speech, language outcomes and implications for parents. *Early Human Development*, 82(6): 379–386.

Sveen, J., Eilegård, A., Steineck, G., & Kreicbergs, U. (2014). They still grieve—a nation-wide follow-up of young adults 2–9 years after losing a sibling to cancer. *Psycho-Oncology*, 23(6): 658–664.

Swanson, P.B., Jillian, G., Pearsall-Jones, J.G., & Hay, D.A. (2002). How mothers cope with the death of a twin or higher multiple. *Twin Research*, 5(3): 156–164.

Szejer, M. (2005). *Talking to babies: Healing with words on a maternity ward*. Boston, MA: Beacon Press.

Talge, N.M., Neal, C., & Glover, V. (2007). The early stress translational research and prevention science network: Fetal and neonatal experience on child and adolescent mental health. *Journal of Child Psychology and Psychiatry*, 48(3/4): 245–261.

Tang, S., Ross, S., & Sauve, R. (2014). Stillbirth in twins, exploring the optimal gestational age for delivery: A retrospective cohort study. *BJOG*, 121(10): 1284–1290.

Teasdale, J.D., Segal, Z., & Williams, M. (2003). Mindfulness training and problem foundation. *Clinical Psychology: Science Practice*, 10(2): 157–160.

Tedeschi, R.G. & Calhoun, I.G. (2004). Posttraumatic growth: Conceptual foundations and empirical evidence. *Psychological Inquiry*, 15: 1–18.

Teixeira, J., Martin, D., Prendiville, O., & Glover, V. (2005). The effects of acute relaxation on indices of anxiety during pregnancy. *Journal of Psychosomatic Obstetrics & Gynaecology*, 26: 237–243.

Tesch, S. (2007). Making the choice and surviving the loss: A qualitative study of the emotional impact of multifetal pregnancy reduction. Unpublished Master's thesis. St. Cloud State University, St. Cloud, MN.

Thachuk, A. (2007). The space in between: Narratives of silence and genetic termination. *Bioethics*, 21(9): 511–514.

Thayer, S. & Hupp, S. (2010). The holding environment as the context for intervention: A case study of two infants. *Emporia State Research Studies*, 46(1): 11–20.

Theut, S.K., Moss, H.A., Zaslow, M.J., & Rabinovich, B.A. (1988). Pregnancy subsequent to perinatal loss: Parental anxiety and depression. *Journal of the American Academy of Child and Adolescent Psychiatry*, 27(3): 289–292.

Theut, S.K., Moss, H.A., Zaslow, M.J., Rabinovich, B.A., Levin, L., & Bartko, J.J. (1992). Perinatal loss and maternal attitudes toward the subsequent child. *Infant Mental Health Journal*, 13(2): 157–166.

Thomas, R. (1996). Reflective dialogue parent education design: Focus on parent development. *Family Relations*, 45(2): 189–200.

Thomson, G. & Downe, S. (2010). Changing the future to change the past: Women's experiences of a positive birth following a traumatic birth experience. *Journal of Reproductive and Infant Psychology*, 28(1): 102–112.

Thomson, P. (2007). "Down will come baby": Prenatal stress, primitive defenses and gestational dysregulation. *Journal of Trauma & Dissociation*, 8(3): 85–113.

Thompson, A., Miller, K., Barrera, M., Davis, B., Foster, T. et al. (2011). A qualitative study of advice from bereaved parents and siblings. *Journal of Social Work End of Life Palliative Care*, 7(2–3): 153–172. DOI: 10.1080/15524256.2011.593153.

Thompson, B. (2012). Mindfulness training. (2012) In R. Neimeyer (Ed.) *Techniques of grief therapy: Creative practices for counseling the bereaved*. New York: Routledge, pp. 39–41.

Timor-Tritsch, I.E., Rebarber, A., MacKenzie, A., Caglione, C.F., & Young, B.K. (2003). Four-dimensional real-time sonographically guided cauterization of the umbilical cord in a case of twin–twin transfusion syndrome. *Journal of Ultrasound Medicine*, 22(7): 741–746.

Tollenaar, M.S., Beijers, R., Jansen, J., Riksen-Walraven, J.M., & de Weerth, C. (2011). Maternal prenatal stress and cortisol reactivity to stressors in human infants. *Stress*, 14(1): 53–65, DOI: 10.3109/10253890.2010.499485.

Toller, P.W. (2005). Negotiation of dialectical contradictions by parents who have experienced the death of a child. *Journal of Applied Communication Research*, 33: 46–66.

Trulsson, O. & Radestad, I. (2004). The silent child–mothers' experiences before, during, and after stillbirth. *Birth*, 31(3): 189–195.

Tsang, H., Chan, E., & Cheung, W. (2010). Effects of mindful and non-mindful exercises on people with depression: A systematic review. *British Journal of Clinical Psychology*, 47(3): 303–322.

Tsartsara, E. & Johnson, M. (2006). The impact of miscarriage on women's pregnancy-specific anxiety and the feelings of prenatal maternal–fetal attachment during the course of a subsequent pregnancy: An exploratory follow-up. *Journal of Psychosomatic Obstetrics and Gynecology*, 27: 17–182.

Tummers, P., DeSutter, P.D., & Dhont, M. (2003). Risk of spontaneous abortion in singleton and twin pregnancies after IVF/ICSI. *Human Reproduction*, 18(8): 1720–1723.

Turton, P., Badenhorst, W., Hughes, P., Ward, J., Riches, S., & White, S. (2006). Psychological impact of stillbirth on fathers in the subsequent pregnancy and puerperium. *British Journal of Psychiatry*, 188: 165–172.

Turton, P., Hughes, P., Evans, C.D., & Fainman, D. (2001). Incidence, correlates and predictors of post-traumatic stress disorder in the pregnancy after stillbirth. *British Journal of Psychiatary*, 178: 556–560.

Umphrey, L.R. & Cacciatore, J. (2011). Coping with the ultimate deprivation: Narrative themes in a parental bereavement support group. *Omega*, 63(2): 141–160.

Urech, C., Fink, N.S., Hoesli, I., Wilhelm, F.H., Blitzer, J., & Alder, J. (2010). Effects of relaxation on psychobiological wellbeing during pregnancy: A randomized controlled trial. *Psychoneuroendocrinology*, 35(9): 1348–1355. DOI: 10.1016/j.psyneuen.2010.03.008.

Vallotton, C.D. (2008). Signs of emotions: What can preverbal children "say" about internal states. *Infant Mental Health Journal*, 29(3): 234–258.

Van den Bergh, B.R.H. (2010). Some societal and historical scientific considerations regarding the mother–fetus relationship and parenthood. *Infant and Child Development*, 19(1), 39–44.

Van den Bergh, B.R.H. & Marcoen, A. (2004). High antenatal maternal anxiety is related to ADHD symptoms, externalizing problems, and anxiety in 8 and 9 year olds. *Child Development*, 75(4): 1085–1097.

Van den Bergh, B.R.H. & Simons, A. (2009). A review of scales to measure the mother–foetus relationship. *Journal of Reproductive and Infant Psychology*, 27(2): 114–126.

Van den Bergh, B.R.H., Mulder, E.J.H., Mennes, M., & Glover, V. (2005). Antenatal maternal anxiety and stress and the neurobehavioral development of the fetus and child: Links and possible mechanisms—a review. *Neuroscience and Biobehavioral Reviews*, 29: 237–258.

Van den Bergh, B.R.H., Van Calster, H., Smits, T., Van Huffel, S., & Lagae, L. (2008). Antenatal maternal anxiety is related to HPA-axis dysregulation and self-reported depressive symptoms in adolescence: A prospective study on the fetal origins of depressed mood. *Neuropsychopharmacology*, 33(3): 536–545.

Van der Gucht, N. & Lewis, K. (2014). Women's experiences of coping with pain during childbirth: A critical review of qualitative research. *Midwifery*, 31(3): 349–358. DOI: 10.1016/j.midw.2014.12.005.

Van Dis, J. (2003). The maternal–fetal relationship. *Journal of the American Medical Association*, 289(13): 1696. DOI: 10.1001/jama.289.13.1696.

Veninga, R. (1985). *A gift of hope: How we survive our tragedies.* Boston, MA: Little, Brown and Co.

Verny, T. (1981). *Secret life of the unborn child.* New York: Summit Books.

Verny, T. (2002). *Tomorrow's baby: The art and science of parenting from conception through infancy.* New York: Simon & Schuster.

Vieten, C. & Astin, J. ((2008). Effects of a mindfulness-based intervention during pregnancy on prenatal stress and mood: Results of a pilot study. *Archives of Women's Mental Health*, 11: 67–74. DOI 10.1007/s00737-008-0214-3.

Voegtline, K., Costigan, K., Pater, H., & DiPietro, J. (2013). Near-term fetal response to maternal spoken voice. *Infant Behavior and Development*, 36: 526–533.

Wachholtz, A.B. & Pargament, K.I. (2005). Is spirituality a critical ingredient of medication? Comparing the effects of spiritual meditation, secular meditation, and relaxation on spiritual, psychological, cardiac, and pain outcomes. *Journal of Behavioral Medicine*, 28: 369–384.

Walsh, D. (2002). Fear of labor and birth. *British Journal of Midwifery*, 10: 78.

Walsh, J. (2010). Definitions matter: If maternal–fetal relationships are not attachment, what are they? *Archives of Women's Mental Health*, 13(5): 449–451. DOI: 10.1007/s00737-010-0152-8.

Walsh, J., Hepper, E.G., Bagge, S.R., Wadephul, F., & Jomeen, J. (2013). Maternal–fetal relationships and psychological health: Emerging research directions. *Journal of Reproductive and Infant Psychology*, 31(5): 490–499. DOI: 10080/02646838.2013.834311.

Walter, T. (1996). A new model of grief: Bereavement and biography. *Mortality*, 1(1): 7–25.

Wang, H.L. & Chao, Y.M.Y. (2006). Lived experience of Taiwanese women and multi-fetal pregnancies who receive fetal reduction. *Journal of Nursing Research*, 14: 143–154.

Warland, J. (2000). *The midwife and the bereaved family.* Melbourne, VT: Ausmed Publications.

Warland, J. & Warland, M. (1996). *Pregnancy after loss.* Self-published.

Warland, J., O'Brien, L.M., Heazell, A.E.P., Mitchell, E.A., & the STARS consortium. (2015). An international internet survey of the experiences of 1,714 mothers with a late still-birth: The STARS cohort study. *BMC Pregnancy and Childbirth*, 15(172). DOI: 10.1186/s12884-015-0602-4.

Warland, J., O'Leary, J., & McCutcheon, H. (2011a). Born after infant loss: The experiences of subsequent children. *Midwifery*, 27(5): 628–633.

Warland, J., O'Leary, J., McCutcheon, H., & Williamson, V. (2011b). Parenting paradox: Parenting after infant loss. *Midwifery*, 27(5): 163–169.

Weatherston, D. (1998). Supporting developmental needs within the context of the family: A relationship-based approach. *IMPrint. Newsletter of the Infant Mental Health Promotion Project*, Vol. 20, Winter.

Weaver-Hightower, M. (2012). Waltzing Matilda: An autoethnography of a father's stillbirth. *Journal of Contemporary Ethnography*, 41(4): 462–491. DOI: 10.1177/0891241611429302.

Wegner, M. (2015). *Embracing Laura: The grief and healing following the death of an infant twin.* Lulu Publishing Services.

Wegner, M. (2015). *Embracing Laura: The grief and healing following the death of an infant twin.* Lulu Publishing Services. ISBN: 978-1-4834-4013-2 (e).

Weinberg, N. (1995). Does apologizing help? The role of self-blame and making amends in recovery from bereavement. *Health and Social Work*, 20: 294–294.

Weinstein, A. (2012). PsyBC seminars: The impact of prenatal and early postnatal experiences over the lifespan. http://www.psybc.com/forums/ubbthreads.php?Cat=0&C=2.

Weiss, R.S. (2001). Grief, bonds, and relationships. In M.S. Stroebe, R.O. Hanssen, W. Stroebe, & H. Schut (Eds) *Handbook of bereavement research: Consequences, coping, and care.* Washington, DC: American Psychological Association, pp. 47–62.

Wheeler, I. (2001). Parental bereavement: The crisis of meaning. *Death Studies*, 25(1): 51–66.

Wiggins, N. (2012). Popular education for health promotion and community empowerment: A review of the literature. *Health Promotion International*, 12: 356–375. DOI: 10.1093/heapro/dar046.

Williams, Z., Zepf, D., Longtine, J., Anchan, R., Boradman, B. et al. (2009). Foreign fetal cells persist in the maternal circulation. *Fertility & Sterility*, 91: 2593–2595.

Wilson, R.E. (2001). Parents' support of their other children after a miscarriage or perinatal death. *Early Human Development*, 61: 55–65.

Wilson, J.F. & Kopitzke, E.J. (2002). Stress and infertility. *Current Women's Health Reports*, 2(3): 194–199.

Wimmer, L. (2013). Defining progress. starlegacyfoundation.org.

Winnicott, D., Winnicott, C., Shepherd, R., & Davis, M. (1987). *Babies and mothers.* Reading, MA: Addison-Wesley.

Wolfelt, A. (1983). *Helping children cope with grief.* New York: Routledge.

Woods, L. & Quenbyn, S. (2010). Women's perceptions of stressful life events in relation to pre-term birth. *British Journal of Midwifery*, 19(2): 350–356.

Woods-Giscombe, C.L., Lobel, M., & Crandell, J. (2010). The impact of miscarriage and parity on patterns of maternal distress in pregnancy. *Research in Nursing and Health*, 33(4): 316–328.

Worden, J.W. (2009). *Grief counseling and grief therapy: A handbook for the mental health practitioner* (4th ed.). New York: Springer Publishing Company.

Worth, N. (1997). Becoming a father to a stillborn child. *Clinical Nursing Research*, 6(1): 71–89.

Wright, P. & Black, B. (2013). Perinatal loss. *International Journal of Childbirth Education*, 28(1): 15–19.

Yalom, I.D. (1970). *The theory and practice of group psychotherapy.* New York: Basic Books.

Yalom, I. (2005). *The theory and practice of group psychotherapy* (5th ed). New York: Basic Books.

Yamazaki, A. (2010). Living with stillborn babies as family members. *Health Care for Women International*, 31: 921–937.

Yehuda, R. (2002). Post-traumatic stress disorder. *New England Journal of Medicine*, 346(2): 108–114.

Young, B. & Papadatou, D. (1997). Childhood death and bereavement. In C. Murray Parkes, P. Laungani, & B. Young (Eds) *Death and bereavement across cultures*. New York: Routledge, pp. 191–205.

Yudin, M.H., Prosen, T.L., & Landers, D.V. (2003). Multiple-marker screening in human immunodeficiency virus-positive pregnant women: Screen positivity rates with the triple and quad screens. *American Journal of Obstetric Gynecology*, 189(4): 973–976.

Zeanah, C.H. & Harmon, R.J. (1995). Perinatal loss and infant mental health: An introduction. *Infant Mental Health Journal*, 16(2): 76–79.

Zeanah, C.H., Danis, B., Hirshberg, L. et al. (1995). Initial adaptation in mothers and fathers following perinatal loss. *Infant Mental Health Journal*, 16: 80–93.

Resources for parents

Axness, M. (2012). *Parenting for peace: Raising the next generation of peacemakers*. Boulder, CO: Sentient Publications.

Carella, M. (1999). *Bonding with your baby before birth*. Fun and enriching activities to create a loving relationship with your unborn child. To order copies, call 314-644-2999 or email mariac@postnet.com. Also available in Spanish.

Chamberlain, D. (1989). *Babies remember birth*. New York: Ballantine Books.

Chamberlain, D. (1998). *The mind of your unborn child* (3rd ed). Berkeley, CA: North Atlantic Books.

Chamberlain, D. (2013). *Windows to the womb: Revealing the conscious baby from conception to birth*. Berkeley, CA: North Atlantic Books.

McCarthy, W. (2009). *Welcoming consciousness: Supporting babies' wholeness from the beginning of life*. Santa Barbara, CA: Wondrous Beginnings.

Schultz, L. (1998). *The diary*. schultz@lm.net.au.

Schultz, L. (2003). *The survivor*. schultz@lm.net.au.

Websites

Vivette Glover: Importance of the Early Years: http://www.educationscotland.gov.uk/video/p/video_tcm4637481.asp.

The womb twin research project: www.wombtwinsurvivors.comCLIMB – Center for Loss in Multiple Births: http://www.climb-support.org/OzMOST: OzMOST@tpg.com.au

INDEX

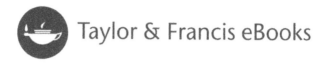